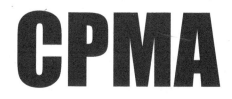

CPMA

Compendium of Products for Minor Ailments

Published by: Canadian Pharmacists Association, Ottawa, Ontario, Canada

Previously titled: *Products for Minor Ailments*

W9-DIM-587

3 9098 02200802 2

CPhA acknowledges the contribution of Carol Repchinsky as former Editor-in-Chief of this publication.

Copyright

Compendium of Products for Minor Ailments was previously titled *Products for Minor Ailments*, First Edition, 2013.

For permission request forms, please email: permissions@pharmacists.ca.

Electronic

The content in the *Compendium of Products for Minor Ailments (CPMA)* is available online in English and French; to subscribe visit **www.pharmacists.ca**. Licensed content is also available for data integration purposes. For more information on data licensing, please call 1-800-917-9489.

Publisher

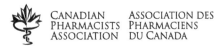

CANADIAN PHARMACISTS ASSOCIATION   ASSOCIATION DES PHARMACIENS DU CANADA

1785 Alta Vista Drive, Ottawa, ON K1G 3Y6 Canada

Comments/Inquiries

Tel: 613-523-7877, 1-800-917-9489 | Fax: 613-523-0445, 1-800-601-1904 | service@pharmacists.ca
Website: www.pharmacists.ca

Printed in Canada

Webcom Inc., 3480 Pharmacy Avenue, Toronto, ON, M1W 2S7 Canada

Website: www.webcomlink.com

Library and Archives Canada Cataloguing in Publication
Compendium of Products for Minor Ailments
ISSN: 2368-0229
ISBN: 978-1-894402-82-8

Continues: Products for Minor Ailments, First Edition
ISSN: 2291-3300
ISBN: 978-1-894402-73-6

1. Drugs, Nonprescription – Canada – Handbooks, manuals etc. 2. Health Products – Canada – Handbooks, manuals, etc. I. Canadian Pharmacists Association. II. Jovaisas, Barbara.

RM671.5   615.5

Table of Contents

Comparative Product Tables

Editorial Advisory Committee

Peter J. McLeod, MD, FRCPC, FACP (Chair)
Professor of Medicine and Pharmacology
McGill University
Montreal, QC

Michael Allen, MD, MSc
Professor, Post-retirement Appointment
Dalhousie University, Continuing Professional Development
Halifax, NS

Shawn Bugden, BSc(Pharm), MSc, PharmD
Associate Professor, Faculty of Pharmacy
University of Manitoba
Winnipeg, MB

John Conly, MD, FRCPC, FACP
Professor of Medicine (Microbiology)
University of Calgary
Medical Officer Infection Prevention and Control
Foothills Hospital
Calgary, AB

Roland Grad, MDCM, MSc, CCFP, FCFP
Associate Professor, McGill University
Herzl Family Practice Centre
Montreal, QC

Muhammad Mamdani, PharmD, MA, MPH
Director, Applied Health Research Centre
Li Ka Shing Knowledge Institute of St. Michael's Hospital
Professor, Faculty of Medicine and Leslie Dan Faculty of Pharmacy
University of Toronto
Toronto, ON

Neil H. Shear, MD, FRCPC
Professor and Head of Dermatology
Faculty of Medicine, University of Toronto
Toronto, ON

Yvonne Shevchuk, BSP, PharmD, FCSHP
Professor of Pharmacy and Director, medSask Medication Information Service
College of Pharmacy and Nutrition
University of Saskatchewan
Saskatoon, SK

Nese Yuksel, BScPharm, PharmD, ACPR, FCSHP, NCMP
Associate Professor
Faculty of Pharmacy and Pharmaceutical Sciences
University of Alberta
Edmonton, AB

Practioner Review Board

Martha Bailkowski, BScPhm, CDE
Bishops Cross Remedy's Rx Pharmacy
Thornhill, ON

Sheldon Baines, BScPharm
BioScript Pharmacy Ltd
St. John's, NL

Kim Cook, BSP
Pharmasave
Melville, SK

Peter Cook, RPh, BScPharm
Regency 6 Medicine Centre
Vancouver, BC

Shera Hanson, BScPharm
Murphy's Pharmacies
Charlottetown, PEI

Pam L. Johnson, BScPharm
Loblaw Pharmacy
Winnipeg, MB

Scott McLeod, BSc(Pharm)
Shoppers Drug Mart
Canmore, AB

Louise Petit, BPharm
J Matte & L Petit Pharmaciens
Quebec, QC

Sandeep Sodhi, BSc, PhC
Village Family Pharmacy Inc.
Truro, NS

Editor's Message

Welcome to the *Compendium of Products for Minor Ailments (CPMA)*, formerly *Products for Minor Ailments*. This year, the Canadian Pharmacists Association (CPhA) has undertaken a strategic rebranding of its products and services. As a result, many of its publications have new names. *CPMA* contains the same unique collection of nonprescription product information published in 2013 under its former name.

This book represents an unrivalled collection of information on formulations and ingredients of nonprescription drugs, natural health products, medical devices and aids to daily living, organized by condition. It is a vital companion to the therapeutic information in the *Compendium of Therapeutics for Minor Ailments (CTMA)*, containing invaluable evidence-based information on managing minor ailments.

This book is the product of diligent research and validation conducted by managing scientific editor Sonal Acharya and scientific editor Gustavo Paguaga, with the support of a dedicated team of editors, graphic designers and content publishing specialists. We trust you will find the information in these pages useful in your daily practice.

Feedback is an essential element in the quality of any publication and we invite you to contact us with any comments or questions.

Barbara Jovaisas,
Editor-in-Chief

Editorial Policy, Description and Limitations of Information

Compendium of Products for Minor Ailments (CPMA) is compiled and produced by the Canadian Pharmacists Association (CPhA) for the benefit of all healthcare providers.

CPhA does not accept funding from pharmaceutical manufacturers for any content that we develop. The inclusion of individual products does not imply that the editors accept, endorse or recommend these preparations as being clinically superior to similar products of any other firm.

Great care has been taken to ensure the accuracy and completeness of the information contained in the product tables. However, the editors and publishers are not responsible for errors or any consequences arising from the use of the information published herein. In cases of error or dispute, it is the user's responsibility to consult the appropriate regulatory instrument.

Drug therapy is constantly changing; consequently, it is the responsibility of the healthcare provider to seek additional and confirmatory information, to evaluate its appropriateness as it relates to the actual clinical situation, and to consider new developments.

Errata

In spite of the rigorous review process, should a major error be identified it will be corrected immediately on www.pharmacists.ca\errata. All errors will be corrected in the next print edition.

How to Use the
Compendium of Products
for Minor Ailments

Compendium of Products for Minor Ailments (CPMA) is the nonprescription companion to *Compendium of Therapeutics for Minor Ailments (CTMA)*. It is an exclusive collection of information about nonprescription products including drugs and natural health products, home tests, medical aids and medical devices.

The user-friendly Comparative Product Tables are designed to be consulted in conjunction with *CTMA*, which discusses drug therapies by generic name. After choosing a drug or ingredient for self-care, the user of *CTMA* can consult this reference to find the brand name and source of the product to be used.

CPMA is composed of 104 Comparative Product Tables (compiled by CPhA). The tables list nonprescription products available in Canada, categorized by use.

CPMA also includes a Directory that contains contact information for Poison Control Centres and pharmaceutical manufacturers.

The Comparative Product Tables are designed for quick consultation in the practice setting. Use the tables to select a product to meet specific consumer health needs and to determine the availability and content of most nonprescription drug products available in Canada. The classification of products is in accordance with labelling standards.

To locate a product for a specific condition or symptom, consult the Table of Contents at the front of the book.

To locate a specific product, consult the Index at the back of the book by the brand or generic name of the product. The Index will guide you to the appropriate product table page number.

Product	Manufacturer	Dosage Form	Methyl Salicylate	Camphor	Menthol	Other Active Ingredients
Absorbine Extreme Gel	W.F. Young	gel			10%	arnica montana 1%
Absorbine Jr Extra Strength Liniment	W.F. Young	liquid			4%	chloroxylenol 0.5%
Absorbine Jr Liniment	W.F. Young	liquid			1.25%	chloroxylenol 0.5%
Absorbine Power Gel	W.F. Young	gel			4%	chloroxylenol 0.5%
Actipatch Back Pain	Bioelectronics Corp	patch				pulsed electromagnetic field dermal patch
Actipatch Foot/Ankle Pain	Bioelectronics Corp	patch				pulsed electromagnetic field dermal patch
Actipatch Knee Pain	Bioelectronics Corp	patch				pulsed electromagnetic field dermal patch
Actipatch Wrist Pain	Bioelectronics Corp	patch				pulsed electromagnetic field dermal patch
Antiphlogistine Rub A-535 Arnica Spray	Church & Dwight	liquid				arnica montana 15%
Antiphlogistine Rub A-535 Arthritis Extra Strength Roll-On	Church & Dwight	liquid			1.25%	035% triethanolamine salicylate 10%
Antiphlogistine Rub A-535 Capsaicin Cream	Church & Dwight	cream				capsaicin 0.05%
Antiphlogistine Rub A-535 Capsaicin Gel	Church & Dwight	gel				capsaicin 0.05%
Antiphlogistine Rub A-535 Extra Strength	Church & Dwight	ointment	18%	1%	0.75%	eucalyptus oil 0.5%
Antiphlogistine Rub A-535 Heat	Church & Dwight	ointment	12.5%	1%	0.75%	eucalyptus oil 0.5%
Antiphlogistine Rub A-535 Ice	Church & Dwight	gel			4%	
Antiphlogistine Rub A-535 No Odour	Church & Dwight	ointment				triethanolamine salicylate 13.3%
Antiphlogistine Rub A-535 Sport Ice	Church & Dwight	gel			5%	
Antiphlogistine Rub A-535 Sport Ultra Heat	Church & Dwight	cream	30%	1%	0.75%	eucalyptus oil 3%
Aspercreme	Chattem	cream				triethanolamine salicylate 10%
Aspercreme Extra Strength	Chattem	cream				triethanolamine salicylate 15%
Ben-Gay Arthritis Extra Strength	Johnson & Johnson	ointment	30%		8%	
Ben-Gay Ultra Strength	Johnson & Johnson	cream	30%	4%	10%	
Capsaicin Cream/Gel 0.025-0.075%	Various Manufacturers	cream/gel				capsaicin 0.025%
Capsaicin Cream 0.025%	Valeo Pharma	cream				capsaicin 0.025%
Capsaicin Cream 0.075%	Valeo Pharma	cream				capsaicin 0.075%
Deep Relief Ultra Joint Pain Gel	Mentholatum	gel			3%	
Deep Relief Sprain & Strain Spray	Mentholatum	spray			8%	
Deep Relief Muscle Ache Ultra Strength Ice Gel	Mentholatum	gel			4%	
Deep Relief Ice Cold Gel	Mentholatum	gel			2%	
Deep Relief Arthritis Pain Patch	Mentholatum	patch	10%			
Deep Relief Dual Action Neck, Shoulder & Back Pain Warming Rub	Mentholatum	lotion	20%		6%	

▶

Product	Manufacturer	Dosage Form	Methyl Salicylate	Camphor	Menthol	Other Active Ingredients
Deep Relief Ultra Strength Neck, Shoulder & Back Pain Patch	Mentholatum	patch	8%			
Deep Relief Muscle Ache Night Time Rub	Mentholatum	cream	12.8%	5.91%		
Deep Relief Muscle Ache Ultra Strength Rub	Mentholatum	cream	30%		8%	
Doctor's Pain Formula Cream	Blue Mountain Springs Wellness	cream			1.4%	
Doctor's Pain Formula Roll-On	Blue Mountain Springs Wellness	liquid			1.4%	
Fast Freeze Gel	Bell-Horn	gel			3.5%	
Fast Freeze Roll-On	Bell-Horn	liquid			3.5%	
Fast Freeze Spray	Bell-Horn	liquid			10%	
Flex-All Extra Strength	Chattem	gel			10%	
Icy Hot Cream	Chattem	cream	30%		10%	
Icy Hot Gel	Chattem	gel			2.5	
Icy Hot Medicated Patch	Chattem	patch			5%	
Icy Hot Medicated Sleeve	Chattem	sleeve			16%	
Kenzen Medicated Cool Pads	Sato Pharma	patch		3%	1.25%	eucalyptus 0.5%
Kenzen Medicated Hot Pads	Sato Pharma	patch				capsaicin 0.025%
LivRelief Nerve Pain Cream	LivCorp	cream				capsaicin 0.075%
LivRelief Pain Relief Cream	LivCorp	cream				rutin 0.4%
Methacin Cream	Mentholatum	cream			4%	capsaicin 0.025%
Mentholatum	Mentholatum	ointment		9%	1.35	
Minard's Liniment	Stella Pharmaceutical	liquid		5%		ammonium hydroxide 2.3% turpentine 10.5%
Myoflex Deep Therapy Patch	Bayer Consumer	patch				triethanolamine salicylate 12.5%
Myoflex Extra Strength	Bayer Consumer	cream				triethanolamine salicylate 15%
Myoflex Maximum Strength	Bayer Consumer	gel				triethanolamine salicylate 20%
Myoflex Regular	Bayer Consumer	cream				triethanolamine salicylate 10%
Redfeather Pain Spray	Premiere Enterprises	liquid			7%	
Salonpas Gel Patch	Hisamitsu Pharmaceutical	patch			1.25%	capsaicin 0.025%
Salonpas Hot Capsicum Patch	Hisamitsu Pharmaceutical	patch				capsaicin 0.025%
Salonpas Pain Relieving Patch	Hisamitsu Pharmaceutical	patch	6.29%	1.24%	5.71%	
Tiger Balm Arthritis Rub	Haw Par	cream		11%	11%	oil of cajeput 13% oil of clove 5% peppermint oil 6%
Tiger Balm Neck & Shoulder Rub	Haw Par	cream		11%	10%	oil of eucalyptus 3%
Tiger Balm Patch	Haw Par	patch		1%	0.3%	capsaicin 0.004% oil of eucalyptus 0.5% peppermint oil 0.6%
Tiger Balm Red Strong	Haw Par	ointment		11%	10%	oil of cajeput 7% oil of cinnamon 5% oil of clove 5% peppermint oil 6%

Product	Manufacturer	Dosage Form	Methyl Salicylate	Camphor	Menthol	Other Active Ingredients
Tiger Balm White Regular	Haw Par	ointment		11%	7.96%	oil of cajeput 12.93% oil of clove 1.49% peppermint oil 15.9%
Tiger Balm Ultra	Haw Par	ointment		11%	11%	oil of cajeput 13% oil of cinnamon 3% oil of clove 2% peppermint oil 6%
TPR20 (Topical Pain Relief)	Trans Research Labs	cream			1%	lidocaine 5%
Ultra Strength Heat Rub	Hyde	cream	30%		8%	
Voltaren Emulgel	Novartis Consumer Health	gel				diclofenac diethylamine 1.16%
Voltaren Emulgel Joint Pain	Novartis Consumer Health	gel				diclofenac diethylamine 1.16%
Watkins Liniment Cream	Watkins	cream		3%		turpentine 9%
Watkins Medicated Ointment	Watkins	ointment		5%	2.8	
Youngflex Massage Ointment 168	Youngflex	ointment			15.5%	eucalyptus oil 3% oil of cajeput 6.5%
Zoderm Cream	Euro-Pharm	cream				capsaicin 0.025%
Zostrix	Medicis	cream				capsaicin 0.025%
Zostrix HP	Medicis	cream				capsaicin 0.075%

4 Analgesic Products: Internal Analgesics and Antipyretics

Product	Manufacturer	Dosage Form	ASA	Acetaminophen	Ibuprofen	Other Active Ingredients
222	Johnson & Johnson Merck	tablet	375 mg			caffeine citrate 30 mg codeine phosphate 8 mg
A.C.&C.	Various Manufacturers	tablet	325-375 mg			caffeine 15 mg codeine phosphate 8 mg
Abenol 120 mg	Pendopharm	suppository		120 mg		
Abenol 325 mg	Pendopharm	suppository		325 mg		
Abenol 650 mg	Pendopharm	suppository		650 mg		
Acetaminophen Children's Tablet	Various Manufacturers	tablet, chewable		80 mg		
Acetaminophen Children's Tablet	Various Manufacturers	tablet, chewable		160 mg		
Acetaminophen Extra Strength Caplet	Various Manufacturers	caplet		500 mg		
Acetaminophen Extra Strength Tablet	Various Manufacturers	tablet		500 mg		
Acetaminophen Extra Strength with Codeine	Various Manufacturers	tablet		500 mg		caffeine 15-30 mg codeine phosphate 8 mg
Acetaminophen Junior Melts Tablets	Tanta	tablet		160 mg		
Acetaminophen Oral Drops	Various Manufacturers	drops		80 mg/mL		
Acetaminophen Oral Solution 16 mg/mL	Various Manufacturers	liquid		16 mg/mL		
Acetaminophen Oral Solution 32 mg/mL	Various Manufacturers	liquid		32 mg/mL		
Acetaminophen Regular Strength Caplet	Various Manufacturers	caplet		325 mg		
Acetaminophen Regular Strength Tablet	Various Manufacturers	tablet		325 mg		
Acetaminophen with Codeine	Various Manufacturers	tablet		300-325 mg		caffeine 15-30 mg codeine phosphate 8 mg
Acetazone Forte	Teva Canada	tablet		300 mg		chlorzoxazone 250 mg
Acetazone Forte C8	Teva Canada	tablet		300 mg		chlorzoxazone 250 mg codeine phosphate 8 mg
Advil Caplets	Pfizer Consumer Healthcare	caplet			200 mg	
Advil Children's Suspension	Pfizer Consumer Healthcare	suspension			20 mg/mL	
Advil Extra Strength Caplets	Pfizer Consumer Healthcare	caplet			400 mg	
Advil Gel Caplet	Pfizer Consumer Healthcare	gelatin caplet			200 mg	
Advil Junior Chewable Tablets	Pfizer Consumer Healthcare	tablet, chewable			100 mg	
Advil Liqui-Gels	Pfizer Consumer Healthcare	capsule			200 mg	
Advil Liqui-Gels Extra Strength	Pfizer Consumer Healthcare	capsule			400 mg	
Advil Nighttime	Pfizer Consumer Healthcare	capsule			200 mg	diphenhydramine 25 mg

Product	Manufacturer	Dosage Form	ASA	Acetaminophen	Ibuprofen	Other Active Ingredients
Advil Pediatric Drops	Pfizer Consumer Healthcare	suspension			40 mg/mL	
Advil Tablets	Pfizer Consumer Healthcare	tablet			200 mg	
Aleve Caplets	Bayer Consumer	caplet				naproxen sodium 220 mg
Aleve Liqui-Gels	Bayer Consumer	capsule				naproxen sodium 220 mg
Aleve Tablets	Bayer Consumer	tablet				naproxen sodium 220 mg
Alka-Seltzer	Bayer Consumer	tablet, effervescent	325 mg			citric acid 1000 mg sodium bicarbonate 1916 mg
Alka-Seltzer Flavored	Bayer Consumer	tablet, effervescent	325 mg			citric acid 1220 mg sodium bicarbonate 1710 mg
Anacin Extra Strength Tablets	Pfizer Consumer Healthcare	tablet	500 mg			caffeine 32 mg
Anacin Tablets	Pfizer Consumer Healthcare	tablet	325 mg			caffeine 32 mg
Apo-Acetaminophen 325 mg Caplets	Apotex	caplet		325 mg		
Apo-Acetaminophen 325 mg Tablets	Apotex	tablet		325 mg		
Apo-Acetaminophen 500 mg Caplets	Apotex	caplet		500 mg		
Apo-Acetaminophen 500 mg Tablets	Apotex	tablet		500 mg		
Apo-ASA 325 mg	Apotex	tablet	325 mg			
Apo-Ibuprofen Caplets	Apotex	caplet			200 mg	
Apo-Ibuprofen Extra Strength Caplets	Apotex	caplet			400 mg	
Apo-Ibuprofen Extra Strength Tablets	Apotex	tablet			400 mg	
Apo-Ibuprofen Tablets	Apotex	tablet			200 mg	
Apo-Ibuprofen 300 mg Tablets	Apotex	tablet			300 mg	
ASA ECT 325 mg	Various Manufacturers	tablet, enteric coated	325 mg			
ASA ECT 650 mg	Various Manufacturers	tablet, enteric coated	650 mg			
ASA Suppositories 150 mg	Pendopharm	suppository	150 mg			
ASA Suppositories 650 mg	Pendopharm	suppository	650 mg			
ASA Tablets 325 mg	Various Manufacturers	tablet	325 mg			
ASA Tablets 80 mg	Various Manufacturers	tablet	80 mg			
Asaphen 81 mg	Pendopharm	tablet, chewable	81 mg			
Asaphen Chewable 80 mg	Pendopharm	tablet, chewable	80 mg			
Asaphen Enteric Coated 80 mg	Pendopharm	tablet, enteric coated	80 mg			
Asaphen Enteric Coated 81 mg	Pendopharm	tablet, enteric coated	81 mg			

Product	Manufacturer	Dosage Form	ASA	Acetaminophen	Ibuprofen	Other Active Ingredients
Aspirin Caplets	Bayer Consumer	caplet	325 mg			
Aspirin Extra Strength Tablets 500 mg	Bayer Consumer	tablet	500 mg			
Aspirin Tablets 325 mg	Bayer Consumer	tablet	325 mg			
Aspirin With Stomach Guard Extra Strength	Bayer Consumer	caplet	500 mg			calcium carbonate 246.2 mg magnesium carbonate 52.3 mg magnesium oxide 96.9 mg
Aspirin With Stomach Guard Regular Strength	Bayer Consumer	tablet	325 mg			calcium carbonate 160 mg magnesium carbonate 34 mg magnesium oxide 63 mg
Atasol Drops	Church & Dwight	drops		80 mg/mL		
Atasol Forte Caplets	Church & Dwight	caplet		500 mg		
Atasol Forte Tablets	Church & Dwight	tablet		500 mg		
Atasol Regular Tablets	Church & Dwight	tablet		325 mg		
Axum	Teva Canada	tablet			200 mg	methocarbamol 500 mg
Children's Feverhalt Chewable Tablet 160 mg	Pendopharm	tablet, chewable		160 mg		
Children's Europrofen	Euro-Pharm	suspension			20 mg/mL	
Children's Feverhalt Drops	Pendopharm	liquid		80 mg/mL		
Children's Little Remedies for Fevers	Prestige Brands`	liquid		32 mg/mL		
Coated Aspirin Arthritis Pain Relief	Bayer Consumer	caplet, enteric coated	325 mg			
Coated Aspirin Arthritis Pain Relief Extra Strength	Bayer Consumer	caplet, enteric coated	500 mg			
Coated Aspirin 81mg	Bayer Consumer	tablet, enteric coated	81 mg			
Dodd's Extra Strength	G.T. Fulford	tablet				sodium salicylate 500 mg
Dom-Acetaminophen Suppositories 120 mg	Dominion Pharmacal	suppository		120 mg		
Dom-Acetaminophen Suppositories 325 mg	Dominion Pharmacal	suppository		325 mg		
Entrophen Extra Strength Tablets	Pendopharm	tablet, delayed release	500 mg			
Entrophen Regular Strength Caplets	Pendopharm	caplet, delayed release	325 mg			
Entrophen Regular Strength Tablets	Pendopharm	tablet, delayed release	325 mg			
Entrophen Super Extra Strength Caplets	Pendopharm	caplet, delayed release	650 mg			
Entrophen Super Extra Strength Tablets	Pendopharm	tablet, delayed release	650 mg			
Equate Daily Low Dose	Pendopharm	tablet, enteric coated	81 mg			
Ibuprofen Caplets 200 mg	Various Manufacturers	caplet			200 mg	
Ibuprofen Caplets 400 mg	Various Manufacturers	caplet			400 mg	
Ibuprofen Liquid Capsules	Tanta	capsule			200 mg	

Product	Manufacturer	Dosage Form	ASA	Acetaminophen	Ibuprofen	Other Active Ingredients
Ibuprofen Tablets 200 mg	Various Manufacturers	tablet			200 mg	
Ibuprofen Tablets 400 mg	Various Manufacturers	tablet			400 mg	
Infant's Little Remedies for Fevers	Prestige Brands	liquid		80 mg/mL		
Instantine	Bayer Consumer	tablet	325 mg			caffeine 65 mg
Lenoltec No 1	Teva	tablet		300 mg		caffeine 15 mg codeine phosphate 8 mg
Lowprin Chewable Tablets	Euro-Pharm	tablet	80 mg			
Lowprin Tablets	Euro-Pharm	tablet	80 mg			
Maxidol Liquid Gels	Bayer Consumer	capsule				naproxen sodium 220 mg
Mersyndol with Codeine	sanofi-aventis	tablet		325 mg		codeine phosphate 8 mg doxylamine succinate 5 mg
Methoxacet	Teva Canada	tablet		325 mg		methocarbamol 400 mg
Methoxacet C1/8	Teva Canada	tablet		325 mg		codeine 8 mg methocarbamol 400 mg
Methoxacet Extra Strength	Teva Canada	tablet		500 mg		methocarbamol 400 mg
Methoxisal	Teva Canada	tablet	325 mg			methocarbamol 400 mg
Methoxisal C1/8	Teva Canada	tablet	325 mg			codeine phosphate 8 mg methocarbamol 400 mg
Methoxisal Extra Strength	Teva Canada	tablet	500 mg			methocarbamol 400 mg
Midol Extra Strength Caplets	Bayer Consumer	caplet		500 mg		caffeine 60 mg pyrilamine maleate 15 mg
Midol PMS Extra Strength	Bayer Consumer	caplet		500 mg		pamabrom 25 mg pyrilamine maleate 15 mg
Midol Teen Complete	Bayer Consumer	caplet		325 mg		caffeine 60 mg pyrilamine maleate 15 mg
Motrin Children's Chewable Tablets	McNeil Consumer Healthcare	tablet			50 mg	
Motrin Children's Suspension Drops	McNeil Consumer Healthcare	drops			40 mg/mL	
Motrin Children's Suspension Liquid Berry/Bubblegum/Grape	McNeil Consumer Healthcare	suspension			20 mg/mL	
Motrin IB Caplets	McNeil Consumer Healthcare	caplet			200 mg	
Motrin IB Extra Strength	McNeil Consumer Healthcare	tablet			300 mg	
Motrin IB Liquid Gels	McNeil Consumer Healthcare	gelcap			200 mg	
Motrin IB Super Strength	McNeil Consumer Healthcare	tablet			400 mg	
Motrin IB Tablets	McNeil Consumer Healthcare	tablet			200 mg	
Motrin Junior Strength Caplets	McNeil Consumer Healthcare	caplet			100 mg	
Motrin Junior Strength Chewable Tablets	McNeil Consumer Healthcare	tablet, chewable			100 mg	
MSD Enteric Coated ASA 325 mg	Merck Frosst	tablet, enteric coated	325 mg			

Product	Manufacturer	Dosage Form	ASA	Acetaminophen	Ibuprofen	Other Active Ingredients
MSD Enteric Coated ASA 650 mg	Merck Frosst	tablet, enteric coated	650 mg			
Multi-gesic	Multi-Pro	tablet		325 mg		
Muscle & Back Pain Relief	Various Manufacturers	tablet		325 mg		methocarbamol 400 mg
Muscle & Back Pain Relief Extra Strength	Various Manufacturers	tablet		500 mg		methocarbamol 400 mg
Naproxen	Pendopharm	tablet				naproxen sodium 220 mg
Novo-Gesic	Novopharm	tablet		325 mg		
Novo-Gesic C8	Novopharm	tablet		300 mg		caffeine 15 mg codeine phosphate 8 mg
Novo-Gesic Forte	Novopharm	tablet		500 mg		
Novo-Profen	Novopharm	tablet			200 mg	
Orfenace	Sterimax	tablet				orphenadrine citrate 100 mg
Pain Aid	Zee Medical	tablet	500 mg			caffeine 32 mg
Pain Aid Free	Zee Medical	tablet		500 mg		
Pediaphen 80 mg Chewable Tablets	Euro-Pharm	tablet		80 mg		
Pediaphen 160 mg Chewable Tablets	Euro-Pharm	tablet		160 mg		
Pediaphen 16 mg/mL	Euro-Pharm	liquid		16 mg/mL		
Pediaphen 32 mg/mL	Euro-Pharm	liquid		32 mg/mL		
Pediaphen 80 mg/mL	Euro-Pharm	liquid		80 mg/mL		
Pediatrix Drops	Teva Canada	drops		80 mg/mL		
Pediatrix Liquid	Teva Canada	liquid		32 mg/mL		
PMS Acetaminophen 325 mg	Pharmascience	tablet		325 mg		
PMS Acetaminophen 500 mg	Pharmascience	tablet		500 mg		
PMS Acetaminophen Solution 16 mg/mL	Pharmascience	liquid		16 mg/mL		
PMS Acetaminophen Solution 32 mg/mL	Pharmascience	liquid		32 mg/mL		
PMS Acetaminophen Solution 80 mg/mL	Pharmascience	liquid		80 mg/mL		
PMS Acetaminophen Suppositories 120 mg	Pharmascience	suppository		120 mg		
PMS Acetaminophen Suppositories 160 mg	Pharmascience	suppository		160 mg		
PMS Acetaminophen Suppositories 325 mg	Pharmascience	suppository		325 mg		
PMS Acetaminophen Suppositories 650 mg	Pharmascience	suppository		650 mg		
Relievol PMS Extra Strength	Tanta	tablet		500 mg		pamabrom 25 mg pyrilamine maleate 15 mg
Robax Platinum	Pfizer Consumer Healthcare	caplet			200 mg	methocarbamol 500 mg
Robaxacet Caplets	Pfizer Consumer Healthcare	caplet		325 mg		methocarbamol 400 mg

Product	Manufacturer	Dosage Form	ASA	Acetaminophen	Ibuprofen	Other Active Ingredients
Robaxacet Caplets Extra Strength	Pfizer Consumer Healthcare	caplet		500 mg		methocarbamol 400 mg
Robaxacet-8	Pfizer Consumer Healthcare	tablet		325 mg		codeine phosphate 8 mg methocarbamol 400 mg
Robaxin	Pfizer Consumer Healthcare	tablet				methocarbamol 500 mg
Robaxin 750	Pfizer Consumer Healthcare	tablet				methocarbamol 750 mg
Robaxisal Extra Strength	Pfizer Consumer Healthcare	caplet	500 mg			methocarbamol 400 mg
Robigesic Elixir	Pfizer Consumer Healthcare	liquid		16 mg/mL		
Sandoz-Orphenadrine 100 mg	Sandoz	tablet				orphenadrine citrate 100 mg
Spasmhalt-8	Pendopharm	tablet		325 mg		codeine phosphate 8 mg methocarbamol 400 mg
Summit Ultra	Pendopharm	tablet			400 mg	methocarbamol 500 mg
Tantaphen Acetaminophen Oral Solution	Tanta	liquid		80 mg/mL		
Tantaphen Extra Strength Caplets	Tanta	caplet		500 mg		
Tempra Children's Double Strength Syrup	Mead Johnson	syrup		32 mg/mL		
Tempra Children's Syrup	Mead Johnson	syrup		16 mg/mL		
Tempra Infant Drops	Mead Johnson	drops		80 mg/mL		
Triatec-8	Trianon	caplet		325 mg		caffeine citrate 30 mg codeine phosphate 8 mg
Triatec-8 Fort	Trianon	tablet		500 mg		caffeine citrate 30 mg codeine phosphate 8 mg
Tylenol Arthritis Pain Extended Release 650 mg	McNeil Consumer Healthcare	caplet, extended release		650 mg		
Tylenol Back Pain	McNeil Consumer Healthcare	caplet		500 mg		methocarbamol 400 mg
Tylenol Body Pain Night	McNeil Consumer Healthcare	caplet		500 mg		methocarbamol 400 mg
Tylenol Children's Suspension	McNeil Consumer Healthcare	suspension		32 mg/mL		
Tylenol Children's Suspension Bubblegum/ Grape	McNeil Consumer Healthcare	suspension		32 mg/mL		
Tylenol Children's Meltaways Bubble Gum/ Grape	McNeil Consumer Healthcare	tablet, dissolving		80 mg		
Tylenol Extra Strength Caplets	McNeil Consumer Healthcare	caplet		500 mg		
Tylenol Extra Strength Gelcaps	McNeil Consumer Healthcare	tablet, gel coated		500 mg		
Tylenol Extra Strength EZ Tabs	McNeil Consumer Healthcare	tablet		500 mg		

Product	Manufacturer	Dosage Form	ASA	Acetaminophen	Ibuprofen	Other Active Ingredients
Tylenol Extra Strength Rapid Release	McNeil Consumer Healthcare	tablet		500 mg		
Tylenol Infants' Suspension Drops Cherry/Dye Free Grape	McNeil Consumer Healthcare	suspension		80 mg/mL		
Tylenol Junior Strength Fastmelts Tutti Fruitti/ Orange	McNeil Consumer Healthcare	tablet, dissolving		80 mg		
Tylenol Junior Strength Meltaways Bubblegum/ Grape	McNeil Consumer Healthcare	tablet, dissolving		160 mg		
Tylenol Menstrual Extra Strength	McNeil Consumer Healthcare	tablet		500 mg		pamabrom 25 mg pyrilamine maleate 15 mg
Tylenol Muscle Aches and Body Pain	McNeil Consumer Healthcare	tablet		650 mg		
Tylenol No 1 Caplets	McNeil Consumer Healthcare	caplet		300 mg		caffeine 15 mg codeine phosphate 8 mg
Tylenol Regular Strength Caplets	McNeil Consumer Healthcare	caplet		325 mg		
Tylenol Regular Strength Tablets	McNeil Consumer Healthcare	tablet		325 mg		
Tylenol Ultra Relief Migraine Pain	McNeil Consumer Healthcare	tablet		500 mg		caffeine 65 mg

Product	Manufacturer	Dosage Form	Active Ingredients
Combantrin Tablets	Pfizer Consumer Healthcare	tablet	pyrantel pamoate 125 mg

Product	Manufacturer	Dosage Form	Active Ingredients
Adidas A3 Antiperspirant	Coty Canada	stick	aluminum zirconium tetrachlorohydrex-glycine 20%
Adidas A3 Antiperspirant Roll-on	Coty Canada	liquid	aluminum zirconium tetrachlorohydrex-glycine 20%
Adidas A3 Dry Max Antiperspirant	Coty Canada	stick	aluminum zirconium tetrachlorohydrex-glycine 20%
Adidas Antiperspirant Cool Gel	Coty Canada	gel	aluminum zirconium tetrachlorohydrex-glycine 20%
Antiperspirant Deodorant	Body Shop	liquid	aluminum chlorohydrate 20%
Antiperspirant Pump Spray	Atlas	aerosol	aluminum chlorohydrate 15%
Antiperspirant Roll-On	Atlas	lotion	aluminum chlorohydrate 20%
Antiperspirant Roll-On Deodorant	Estee Lauder	liquid	aluminum chloride 2% aluminum chlorohydrate 20%
Arm & Hammer Advance Antiperspirant	Church & Dwight	stick	aluminum zirconium tetrachlorohydrex-glycine 19%
Arm & Hammer Advance Antiperspirant Clear Gel	Church & Dwight	gel	aluminum zirconium tetrachlorohydrex-glycine 16%
Arm & Hammer Advance Antiperspirant Invisible	Church & Dwight	stick	aluminum zirconium tetrachlorohydrex-glycine 19%
Arrid Extra Dry Aerosol	Church & Dwight	aerosol	aluminum chlorohydrate 10%
Arrid Extra Dry Invisible	Church & Dwight	stick	aluminum zirconium trichlorohydrex-glycine 19%
Arrid Extra Dry Roll-On Unscented	Church & Dwight	lotion	aluminum chlorohydrate 16%
Arrid Total Gel	Church & Dwight	gel	aluminum zirconium tetrachlorohydrex-glycine 16%
Arrid Total Solid Invisible	Church & Dwight	stick	aluminum zirconium tetrachlorohydrex-glycine 19%
Avon Roll-On Antiperspirant Deodorant Cool Confidence/Feelin' Fresh/Skin So Soft	Avon	lotion	aluminum chlorohydrate 25%
Avon Roll-On Antiperspirant Deodorant/Lumieres/Skin So Soft/Soft & Sensual	Avon	lotion	aluminum chlorohydrate 17.5%
AXE Dry Gel	Unilever Canada	gel	aluminum zirconium tetrachlorohydrex-glycine 18.6%
AXE Invisible Deodorant Stick	Unilever Canada	stick	aluminum zirconium tetrachlorohydrex-glycine 17.8%
Ban Antiperspirant Roll-On	Kao Brands	liquid	aluminum chlorohydrate 18%
Ban Invisible Antiperspirant Stick	Kao Brands	stick	aluminum zirconium tetrachlorohydrex-glycine 24%
Brut Antiperspirant Aerosol	Idelle Labs	aerosol	aluminum chlorohydrate 10.95%
Brut Antiperspirant Stick	Idelle Labs	stick	aluminum zirconium tetrachlorohydrex-glycine 24%
Certain Dri Anti-Perspirant Roll-On	Numark Laboratories	liquid	aluminum chloride 12% aqueous solution
Certain Dri A.M. Anti-perspirant Roll-On	Numark Laboratories	liquid	aluminum zirconium trichlorohydrex-glycine 17.8%
Cool Confidence Deodorant Stick	Avon	stick	aluminum chlorohydrate 20.7%
Cool Confidence Roll-On Antiperspirant	Avon	liquid	aluminum chlorohydrate 20.7%
Crystal Body Deodorant Roll-On	Crystal	liquid	natural mineral salts potassium alum
Crystal Body Deodorant Spray	Crystal	liquid	natural mineral salts potassium alum
Crystal Body Deodorant Stick	Crystal	stick	natural mineral salts ammonium alum
Degree Antiperspirant Aerosol	Unilever Canada	aerosol	aluminum chlorohydrate 8.8%
Degree Clinical Solid	Unilever Canada	stick	aluminum zirconium tetrachlorohydrex-glycine 20%
Degree Deodorant Stick	Unilever Canada	stick	aluminum zirconium tetrachlorohydrex-glycine 17.8%
Degree Invisible Solid	Unilever Canada	stick	aluminum zirconium tetrachlorohydrex-glycine 17.8%
Degree Ultra Clear Antiperspirant	Unilever Canada	stick	aluminum zirconium tetrachlorohydrex-glycine 14.8%
Dove Antiperspirant Clear Supreme	Unilever Canada	stick	aluminum zirconyl hydroxychloride complex 17.8%
Dove Antiperspirant Invisible	Unilever Canada	stick	aluminum zirconyl hydroxychloride complex 17.8%
Dove Clinical Protection	Unilever Canada	stick	aluminum zirconyl hydroxychloride complex 20%

Product	Manufacturer	Dosage Form	Active Ingredients
Dove Invisible Antiperspirant	Unilever Canada	stick	aluminum zirconium tetrachlorohydrex-glycine 18.5%
Dove Pro-Age Antiperspirant/Deodorant	Unilever Canada	stick	aluminum zirconyl hydroxychloride complex 17.8%
Dove Pro-Age Antiperspirant/Deodorant Roll-On	Unilever Canada	liquid	aluminum chlorohydrate 15%
Dove Ultimate Clear Invisible	Unilever Canada	stick	aluminum zirconium tetrachlorohydrex-glycine 14.8%
Dry Idea Clinical Anti-Perspirant & Deodorant	Dial Canada	aerosol	aluminum chlorohydrate 11%
Dry Idea Clinical Complete Invisible Solid	Dial Canada	stick	aluminum zirconium pentachlorohydrex-glycine 20%
Dry Idea Clinical Complete Roll-On	Dial Canada	liquid	aluminum zirconium pentachlorohydrex-glycine 16.3%
Dry Idea Gel Antiperspirant	Dial Canada	gel	aluminum zirconyl hydroxychloride complex 23.5%
Dry Idea Roll-On Antiperspirant Baby Powder	Dial Canada	lotion	aluminum zirconyl hydroxychloride complex 20%
Drysol	Seaford	liquid	alcohol denatured 80% aluminum chloride 20%
Drysol Dab-O-Matic	Seaford	liquid	alcohol denatured 80% aluminum chloride 20%
Drysol Dab-O-Matic Extra Strong	Seaford	liquid	alcohol denatured 80% aluminum chloride 20%
Drysol Dab-O-Matic Mild	Seaford	liquid	aluminum chloride 6.25% ethyl alcohol 93.75%
Gillette 3X Antiperspirant Clear Gel	Dial Canada	gel	aluminum zirconium octachlorohydrex-glycine 16%
Gillette 3X Clear Gel Power Beads	Dial Canada	gel	aluminum zirconium octachlorohydrex-glycine 16%
Gillette 3X Invisible Stick	Dial Canada	stick	aluminum zirconium trichlorohydrex-glycine 19%
Gillette Clear Shield	Procter & Gamble	stick	aluminum chlorohydrate 16.2%
Gillette Clinical Strength Antiperspirant	Gillette	stick	aluminum zirconium trichlorohydrex-glycine 20%
Happy for Men Antiperspirant Deodorant	Clinique	stick	aluminum zirconium tetrachlorohydrex-glycine 18.6%
Hydrosal Gel	Valeo Pharma	gel	aluminum chloride 15%
Ladies Antiperspirant Invisible	H.J. Sutton	stick	aluminum zirconium tetrachlorohydrex-glycine 20%
Lady Speed Stick 24/7	Colgate-Palmolive	stick	aluminum zirconium tetrachlorohydrex-glycine 22%
Lady Speed Stick 24/7 Gel	Colgate-Palmolive	gel	aluminum zirconium tetrachlorohydrex-glycine 22%
Lady Speed Stick Antiperspirant	Colgate-Palmolive	stick	aluminum zirconium tetrachlorohydrex-glycine 20%
Lady Speed Stick Clinical Proof	Colgate-Palmolive	stick	aluminum zirconium tetrachlorohydrex-glycine 17%
Lady Speed Stick Invisible Antiperspirant	Colgate-Palmolive	stick	aluminum zirconium tetrachlorohydrex-glycine 22%
Men's Antiperspirant	H.J. Sutton	stick	aluminum zirconium tetrachlorohydrex-glycine 22%
Mitchum Antiperspirant & Deodorant Clear Gel	Revlon	lotion	aluminum sesquichlorohydrate 25%
Mitchum Antiperspirant & Deodorant Super Sport	Revlon	stick/gel	aluminum sesquichlorohydrate 24%
Mitchum Antiperspirant Super Dry Roll-On	Revlon	lotion	aluminum zirconium tetrachlorohydrex-glycine 25%
Mitchum Clear Roll-On	Revlon	lotion	aluminum zirconium tetrachlorohydrex-glycine 24%
Mitchum for Women Clear Gel Antiperspirant	Revlon	gel	aluminum zirconium tetrachlorohydrex-glycine 20%
Mitchum for Women Clear Roll-On Antiperspirant	Revlon	lotion	aluminum zirconium tetrachlorohydrex-glycine 20%
Mitchum for Women Super Dry Roll-On Antiperspirant	Revlon	liquid	aluminum zirconium tetrachlorohydrex-glycine 20%
Mitchum for Women Wide Solid Powder Fresh	Revlon	stick	aluminum zirconium tetrachlorohydrex-glycine 20%
Mitchum Powergel	Revlon	lotion	aluminum sesquichlorohydrate 25%
Mitchum Wide Antiperspirant	Revlon	stick	aluminum zirconium tetrachlorohydrex-glycine 25%
No Sweat Antiperspirant	Aurium	liquid	aluminum chloride 10% aluminum lactate 10%
Old Spice Antiperspirant Solid	Procter & Gamble	stick	aluminum zirconium trichlorohydrex-glycine 20%
Old Spice Ever Clear	Procter & Gamble	stick	aluminum chlorohydrate 16.2%

Product	Manufacturer	Dosage Form	Active Ingredients
Old Spice High Endurance Clear Gel	Procter & Gamble	stick	aluminum zirconium octachlorohydrex-glycine 16%
Old Spice High Endurance Invisible	Procter & Gamble	stick	aluminum zirconium trichlorohydrex-glycine 17.8%
Old Spice High Endurance Red Zone	Procter & Gamble	stick	aluminum zirconium octachlorohydrex-glycine 16%
Old Spice Pro-Strength Antiperspirant/Deodorant	Procter & Gamble	stick	aluminum zirconium trichlorohydrex-glycine 20%
Old Spice Red Zone Invisible	Procter & Gamble	stick	aluminum zirconium trichlorohydrex-glycine 17.8%
On Duty 24 Plus	Avon	lotion	aluminum chlorohydrate 25%
Perspirex	Riemann & Co	gel	aluminum chloride 10%
Polo Baton Antiperspirant	Cosmair	stick	aluminum zirconium tetrachlorohydrex-glycine 20%
Protegel	Nutrimmune Technologies	gel	aluminum chloride 15%
Right Guard Antiperspirant Aerosol	Dial Canada	aerosol	aluminum chlorohydrate 9.5%
Right Guard Antiperspirant Gel	Dial Canada	gel	aluminum zirconyl hydroxychloride complex 23.5%
Right Guard Antiperspirant Sport	Dial Canada	stick	aluminum zirconyl hydroxychloride complex 11%
Right Guard Clinical Invisible Solid	Dial Canada	stick	aluminum zirconium pentachlorohydrex-glycine 20%
Right Guard Extreme	Dial Canada	stick	aluminum zirconium tetrachlorohydrex-glycine 14.8%
Right Guard Professional Strength Invisible Solid	Dial Canada	stick	aluminum zirconium pentachlorohydrex-glycine 20%
Secret Antiperspirant Dry Roll-On	Procter & Gamble	lotion	aluminum zirconium trichlorohydrex-glycine 22.5%
Secret Antiperspirant Solid	Procter & Gamble	stick	aluminum zirconium trichlorohydrex-glycine 20%
Secret Clean Antiperspirant Aerosol	Procter & Gamble	aerosol	aluminum chlorohydrate 12%
Secret Clinical Strength Antiperspirant	Gillette	stick	aluminum zirconium trichlorohydrex-glycine 20%
Secret Flawless Crystal Clear Gel	Procter & Gamble	stick	aluminum zirconium octachlorohydrex-glycine 16%
Secret Gentle Care Antiperspirant Stick and Deodorant	Procter & Gamble	stick	aluminum zirconium trichlorohydrex-glycine 23%
Secret Platinum Protection	Procter & Gamble	stick	aluminum zirconium octachlorohydrex-glycine 16%
Secret Roll-On Antiperspirant	Procter & Gamble	lotion	aluminum zirconium trichlorohydrex-glycine 25%
Secret Sheer Dry Antiperspirant	Procter & Gamble	stick	aluminum zirconium trichlorohydrex-glycine 22.7%
Skin So Soft Roll-On Antiperspirant	Avon	lotion	aluminum chlorohydrate 17.5%
Skin Supplies for Men Antiperspirant & Deodorant	Clinique	stick	aluminum zirconium trichlorohydrex-glycine 18.4%
Soft & Dri Antiperspirant Aerosol	Dial Canada	aerosol	aluminum chlorohydrate 8.2%
Soft & Dri Antiperspirant Gel	Dial Canada	gel	aluminum zirconyl tetrachlorohydrex-glycine 23.5%
Soft & Dri For Women Invisible Solid	Dial Canada	stick	aluminum zirconium trichlorohydrex-glycine 22.8%
Soft & Dri Roll-On	Dial Canada	liquid	aluminum zirconium pentachlorohydrex-glycine 16.3%
Speed Stick Clear	Colgate-Palmolive	stick	aluminum zirconium tetrachlorohydrex-glycine 8.4%
Speed Stick Gel	Colgate-Palmolive	gel	aluminum zirconium tetrachlorohydrex-glycine 22%
Speed Stick Plus	Colgate-Palmolive	stick	aluminum zirconium tetrachlorohydrex-glycine 22%
Speed Stick Ultimate	Colgate-Palmolive	stick	aluminum zirconium tetrachlorohydrex-glycine 22%
Youth Dew Roll-On Antiperspirant Deodorant	Estee Lauder	lotion	aluminum chlorohydrate 20%

Product	Manufacturer	Dosage Form	Active Ingredients
Abenol 120 mg	Pendopharm	suppository	acetaminophen 120 mg
Acetaminophen Children's Tablet	Various Manufacturers	tablet, chewable	acetaminophen 80 mg
Acetaminophen Children's Tablet	Various Manufacturers	tablet, chewable	acetaminophen 160 mg
Acetaminophen Oral Drops	Various Manufacturers	drops	acetaminophen 80 mg/mL
Acetaminophen Oral Solution 16 mg/mL	Various Manufacturers	liquid	acetaminophen 16 mg/mL
Acetaminophen Oral Solution 32 mg/mL	Various Manufacturers	liquid	acetaminophen 32 mg/mL
Advil Children's Suspension	Wyeth Consumer	liquid	ibuprofen 20 mg/mL
Advil Junior Chewable Tablets	Wyeth Consumer	chewable tablets	ibuprofen 100 mg
Advil Pediatric Drops	Wyeth Consumer	liquid	ibuprofen 40 mg/mL
Atasol Drops	Church & Dwight	drops	acetaminophen 80 mg/mL
Children's Accudial Pain & Fever	Accudial	liquid	acetaminophen 32 mg/mL
Children's Feverhalt Chewable Tablet 160 mg	Pendopharm	tablet, chewable	acetaminophen 160 mg
Children's Feverhalt Drops	Pendopharm	liquid	acetaminophen 80 mg/mL
Children's Little Remedies for Fevers	Prestige Brands	liquid	acetaminophen 32 mg/mL
Dom-Acetaminophen Suppositories	Dominion Pharmacal	suppository	acetaminophen 120 mg
Infant's Little Remedies for Fevers	Prestige Brands	liquid	acetaminophen 80 mg/mL
Motrin Infants Suspension Drops	McNeil Consumer Healthcare	drops	ibuprofen 40 mg/mL
Pediaphen 80 mg Chewable Tablets	Euro-Pharm	chewable tablets	acetaminophen 80 mg
Pediaphen 160 mg Chewable Tablets	Euro-Pharm	chewable tablets	acetaminophen 160 mg
Pediaphen16 mg/mL	Euro-Pharm	liquid	acetaminophen 16 mg/mL
Pediaphen 32 mg/mL	Euro-Pharm	liquid	acetaminophen 32 mg/mL
Pediaphen 80 mg/mL	Euro-Pharm	drops	acetaminophen 80 mg/mL
Pediatrix Drops	Teva Canada	drops	acetaminophen 80 mg/mL
Pediatrix Liquid	Teva Canada	liquid	acetaminophen 32 mg/mL
PMS Acetaminophen Solution 16 mg/mL	Pendopharm	liquid	acetaminophen 16 mg/mL
PMS Acetaminophen Solution 32 mg/mL	Pendopharm	liquid	acetaminophen 32 mg/mL
PMS Acetaminophen Solution 80 mg/mL	Pendopharm	liquid	acetaminophen 80 mg/mL
PMS Acetaminophen Suppositories 120 mg	Pendopharm	suppository	acetaminophen 120 mg
Tantaphen Acetaminophen Oral Solution	Tanta	liquid	acetaminophen 80 mg/mL
Tempra Children's Syrup	Mead Johnson	syrup	acetaminophen 16 mg/mL
Tempra Infant Drops	Mead Johnson	drops	acetaminophen 80 mg/mL
Tylenol Children's Soft Chews	McNeil Consumer Healthcare	tablet	acetaminophen 80 mg
Tylenol Children's Suspension	McNeil Consumer Healthcare	liquid	acetaminophen 32 mg/mL
Tylenol Infants' Suspension Drops	McNeil Consumer Healthcare	liquid	acetaminophen 80 mg/mL
Tylenol Junior Strength Meltaways	McNeil Consumer Healthcare	tablet, dissolving	acetaminophen 160 mg

Product	Manufacturer	Dosage Form	Active Ingredients
Hydrasense Easy Dose	Schering Plough	nasal drops	natural source sea water 100%
Hydrasense Ultra Gentle Mist	Schering Plough	nasal spray	natural source sea water 100%
Little Noses Saline Spray	Little Remedies	nasal drops	sodium chloride 0.65% solution
Nasadrops Single Use Saline Ampoules	NeilMed Pharmaceutical	nasal drops	sodium chloride 0.9% solution
Otrivin Saline Pediatric Nose Drops	Novartis Consumer Health	nasal drops	sodium chloride 0.7% solution
Rhinaris Lubricating Nasal Gel	Pendopharm	nasal gel	polyethylene glycol 15% propylene glycol 20%
Rhinaris Pediatric Solution	Pendopharm	nasal drops	sodium chloride 0.9% solution
Salinex Nasal Drops	Sandoz	nasal drops	sodium chloride 0.9% solution
Salinex Nasal Lubricant Gel	Sandoz	nasal gel	polyethylene glycol 15% propylene glycol 20% sodium chloride 0.9%
Salinex Nasal Lubricant Solution	Sandoz	nasal spray	polyethylene glycol 5% propylene glycol 16% sodium chloride 0.9%
Simply Saline	Church & Dwight	nasal mist	sodium chloride 0.9% solution

Product	Manufacturer	Dosage Form	Active Ingredients
Aveeno Diaper Rash Cream	Johnson & Johnson	cream	zinc oxide 13%
Barriere	WellSpring	cream	dimethylpolysiloxane 20%
Boudreaux's Butt Paste	Blairex	ointment	zinc oxide 16%
Canesten Topical	Bayer Consumer	cream	clotrimazole 1%
Clotrimazole 1% Cream	Various Manufacturers	cream	clotrimazole 1%
Cortate 0.5 % Cream	Schering-Plough	cream	hydrocortisone 0.5%
Cortate 0.5 % Ointment	Schering-Plough	ointment	hydrocortisone 0.5%
Desitin Diaper Rash Ointment	Pfizer Consumer Healthcare	ointment	cod liver oil 13.5% zinc oxide 40%
Diaper Rash Ointment	D.C. Labs	ointment	zinc oxide 15%
Hydrocortisone 0.5% Cream	Various Manufacturers	cream	hydrocortisone 0.5%
Hydrocortisone 0.5% Ointment	Various Manufacturers	ointment	hydrocortisone 0.5%
Ihle paste	Atlas	ointment	zinc oxide 25%
Ihle's paste	Teva	ointment	zinc oxide 25%
Infazinc	Atlas	ointment	zinc oxide 15%
Li'l Goat's Milk Zinc Oxide Ointment	Canus Goat's Milk	ointment	petrolatum 49.5% zinc oxide 40%
Micatin Derm Cream	McNeil Consumer Healthcare	cream	miconazole nitrate 2%
Moisturel Cream	Novartis Consumer Health	cream	dimethicone 1% white petrolatum 30%
Monistat Derm Cream	Johnson & Johnson	cream	miconazole nitrate 2%
Nyaderm Cream	Taro	cream	nystatin 100 000 IU/g
Nystatin Cream	Various Manufacturers	cream	nystatin 100 000 IU/g
Nystatin Ointment	Various Manufacturers	ointment	nystatin 100 000 IU/g
Penaten Medicated Cream	Johnson & Johnson	cream	zinc oxide 18%
Petroleum jelly	Various Manufacturers	ointment	petrolatum 100%
ratio-Nystatin cream	Teva	cream	nystatin 100 000 IU/g
ratio-Nystatin ointment	Teva	ointment	nystatin 100 000 IU/g
Sudocrem Diaper Rash Cream	Leda Health	cream	zinc oxide 15.25%
Vaseline Petroleum Jelly Baby Fresh	Unilever Canada	jelly	petrolatum 99.9%
Vaseline Petroleum Jelly	Unilever Canada	jelly	petrolatum 100%
Zinaderm Cream	Teva	cream	zinc oxide 15%
Zinc Cream 15%	Various Manufacturers	cream	zinc oxide 15%
Zinc Ointment 15%	Various Manufacturers	ointment	zinc oxide 15%
Zinc Ointment 20%	Various Manufacturers	ointment	zinc oxide 20%
Zincofax Extra Strength	Pendopharm	ointment	zinc oxide 40%
Zincofax Original/Fragrance-Free	Pendopharm	ointment	zinc oxide 15%

Product	Manufacturer	Dosage Form	Active Ingredients
BioGaia Drops	Ferring	drops	lactobacillus reuteri active culture 20 million/drop
Chase Kolik Gripe Water	Stella	liquid	alcohol anhydrous 0.039 mL/mL ginger 0.01 mL/mL oil of dill 0.0004 mL/mL sodium bicarbonate 10 mg/mL
Chase Kolik Gripe Water Alcohol-Free	Stella	liquid	oil of fennel 0.5 mg/mL sodium bicarbonate 10 mg/mL
Glycerin Suppositories for Infants & Children	Teva Canada	suppository	glycerin 1.62 g
Glycerin Suppositories for Infants & Children	Various Manufacturers	suppository	glycerin 1.44 g
Gripe Water	Various Manufacturers	liquid	sodium hydrogen carbonate 10 mg/mL
Infacol	Forest Laboratories	drops	simethicone 40 mg/mL
Little Tummys Gas Relief Drops	Prestige Brands	liquid	simethicone 66 mg/mL
Ovol Drops	Church & Dwight	drops	simethicone 40 mg/mL
Pediacol	Euro-pharm	drops	simethicone 40 mg/mL

Product	Manufacturer	Supplied	Comment
Lansinoh Freezer bags	Lansinoh	25/box	Leak proof zipper design Self-standing
Milk Storage Set	Hollister	2 polycarbonate bottles with caps and closures	Breast milk can be frozen in these bottles
Mother's Milk Freezer Bags	Hollister	20 bags in 5 sterile inner packs Includes sealing ties, sealing clip	Extra strong, multi-ply construction prevents splitting or cracking as milk freezes Clip sealer squeezes air from bag to prevent freezer burn
One-Hand HygieniKit Collection System Adapter	Hollister	Single collection kit with instructions	Sterile Converts to manual pump
One-Hand: Handle Assembly	Hollister	Handle assembly with piston Piston seal Instructions	Converts collection kit to manual pump
Pump & Save Bags	Medela	20/50/pack	Collect, store and freeze breastmilk Double-walled, pre-sterilized, zipper closure, self-standing Pump directly into bag
Seal N Go Breast Milk Storage Bag	Gerber	25/45/box	Leak proof zipper design Self-standing
Single and Dual HygieniKit Collection System	Hollister	Single and dual kit with instructions	Compatible with every Ameda electric breast pump

[a]All products in this table are BPA free.

Product	Manufacturer	Supplied	Comment
Bra Pads	Medela	4 washable bra pads	100% cotton
Breast Shell System	Hollister	2 aerated shell fronts 2 sets of shell backs for prenatal and postnatal use 10 cotton roll inserts 6 comfort pads	Aeration system with holes on top 2 different-sized backs: one has small hole for inverted or flat nipple The other has larger opening for sore or sensitive nipples Includes shells with two sized backs and 5 pair of absorbent pads and 3 pair of comfort pads
Breast Shells	Hollister	2 aerated shell fronts 2 sets of shell backs for prenatal and postnatal use	Aeration system with holes only at top 2 different-sized backs: one back has small hole which is used for inverted or flat nipples The other back with the larger opening can be used for sore or sensitive nipples
Comfort Breast Shell Set	Philips Avent	2 sets Ventilated and nonventilated	
Comfort Pads	Hollister	10/box	Adhesive-backed fibre pads
Contact Nipple Shield	Medela	Set of 2	Available in 3 sizes
Custom Breast Flange XL	Hollister	2/box	X-large flange allows for larger opening 28.5-30.5 mm
Custom Breast Flange XXL	Hollister	2/box	XX-large flange allows for larger opening 32.5-36 mm
Disposable Bra Pads	Medela	30/60/box	Individually wrapped
Disposable Breast Pads	Philips Avent	40/100 count	Anti-slip backing
Flexishield Areola Stimulator	Hollister	1/box	Flexible insert, fits any Ameda breast shield Reduced shield size for max effectiveness with smaller breasts
Heavy Flow Nursing Pads	Gerber	24/box	Overnight protection Natural contoured shape No-slip adhesive strip
Lansinoh	Lansinoh	2 oz (56 g)	100% lanolin, safe and nontoxic for baby and mother
Lansinoh Disposable nursing pads	Lansinoh	36/60 count	Ultra-thin, very absorbent
Light Flow Nursing Pads	Gerber	36/box	Natural contoured shape, no-slip adhesive strip
Medium Flow Nursing Pads	Gerber	30/box	Natural contoured shape, no-slip adhesive strip
Niplette	Philips Avent	Set of 2 2 breast pads included	
Nipple Protectors	Philips Avent	sets of 2	Available in small (15 mm) and standard (21 mm) sizes
Nipple Shield	Hollister	1 ultra-thin flexible shield	Short-term use only
Reusable Breast Pads	Philips Avent	6/pack	Washable cotton pads Includes mesh laundry bag Anti-slip outer layer
Reusable Nursing Pads	Gerber	6/box	100% cotton inner layer Machine washable
Reusable Nursing Pads	Hollister	6/box	100% cotton Multi-layered (7 ply) Machine washable
Softshells for Sore/Inverted Nipples	Medela	2 shells 2 backs for inverted nipples 2 backs for sore nipples	
Tender Care Hydrogel Pads	Medela	Individually packaged	Reusable for up to 24 hours
Tender Care Lanolin Cream	Medela	59 mL	100% lanolin No need to remove to nurse baby
Thera Breast Shells	Medela	Individually packaged	

Product	Manufacturer	Supplied	Comment
Ultra Thin Nursing Pads	Gerber	60/box	Disposable pads Breathable moisture barrier draws moisture away from skin
Washable Bra Pads	Medela	6/pack	Washable cotton pads Includes mesh laundry bag

Product	Manufacturer	Warranty	Power Source	Weight	Suction Settings
Ameda Elite Electric Breast Pump	Hollister	2 year (pump mechanism)	AC adapter Car adapter Built-in rechargeable battery	13.2 kg	Fully adjustable
Ameda One-Hand Breast Pump	Hollister		Manual	<2.2 kg	Manual
Ameda Purely Yours Electric Personal Breast Pump	Hollister	One year (pump mechanism) 90 days (parts)	AA batteries AC adapter Car adapter	2.2 kg	Fully adjustable: 8 suction levels available
Ameda Purely Yours Electric Personal Pump - Backpack	Hollister	One year (pump mechanism) 90 days (parts)	AA batteries AC adapter Car adapter	2.2 kg	Fully adjustable: 8 suction levels available
Ameda Purely Yours Electric Personal Pump - Tote	Hollister	One year (pump mechanism) 90 days (parts)	AA batteries AC adapter Car adapter	2.2 kg	Fully adjustable: 8 suction levels available
Avent Isis Manual Breast Pump	Philips Avent		Manual		
Cylinder Hand Breast Pump	Hollister		Manual	<2.2 kg	Manual
FreeStyle Breastpump	Medela	One year (pump mechanism) 90 days (parts)	AA batteries AC adapter Car adapter	2.6 kg	2-phase expression
Harmony	Medela	30 days	Manual	<1 kg	Manual
Lactina	Medela	3-year limited	Electric or battery Car adapter available	4.5 kg	Fully adjustable
Lansinoh Manual Breast Pump	Lansinoh		Manual	<1 kg	Manual
Medela MiniElectric	Medela	90 days	AA batteries AC adapter Manual	3.3 kg	Fully adjustable
Pump-In-Style Advanced	Medela	90 days	AC adapter AC/car adapter Optional rechargeable battery pack	4 kg	Fully adjustable
SpringExpress	Medela	90 days	Manual	2.2 kg	Fully adjustable
Symphony	Medela	3-year limited	Electric or battery	3.2 kg	2-phase expression
Swing	Medela	One year (pump mechanism) 90 days (parts)	Electric or AA batteries	1 kg	2-phase expression

Cycle Setting	Single or Dual Pumping Options	Tote/Cooler bag	Comments
Fully adjustable	Both	Hard plastic protective carrying case	Hospital grade piston pump Available for sale or rent
Manual	Both: two hand pumps can be used to pump both breasts at the same time	Not included	Compact- fits into a purse
Adjustable: 4 cycle speeds available	Both		Clean collection kit parts except for tubing, white cap and white pump connector These 3 items do not need to be cleaned because they do not come in contact with collected milk Other parts should be hand washed and rinsed with hot clean water
Adjustable: 4 cycle speeds available	Both	Black backpack includes insulated freezer compartment and freezer packs, cotton nursing pads and manual handle assembly	Clean collection kit parts except for tubing, white cap and white pump connector These 3 items do not need to be cleaned because they do not come in contact with collected milk Other parts should be hand washed and rinsed with hot clean water
Adjustable: 4 cycle speeds available	Both	Black tote bag with insulated freezer compartment and freezer packs	Clean collection kit parts except for tubing, white cap and white pump connector These 3 items do not need to be cleaned because they do not come in contact with collected milk Other parts should be hand washed and rinsed with hot clean water
Manual	Both	Optional On-the-Go Set (includes insulated travel bag and cool packs)	4 oz & 9 oz capacity
Manual	Single		Reducing insert (for smaller breasts)
2-phase expression	Dual	Hands-free accessories, rechargeable battery, tote bag	2-phase expression LCD screen Memory button to record breastfeeding pumping patterns
Manual	Single		2-phase expression Manual, but upgradeable to electric with conversion kit
Fully adjustable	Both		Ideal for long-term daily use For multi-users with personal double pumping kit Accesory set can be used as manual breastpump Available only for rent
Manual	Single		ComfortSeal Cushion
Fully adjustable	Single	Not included	
Fully adjustable	Both	Soft-sided black designer shoulder bag with separate compartments for kit and milk storage	Fully automatic, portable professional grade breast-pump
Manual	Single	Not included	Can be upgraded to MiniElectric Breastpump
2-phase expression	Both	Container stand	Hospital-grade double pump 2-phase expression pumping for long-term use For multiple users with personal double pumping kit with overflow protection Available for sale or rent
2-phase expression	Single	Carry bag	Single electric, personal-use pump 2-phase expression Suitable for occasional or frequent use

Product	Manufacturer	Use	Type of Lens	Ingredients	Preservatives
AOSept	CIBA Vision	disinfecting	soft	hydrogen peroxide 3% sodium chloride 0.85% buffered with phosphates	none
AQuify Long Lasting Comfort Drops	CIBA Vision	lubricant	all	sodium hyaluronate sodium chloride sodium perborate	phosphonic acid
Boston Advance Cleaner	Bausch & Lomb	daily cleaning	rigid gas permeable	alkyl ether sulfate ethoxylated alkyl phenol tri-quatenary cocoa-based phospholipid titanium dioxide nonionic alcohol surfactant, silica gel	none
Boston Advance Comfort Formula Conditioning Solution	Bausch & Lomb	wetting soaking disinfecting	rigid gas permeable	not stated	polyaminopropyl biguanide 0.0005% EDTA 0.05% chlorhexidine gluconate 0.003%
Boston One Step Liquid Enzymatic Cleaner	Bausch & Lomb	protein removal	rigid gas permeable	subtilisin A glycerol	none
Boston Rewetting Drops	Bausch & Lomb	lubricant	rigid gas permeable	not stated	chlorhexidine gluconate 0.006% EDTA 0.05%
Boston Simplus Multi-Action Solution	Bausch & Lomb	daily cleaning rinsing disinfecting conditioning	rigid gas permeable	poloxamine hydroxyalkylphosphonate boric acid sodium borate sodium chloride hydroxypropyl methylcellulose	polyaminopropyl biguanide 0.0005% chlorhexidine gluconate 0.003%
Clear Care Cleaning & Disinfecting Solution	CIBA Vision	cleaning disinfecting protein removal	soft rigid gas permeable	hydrogen peroxide 3% sodium chloride 0.79% buffered with phosphates pluronic 17R4	phosphonic acid
Clens-100	Alcon	protein removal	soft rigid gas permeable	RLM-100 poloxamine citrate	polyquad 0.001% EDTA 0.05%
Complete Blink & Clean Drops	AMO Canada	daily cleaning lubricating protein removal	soft	polyhexamethylene biguanide hydrochloride (trischem) 0.0001% tromethamine tyloxapol	EDTA
Complete Multi Purpose Solution Easy Rub Formula	AMO Canada	cleaning disinfecting protein removal	soft	poloxamer 237	EDTA
Multi-Purpose Lens Drops	Bausch & Lomb	wetting	soft	poloxamine sodium chloride boric acid sodium borate	sorbic acid 0.15% EDTA 0.1%
Opti-Clean II Daily Cleaner	Alcon	daily cleaning	all	polymeric beads nonionic surfactant	disodium edetate 0.1% polyquad 0.001%
Opti-Free Replenish Multi-Purpose Disinfecting Solution	Alcon	wetting soaking disinfecting	soft	myristamidopropyl dimethylamine 0.0005%	polyquaternium 0.001%
Opti-Free Daily Cleaner	Alcon	daily cleaning	soft	polymeric beads nonionic surfactant	disodium edetate 0.1% polyquad 0.001%
Opti-Free Enzymatic Cleaner	Alcon	protein removal	soft	pancreatin	none

Product	Manufacturer	Use	Type of Lens	Ingredients	Preservatives
Opti-Free Express Multi-Purpose Disinfecting Solution-No Rub Formula	Alcon	cleaning rinsing lubricating disinfecting storage protein removal	soft	myristamidopropyl dimethylamine	polyquaternium 0.001% EDTA 0.05%
Opti-Free Multi-Action Solution	Alcon	cleaning rinsing disinfecting storage	soft	citric acid sodium chloride sodium citrate in sterile buffered aqueous solution	polyquaternium 0.001% EDTA 0.05%
Opti-Free Rewetting Drops	Alcon	wetting	soft	sterile buffered aqueous solution	polyquad 0.001%
Opti-Free SupraClens Daily Protein Remover	Alcon	protein removal	all	pancreatin	none
ReNu MultiPlus, Lubricating Drops	Bausch & Lomb	lubricating wetting	soft	poloxamine boric acid sodium borate sodium chloride	EDTA 0.1% sorbic acid 0.1%
ReNu MultiPlus, Multi-Purpose Solution No Rub Formula	Bausch & Lomb	protein removal cleaning rinsing disinfecting lubricating storage	soft	hydranate poloxamine boric acid sodium chloride sodium borate	DYMED 0.0001% EDTA 0.1%
Sensitive Eyes Daily Cleaner	Bausch & Lomb	daily cleaning	soft	poloxamine sodium chloride sodium borate hydroxypropyl methylcellulose	EDTA 0.5% sorbic acid 0.25%
Sensitive Eyes Effervescent Cleaning Tablets	Bausch & Lomb	protein removal	soft	subtilisin A sodium carbonate sodium chloride boric acid	none
Sensitive Eyes Lens Lubricant	Bausch & Lomb	lubricant wetting	soft	sodium chloride sodium borate boric acid	EDTA 0.025% sorbic acid 0.1%
Sensitive Eyes Multi-Purpose Solution	Bausch & Lomb	daily cleaning rinsing disinfecting storage	soft	poloxamine boric acid sodium borate sodium chloride	DYMED 0.00005% EDTA 0.1%
Sensitive Eyes Saline Plus Solution	Bausch & Lomb	rinsing	soft	boric acid sodium borate potassium chloride	DYMED 0.00003% EDTA 0.025%
SOLO-Care Aqua	CIBA Vision	daily cleaning rinsing disinfecting storage	soft	sorbitol tromethamine pluronic F127 sodium phosphate dihydrogen dexpanthenol	polyhexamide HCl 0.0001% EDTA
UltraCare Daily Cleaner	Allergan	daily cleaning	soft	trisurfactant plus alcohol	none
Ultrazyme Enzymatic Cleaner	AMO Canada	protein removal	soft	subtilisin A	none
Unizyme Enzymatic Cleaner	CIBA Vision	protein removal	soft rigid gas permeable	subtilisin A	none
Visine True Tears Eye Drops	Pfizer Consumer Healthcare	lubricant	soft	glycerin 0.2% hypromellose 0.2%	none

Manufacturer	Lubricant	Cleaner	Wetting	Soaking	Enzymatic Cleaners
Alcon	Opti-Free Rewetting Drops	Opti-Clean II			Opti-Free SupraClens Daily Protein Remover
Bausch and Lomb	Boston Rewetting Drops	Boston Advance Cleaner	Boston Advance Comfort Formula Conditioning Solution	Boston Advance Comfort Formula Conditioning Solution	
Bausch and Lomb		Boston Simplus Multi-Action Solution	Boston Simplus Multi-Action Solution	Boston Simplus Multi-Action Solution	Boston One Step Liquid Enzymatic Cleaner
CIBA Vision	Aquify Long Lasting Comfort Drops	AOFlow			Unizyme Enzymatic Cleaner
CIBA Vision	SOLO-Care Aqua	SOLO-Care Aqua	SOLO-Care Aqua	SOLO-Care Aqua	

Manufacturer	System	Lubricant	Cleaner (Daily)	Cleaner (Weekly)	Rinsing Solution	Disinfecting Medium	Soaking (Storage) Solution
Alcon	Opti-Free	Opti-Free Rewetting Drops	Opti-Free Multi-Action Solution or, Opti Free Daily Cleaner or, Opti-Free SupraClens Daily Protein Remover[a]	Opti-Free Enzymatic Cleaner	Opti-Free Multi-Action Solution	Opti-Free Multi-Action Solution	Opti-Free Multi-Action Solution
Alcon	Opti-Free Express	Opti-Free Express Multi-Purpose Disinfecting Solution No Rub Formula (MPDS-NRF), Opti-Free Rewetting Drops	Opti-Free Express MPDS-NRF		Opti-Free Express MPDS-NRF	Opti-Free Express MPDS-NRF	Opti-Free Express MPDS-NRF
AMO Canada	Complete Multi Purpose Solution Easy Rub Formula		Complete Multi Purpose Solution Easy Rub Formula	Complete Multi Purpose Solution Easy Rub Formula		Complete Multi Purpose Solution Easy Rub Formula	
Abbott	Complete Blink & Clean Drops	Complete Blink & Clean Drops	Complete Blink & Clean Drops	Ultrazyme Enzymatic Cleaner			
Bausch & Lomb	ReNu MultiPlus	ReNu MultiPlus Lubricating Drops	ReNu MultiPlus[b]		ReNu MultiPlus	ReNu MultiPlus	ReNu MultiPlus
Bausch & Lomb	Sensitive Eyes	Sensitive Eyes Lens Lubricant or, Multi-Purpose Lens Drops	Sensitive Eyes Multi-Purpose Solution, or Sensitive Eyes Daily Cleaner	Sensitive Eyes Effervescent Cleaning Tablets	Sensitive Eyes Multi-Purpose Solution	Sensitive Eyes Multi-Purpose Solution	Sensitive Eyes Multi-Purpose Solution
CIBA Vision	SOLO-Care Aqua	SOLO-Care Aqua	SOLO-Care Aqua	Unizyme	SOLO-Care Aqua	SOLO-Care Aqua	SOLO-Care Aqua
Johnson & Johnson		Visine Contact Lens Eye Drops					

[a] Enzymatic

[b] No separate weekly cleaner required when used daily

Manufacturer	System	Lubricant	Cleaner (Daily)	Cleaner (Weekly)	Rinsing Solution	Disinfecting, Medium	Soaking, (Storage) Solution
Allergan	UltraCare B12		UltraCare Daily Cleaner	Ultrazyme	UltraCare B12 Neutralizing Tablets	UltraCare Solution	
Bausch & Lomb	HP	Sensitive Eyes Lens Lubricant or Multi-Purpose Lens Drops	Sensitive Eyes Daily Cleaner	Efferzyme Protein Remover Tablets	Sensitive Eyes Saline Plus Solution		
CIBA Vision	AOSept	AODrops	AOFlow	Unizyme		AOSept	AOSept or Softwear Saline
CIBA Vision	Clear Care Cleaning & Disinfecting Solution		Clear Care Cleaning & Disinfecting Solution			Clear Care Cleaning & Disinfecting Solution	
CIBA Vision	In A Wink	In A Wink Refreshing Drops	In A Wink Daily Cleaner	Unizyme	In A Wink Neutralizing Rinse	In A Wink Disinfectant	In A Wink Neutralizing Rinse

Contact Lens Products: Soft Contact Lens Thermal Cleaning Systems

Manufacturer	System	Lubricant	Cleaner (Daily)	Cleaner (Weekly)	Rinsing Solution	Disinfecting Medium	Soaking, (Storage) Solution
Bausch & Lomb		Sensitive Eyes Lens Lubricant or Multi-Purpose Lens Drops	Sensitive Eyes Daily Cleaner		Sensitive Eyes Saline Plus Solution	Sensitive Eyes Saline Plus Solution	Sensitive Eyes Saline Plus Solution

Product	Manufacturer	Dosage Form	Active Ingredient
Next Choice	Cobalt	tablet	levonorgestrel 0.75 mg
NorLevo	HRA Pharma	tablet	levonorgestrel 0.75 mg
Plan B	Duramed Pharmaceuticals	tablet	levonorgestrel 0.75 mg

Product	Manufacturer	Comments
Durex Avanti Lub	Durex Canada	Lubricated, polyurethane material thinner than latex Non-allergenic, suitable for latex sensitive users
Durex Comfort Shaped Lub	Durex Canada	Lubricated
Durex Intense Sensation Lub	Durex Canada	Lubricated, studded texture for extra pleasure
Durex Love Lubricated	Durex Canada	Lubricated
Durex Maximum Thin X-Lub	Durex Canada	Extra lubricant
Durex Play Lubricated	Durex Canada	Lubricated, thicker wall
Durex Play Sensations Thin	Durex Canada	Thin latex, lubricated
Durex Sheik Non-Lubricated	Durex Canada	Dry, no lubricant
Durex Sheik Sensi-Creme Lub	Durex Canada	Lubricated
Durex Sheik Sensi-Thin Lub	Durex Canada	Lubricated
Durex Sheik Sensi-Thin Ribbed Lub	Durex Canada	Lubricated
Durex Tropical Colours & Scents Lub	Durex Canada	Lubricated
LifeStyles 4Play	Ansell	Lubricated, natural latex Available with variety of accessories
LifeStyles Endurance (climax control lubricant)	Ansell	Natural latex Active ingredient: benzocaine 4.5% in the lubricant
LifeStyles Excite Combo	Ansell	Lubricated, natural latex, studded with accessories
LifeStyles Her Passion (lubricated)	Ansell	Natural latex, slightly flared and studded
LifeStyles Large (lubricated)	Ansell	Natural latex, flare shaped and larger 56mm
LifeStyles Lubricated	Ansell	Natural latex, flare shaped
LifeStyles Luscious Flavours (lubricated)	Ansell	Flare shaped Variety of flavours
LifeStyles Mr. Big (lubricated)	Ansell	Natural latex, flare shaped and larger 56mm Economy pack
LifeStyles Natural Feeling (lubricated)	Ansell	Natural latex, flare shaped and ultimate thinness
LifeStyles Skin (lubricated)	Ansell	Polyisoprene synthetic membrane suitable for natural latex sensitive users More elastic and smoother than other non-latex products
LifeStyles Spermicidally Lubricated	Ansell	Natural latex Active ingredient: nonoxynol-9 (25 mg minimum) in the lubricant
LifeStyles Studded (lubricated)	Ansell	Natural latex, slightly flared and studded
LifeStyles Trio (lubricated)	Ansell	Variety pack with different kinds of condoms
LifeStyles True-Fit (lubricated)	Ansell	Contour shaped
LifeStyles Ultra Sensitive (lubricated)	Ansell	Natural latex, flare shaped, thinner
LifeStyles Ultra Sensitive with Warming Lubricant	Ansell	Flare shaped, thinner, with warming lubricant
LifeStyles Ultrathin (lubricated)	Ansell	Natural latex, straight shaped and ultimate thinness
LifeStyles Ultrathin Large (lubricated)	Ansell	Natural latex, flare shaped, larger and thinner 56mm
LifeStyles Xtra Pleasure (lubricated)	Ansell	Extra flared
LifeStyles Xtra Pleasure with Ribs (lubricated)	Ansell	Extra flared
Trojan Extended Pleasure Lubricated	Church & Dwight	Lubricated, thicker wall
Trojan Her Pleasure Ultra	Church & Dwight	Lubricated, thin, ribbed walls
Trojan Intense Ribbed Ultra Smooth	Church & Dwight	Lubricated, thin, ribbed walls
Trojan Large Lubricated	Church & Dwight	Lubricated
Trojan Lubricated	Church & Dwight	Lubricated
Trojan Luscious Flavours	Church & Dwight	Vanilla-gold, tutti-frutti, strawberry, chocolate

Product	Manufacturer	Comments
Trojan Magnum Lubricated	Church & Dwight	Larger sized condom, lubricated
Trojan NaturaLamb	Church & Dwight	Lambskin, lubricated
Trojan Non-Lubricated	Church & Dwight	Dry, no lubricant
Trojan Shared Sensation Lubricated	Church & Dwight	Lubricated
Trojan Spermicidal	Church & Dwight	Latex, lubricated with nonoxynol-9
Trojan Thin Lubricated	Church & Dwight	Lubricated
Trojan Ultra Fit Lubricated	Church & Dwight	Lubricated
Trojan Ultra Pleasure Lubricated	Church & Dwight	Lubricated, bulbous end
Trojan Ultra Texture Lubricated	Church & Dwight	Lubricated, micro-dot texture

Product	Manufacturer	Active Ingredient
VCF Contraceptive Film	Apothecus	nonoxynol-9 28%
VCF Contraceptive Foam	Apothecus	nonoxynol-9 12.5%

Product	Manufacturer	Supplied	Size	Comments
FC2 Female Condom	Female Health	condom	one size	Synthetic nitrile
FemCap Cervical Cap	FemCap	cervical cap	22, 26, 30 mm	Silicone rubber (non-latex) Size is determined by obstetrical history
Milex Arcing Diaphragm	Cooper Surgical	diaphragm	60, 65, 70, 75, 80, 85, 90, 95 mm	Latex-free diaphragm Wide-seal silicone Arcing spring diaphragm: folds into arc shape when sides are compressed Must be fitted individually
Milex Omniflex Diaphragm	Cooper Surgical	diaphragm	60, 65, 70, 75, 80, 85, 90, 95 mm	Latex-free diaphragm Wide-seal silicone Omniflex diaphragm contains a coil spring which flattens into an oval shape when sides are compressed Must be fitted individually
Today Sponge	Mayer	sponge	one size	Polyurethane Contains nonoxynol-9

Product	Manufacturer	Dosage Form	Decongestant
Advil Cold & Sinus Liqui-Gels	Pfizer Consumer Healthcare	liquid capsule	pseudoephedrine hydrochloride 30 mg
Advil Cold & Sinus Nighttime	Pfizer Consumer Healthcare	tablet	pseudoephedrine hydrochloride 30 mg
Advil Cold & Sinus Plus	Pfizer Consumer Healthcare	tablet	pseudoephedrine hydrochloride 30 mg
Aerius	Schering-Plough	tablet	
Aerius Dual Action	Schering-Plough	tablet, extended release	pseudoephedrine sulfate 120 mg
Aerius Kids	Schering-Plough	liquid	
Allegra 24 Hour	sanofi-aventis	tablet	
Allegra Tablets	sanofi-aventis	tablet	
Allegra-D	sanofi-aventis	tablet, sustained release	pseudoephedrine hydrochloride 120 mg
Allergy Elixir	Tanta	elixir	
Allergy Tablets	Tanta	tablet	
Allergy Tablets Extra Strength	Tanta	tablet	
Allernix	Teva	caplet	
Allernix Elixir	Teva	elixir	
Allernix Extra Strength	Teva	caplet	
Apo-Cetirizine 10 mg	Apotex	tablet	
Apo-Loratadine	Apotex	tablet	
Balminil Cough & Flu	Teva	syrup	pseudoephedrine hydrochloride 2 mg/mL
Balminil DM	Teva	syrup	
Balminil DM + Decongestant + Expectorant	Teva	liquid	pseudoephedrine hydrochloride 6 mg/mL
Balminil DM + Decongestant + Expectorant Extra Strength	Teva	syrup	pseudoephedrine hydrochloride 6 mg/mL
Balminil DM + Expectorant Sucrose-Free	Teva	syrup	
Balminil DM + Expectorant Extra Strength Sucrose Free	Teva	syrup	
Balminil DM Children	Teva	syrup	
Balminil DM Sucrose-Free	Teva	liquid	
Balminil Expectorant	Teva	syrup	
Balminil Expectorant Sucrose-Free	Teva	syrup	
Balminil Nasal Decongestant	Teva	spray	xylometazoline hydrochloride 0.1%
Balminil Night-Time	Teva	syrup	
Benadryl Allergy	McNeil Consumer Healthcare	caplet	
Benadryl Allergy Sinus Headache Caplets	McNeil Consumer Healthcare	caplet	pseudoephedrine hydrochloride 30 mg
Benadryl Children's Allergy Tablet	McNeil Consumer Healthcare	tablet, chewable	
Benadryl Children's Liquid	McNeil Consumer Healthcare	liquid	
Benadryl Elixir	McNeil Consumer Healthcare	elixir	
Benadryl Extra Strength Nightime Caplets	McNeil Consumer Healthcare	caplet	
Benadryl Total Allergy Regular Strength	McNeil Consumer Healthcare	caplet	pseudoephedrine hydrochloride 30 mg

Antihistamine	Antitussive	Expectorant	Other Active Ingredients
			ibuprofen 200 mg
chlorpheniramine maleate 2 mg			ibuprofen 200 mg
chlorpheniramine maleate 2 mg			ibuprofen 200 mg
desloratadine 5 mg			
desloratadine 5 mg			
desloratadine 0.5 mg/mL			
fexofenadine hydrochloride 120 mg			
fexofenadine hydrochloride 60 mg			
fexofenadine hydrochloride 60 mg			
diphenhydramine hydrochloride 2.5 mg/mL			
diphenhydramine hydrochloride 25 mg			
diphenhydramine hydrochloride 50 mg			
diphenhydramine hydrochloride 25 mg			
diphenhydramine hydrochloride 2.5 mg/mL			
diphenhydramine hydrochloride 50 mg			
cetirizine hydrochloride 10 mg			
loratadine 10 mg			
	dextromethorphan hydrobromide 1 mg/mL	guaifenesin 6.7 mg/mL	acetaminophen 21.7 mg/mL
	dextromethorphan hydrobromide 3 mg/mL		
	dextromethorphan hydrobromide 3 mg/mL	guaifenesin 20 mg/mL	
	dextromethorphan hydrobromide 3 mg/mL	guaifenesin 40 mg/mL	
	dextromethorphan hydrobromide 3 mg/mL	guaifenesin 20 mg/mL	
	dextromethorphan hydrobromide 3 mg/mL	guaifenesin 40 mg/mL	
	dextromethorphan hydrobromide 1.5 mg/mL		
	dextromethorphan hydrobromide 3 mg/mL		
		guaifenesin 20 mg/mL	
		guaifenesin 20 mg/mL	
diphenhydramine hydrochloride 2.5 mg/mL	dextromethorphan hydrobromide 3 mg/mL	ammonium chloride 25 mg/mL	
diphenhydramine hydrochloride 25 mg			
diphenhydramine hydrochloride 12.5 mg			acetaminophen 500 mg
diphenhydramine hydrochloride 12.5 mg			
diphenhydramine hydrochloride 1.25 mg/mL			
diphenhydramine hydrochloride 2.5 mg/mL			
diphenhydramine hydrochloride 50 mg			
diphenhydramine hydrochloride 12.5 mg			acetaminophen 500 mg

Product	Manufacturer	Dosage Form	Decongestant
Benadryl Total Allergy Extra Strength	McNeil Consumer Healthcare	caplet	pseudoephedrine hydrochloride 30 mg
Bentasil Black Current Lozenges	Leaf Sweden	lozenge	
Bentasil Cherry Lozenges	Leaf Sweden	lozenge	
Bentasil Honey-Lemon Lozenges	Leaf Sweden	lozenge	
Benylin 2 All-in-One Cold and Flu with Codeine	McNeil Consumer Healthcare	syrup	pseudoephedrine hydrochloride 5 mg/mL
Benylin All-in-One Cold and Flu Extra Strength	McNeil Consumer Healthcare	caplet	pseudoephedrine hydrochloride 30 mg
Benylin All-in-One Cold and Flu Extra Strength	McNeil Consumer Healthcare	syrup	pseudoephedrine hydrochloride 2 mg/mL
Benylin All-in-One Cold and Flu Liquid Gels	McNeil Consumer Healthcare	capsule	pseudoephedrine hydrochloride 30 mg
Benylin All-In-One Cold and Flu Night Extra Strength	McNeil Consumer Healthcare	caplet	pseudoephedrine hydrochloride 30 mg
Benylin All-in-One Cold and Flu Night Extra Strength	McNeil Consumer Healthcare	syrup	pseudoephedrine hydrochloride 2 mg/mL
Benylin Cold and Sinus	McNeil Consumer Healthcare	caplet	phenylephrine hydrochloride 5 mg
Benylin Cold and Sinus Night	McNeil Consumer Healthcare	caplet	phenylephrine hydrochloride 5 mg
Benylin DM	McNeil Consumer Healthcare	syrup	
Benylin DM for Children (Dry Cough)	McNeil Consumer Healthcare	liquid	
Benylin DM-D for Children (Cough and Cold)	McNeil Consumer Healthcare	syrup	pseudoephedrine hydrochloride 3 mg/mL
Benylin DM-D-E	McNeil Consumer Healthcare	syrup	pseudoephedrine hydrochloride 6 mg/mL
Benylin DM-D-E Extra Strength Cough and Cold	McNeil Consumer Healthcare	syrup	pseudoephedrine hydrochloride 6 mg/mL
Benylin DM-E	McNeil Consumer Healthcare	syrup	
Benylin DM-E Extra Strength	McNeil Consumer Healthcare	syrup	
Benylin E Menthol Extra Strength	McNeil Consumer Healthcare	syrup	
Benylin Extra Strength Mucus & Phlegm	McNeil Consumer Healthcare	syrup	
Benylin Extra Strength Mucus & Phlegm Relief plus Cough Control	McNeil Consumer Healthcare	syrup	
Benylin Extra Strength Mucus & Phlegm plus Cold Relief Caplets	McNeil Consumer Healthcare	caplet	pseudoephedrine hydrochloride 30 mg
Benylin Extra Strength Mucus & Phlegm plus Cold Relief Liquid	McNeil Consumer Healthcare	syrup	pseudoephedrine hydrochloride 2 mg/mL
Benylin Extra Strength Mucus & Phlegm plus Cold Relief Night	McNeil Consumer Healthcare	syrup	pseudoephedrine hydrochloride 2 mg/mL
Benylin Extra Strength All-in-One Cold and Flu with Warming Sensation	McNeil Consumer Healthcare	syrup	pseudoephedrine hydrochloride 2 mg/mL

Antihistamine	Antitussive	Expectorant	Other Active Ingredients
diphenhydramine hydrochloride 25 mg			acetaminophen 500 mg
			menthol 0.15%
			anethole 0.1% menthol 0.17%
			anethole 0.12% menthol 0.07%
		guaifenesin 20 mg/mL	codeine phosphate 0.66 mg/mL
	dextromethorphan hydrobromide 15 mg	guaifenesin 100 mg	acetaminophen 500 mg
	dextromethorphan hydrobromide 1 mg/mL	guaifenesin 6.67 mg/mL	acetaminophen 33.3 mg/mL
	dextromethorphan hydrobromide 10 mg	guaifenesin 100 mg	acetaminophen 250 mg
diphenhydramine hydrochloride 25 mg			acetaminophen 500 mg
chlorpheniramine maleate 0.13 mg/mL	dextromethorphan hydrobromide 1 mg/mL	guaifenesin 6.67 mg/mL	acetaminophen 33.3 mg/mL
			acetaminophen 500 mg
chlorpheniramine maleate 2 mg			acetaminophen 500 mg
	dextromethorphan hydrobromide 3 mg/mL		
	dextromethorphan hydrobromide 1.5 mg/mL		
	dextromethorphan hydrobromide 1.5 mg/mL		
	dextromethorphan hydrobromide 3 mg/mL	guaifenesin 20 mg/mL	
	dextromethorphan hydrobromide 3 mg/mL	guaifenesin 40 mg/mL	menthol 3 mg/mL
	dextromethorphan hydrobromide 3 mg/mL	guaifenesin 20 mg/mL	
	dextromethorphan hydrobromide 3 mg/mL	guaifenesin 40 mg/mL	menthol 3 mg/mL
		guaifenesin 40 mg/mL	menthol 3 mg/mL
		guaifenesin 40 mg/mL	menthol 3 mg/mL
	dextromethorphan hydrobromide 3 mg/mL	guaifenesin 40 mg/mL	menthol 3 mg/mL
	dextromethorphan hydrobromide 15 mg	guaifenesin 100 mg	acetaminophen 500 mg
	dextromethorphan hydrobromide 1 mg/mL	guaifenesin 20 mg/mL	acetaminophen 500 mg
chlorpheniramine maleate 2 mg	dextromethorphan hydrobromide 1 mg/mL	guaifenesin 20 mg/mL	acetaminophen 500 mg
	dextromethorphan hydrobromide 1 mg/mL	guaifenesin 6.67 mg/mL	acetaminophen 33.3 mg/mL

Product	Manufacturer	Dosage Form	Decongestant
Benylin for Children All-in-One Cold and Fever	McNeil Consumer Healthcare	syrup	pseudoephedrine hydrochloride 3 mg/mL
Benylin for Children All-in-One Cold and Fever	McNeil Consumer Healthcare	tablet, chewable	pseudoephedrine hydrochloride 15 mg
Benylin for Children All-in-One Cold and Fever Nightime	McNeil Consumer Healthcare	syrup	
Benylin Tickly Throat Cough	McNeil Consumer Healthcare	syrup	
Bionet Lozenge	Church & Dwight	lozenge	
Bradosol Extra Strength Cherry/ Honey-Eucalyptus/ Mint	Columbia	lozenge	
Bronchophan Expectorant (sugar/alcohol free)	Atlas	syrup	
Bronchophan Forte DM (sugar/alcohol free)	Atlas	syrup	
Buckley's Cold & Sinus Liquid Gels - Day	W.K. Buckley	liquid capsule	pseudoephedrine hydrochloride 30 mg
Buckley's Complete Cough Cold and Flu	W.K. Buckley	liquid	
Buckley's Complete + Extra Strength Mucus Relief Cough Cold & Flu	W.K. Buckley	liquid	
Buckley's Complete Liquid Gels Nighttime Relief	W.K. Buckley	liquid capsule	pseudoephedrine hydrochloride 30 mg
Buckley's Complete Liquid Gels plus Mucus Relief	W.K. Buckley	liquid capsule	pseudoephedrine hydrochloride 30 mg
Buckley's Complete Nighttime Cough Cold and Flu	W.K. Buckley	liquid	
Buckley's Cough Chest Congestion	W.K. Buckley	liquid	
Buckley's Complete Cough, Cold & Flu Extra-Strength Day Caplets	W.K. Buckley	caplet	pseudoephedrine hydrochloride 30 mg
Buckley's Complete Cough, Cold & Flu Extra-Strength Night Caplets	W.K. Buckley	caplet	pseudoephedrine hydrochloride 30 mg
Buckley's Cough Mucus and Phlegm	W.K. Buckley	liquid	
Buckley's Daytime Cold & Sinus	W.K. Buckley	tablet	pseudoephedrine hydrochloride 30 mg
Buckley's DM Cough Control	W.K. Buckley	liquid	
Buckley's DM Decongestant Cough, Cold & Sinus	W.K. Buckley	liquid	pseudoephedrine hydrochloride 6 mg/mL
Buckley's Original Mixture	W.K. Buckley	liquid	
Buckley's Original Mixture Nighttime	W.K. Buckley	liquid	
Buckley's Nighttime Cold & Sinus	W.K. Buckley	tablet	pseudoephedrine hydrochloride 30 mg
Calmylin	Teva	liquid	
Calmylin with Codeine	Teva	liquid	pseudoephedrine hydrochloride 6 mg/mL
Cepacol Extra Strength Lozenges	Combe	lozenge	
Cepacol Lozenges	Combe	lozenge	
Cepacol Sore Throat Extra Strength Spray	Combe	spray	
Cepacol Sore Throat Spray	Combe	spray	

Antihistamine	Antitussive	Expectorant	Other Active Ingredients
chlorpheniramine maleate 0.2 mg/mL	dextromethorphan hydrobromide 1.5 mg/mL		acetaminophen 32 mg/mL
chlorpheniramine maleate 1 mg	dextromethorphan hydrobromide 7.5 mg		acetaminophen 32 mg/mL
diphenhydramine hydrochloride 1.25 mg/mL	dextromethorphan hydrobromide 1 mg/mL		acetaminophen 32 mg/mL
	dextromethorphan hydrobromide 3 mg/mL		
			benzocaine 7.5 mg cetalkonium chloride 5 mg
			4-hexylresorcinol 3.5 mg
		guaifenesin 20 mg/mL	
	dextromethorphan hydrobromide 3 mg/mL		
	dextromethorphan hydrobromide 15 mg		acetaminophen 325 mg
			acetaminophen 65 mg/mL menthol 4 mg/mL
		guaifenesin 40 mg/mL	acetaminophen 65 mg/mL menthol 4 mg/mL
doxylamine succinate 6.25 mg	dextromethorphan hydrobromide 15 mg		acetaminophen 325 mg
	dextromethorphan hydrobromide 10 mg	guaifenesin 100 mg	acetaminophen 250 mg
diphenhydramine hydrochloride 5 mg/mL			acetaminophen 65 mg/mL menthol 4 mg/mL
		guaifenesin 20 mg/mL	menthol 2 mg/mL
	dextromethorphan hydrobromide 15 mg		acetaminophen 500 mg
chlorpheniramine maleate 2 mg	dextromethorphan hydrobromide 15 mg		acetaminophen 500 mg
		guaifenesin 20 mg/mL	menthol 2 mg/mL
	dextromethorphan hydrobromide 15 mg		acetaminophen 325 mg
	dextromethorphan hydrobromide 2.5 mg/mL		
	dextromethorphan hydrobromide 2.5 mg/mL		
			ammonium carbonate 30.7 mg/mL camphor 0.44 mg/mL menthol 4.44 mg/mL potassium bicarbonate 53.4 mg/mL
diphenhydramine hydrochloride 2.5 mg/mL			menthol 4.44 mg/mL
	dextromethorphan hydrobromide 15 mg		acetaminophen 325 mg
diphenhydramine hydrochloride 2.5 mg/mL	codeine phosphate 0.66 mg/mL	ammonium chloride 25 mg/mL	
	codeine phosphate 0.66 mg/mL	guaifenesin 20 mg/mL	
			benzocaine 10 mg cetylpyridinium chloride 2 mg
			cetylpyridinium chloride 1.4 mg
			benzocaine 10 mg cetylpyridinium chloride 1.5 mg
			diclonine hydrochloride 0.1%

Product	Manufacturer	Dosage Form	Decongestant
Children's Accudial Allergy	Accudial Pharmaceutical	liquid	
Children's Accudial Cold & Stuffy Nose	Accudial Pharmaceutical	liquid	phenylephrine hydrochloride 0.5 mg/mL
Children's Accudial Chest Congestion	Accudial Pharmaceutical	liquid	
Children's Accudial Cough & Cold	Accudial Pharmaceutical	liquid	
Children's Accudial Daytime Cough & Cold	Accudial Pharmaceutical	liquid	phenylephrine hydrochloride 0.5 mg/mL
Children's Accudial Nite Time Cold & Cough	Accudial Pharmaceutical	liquid	phenylephrine hydrochloride 0.5 mg/mL
Children's Accudial Runny Nose & Cough	Accudial Pharmaceutical	liquid	phenylephrine hydrochloride 0.5 mg/mL
Chloraseptic Lozenges Liquid Filled Various Flavours	Prestige Brands	lozenge	
Chloraseptic Lozenges Various Flavours	Prestige Brands	lozenge	
Chloraseptic Sore Throat Spray Various Flavours	Prestige Brands	spray	
Chlorpheniramine Tablets	Various Manufacturers	tablet	
Chlor-Tripolon Tablets 4 mg	Schering-Plough	tablet	
Claritin Allergy Decongestant	Schering-Plough	spray	oxymetazoline hydrochloride 0.05%
Claritin Allergy & Sinus	Schering-Plough	tablet	pseudoephedrine hydrochloride 120 mg
Claritin Allergy & Sinus Extra Strength	Schering-Plough	tablet	pseudoephedrine hydrochloride 240 mg
Claritin Kids Syrup	Schering-Plough	syrup	
Claritin Rapid Dissolve	Schering-Plough	tablet	
Claritin Tablets	Schering-Plough	tablet	
Cold-A-Tak	WN Pharmaceuticals	softgel	
Cold-FX	Afexa Life Sciences	tablet	
Contac Cold & Sore Throat Extra Strength	Meda Valeant	caplet	phenylephrine hydrochloride 5 mg
Contac Complete Extra Strength Cough, Cold & Flu	Meda Valeant	caplet	phenylephrine hydrochloride 5 mg
Contac Complete Extra Strength Cough, Cold & Flu Nighttime	Meda Valeant	caplet	phenylephrine hydrochloride 5 mg
Coricidin II Cold & Flu	Schering-Plough	tablet	
Coricidin II Cough & Cold	Schering-Plough	tablet	
Coricidin II Extra Strength Cold & Flu	Schering-Plough	tablet	
Cough Lozenges Cherry Menthol	H.J. Sutton	lozenge	
Cough Lozenges Honey-Lemon Menthol	H.J. Sutton	lozenge	
Cough Lozenges Menthol	H.J. Sutton	lozenge	
Cough Lozenges Spearmint Menthol	H.J. Sutton	lozenge	
Cough Syrup Dextromethorphan	Tanta	syrup	
Cough Syrup with Guaifenesin & Dextromethorphan	Tanta	liquid	
Creo-Rectal Adults	Sandoz	suppository	
Creo-Rectal Children	Sandoz	suppository	
Custom Care Cough & Cold PM	Procter & Gamble	liquid	
Custom Care Dry Cough Suppressant	Procter & Gamble	liquid	
Custom Care Chesty Cough Medicine			
DayQuil Cold & Flu Liquicaps	Procter & Gamble	capsule	
DayQuil Cold & Flu Multi-symptom Relief Liquid Medicine	Procter & Gamble	syrup	phenylephrine hydrochloride 0.33 mg/mL
DayQuil Cough Medicine	Procter & Gamble	syrup	

Antihistamine	Antitussive	Expectorant	Other Active Ingredients
diphenhydramine hydrochloride 2.5 mg/mL			
chlorpheniramine maleate 0.2 mg/mL			
		guaifenesin 20 mg/mL	
chlorpheniramine maleate 0.2 mg/mL	dextromethorphan hydrobromide 1.5 mg/mL		
	dextromethorphan hydrobromide 1 mg/mL		
diphenhydramine hydrochloride 1.25 mg/mL			
brompheniramine maleate 0.2 mg/mL	dextromethorphan hydrobromide 1 mg/mL		
			benzocaine 6 mg menthol 10 mg
			benzocaine 6 mg menthol 10 mg
			phenol 1.4%
chlorpheniramine maleate 4 mg			
chlorpheniramine maleate 4 mg			
loratadine 5 mg			
loratadine 10 mg			
loratadine 1 mg/mL			
loratadine 10 mg			
loratadine 10 mg			
			echinacea purpurea 250 mg
			CVT-E002 (North American ginseng root extract) 200 mg
			acetaminophen 500 mg
	dextromethorphan hydrobromide 15 mg		acetaminophen 500 mg
chlorpheniramine maleate 2 mg	dextromethorphan hydrobromide 15 mg		acetaminophen 500 mg
chlorpheniramine maleate 2 mg			acetaminophen 325 mg
chlorpheniramine maleate 2 mg	dextromethorphan hydrobromide 30 mg		
chlorpheniramine maleate 2 mg	dextromethorphan hydrobromide 15 mg		acetaminophen 500 mg
			menthol 7.6 mg
			menthol 8.6 mg
			menthol 7 mg
			menthol 5 mg
	dextromethorphan hydrobromide 3 mg/mL		
	dextromethorphan hydrobromide 3 mg/mL	guaifenesin 20 mg/mL	
diphenylpyraline hydrochloride 1.5 mg		guaiacol 600 mg (as carbonate)	camphor 5 mg
diphenylpyraline hydrochloride 0.5 mg		guaiacol 200 mg (as carbonate)	camphor 2 mg
chlorpheniramine maleate 0.27 mg/mL	dextromethorphan hydrobromide 0.5 mg/mL		acetaminophen 43.3 mg/mL
	dextromethorphan hydrobromide 0.5 mg/mL		
	dextromethorphan hydrobromide 1.3 mg/mL	guaifenesin 13.3 mg/mL	
	dextromethorphan hydrobromide 10 mg		acetaminophen 250 mg
	dextromethorphan hydrobromide 0.67 mg/mL		acetaminophen 21.7 mg/mL
	dextromethorphan hydrobromide 1 mg/mL		

Product	Manufacturer	Dosage Form	Decongestant
DayQuil Sinus Liquicaps	Procter & Gamble	capsule	phenylephrine hydrochloride 5 mg
Decongestant Nasal Spray 0.1%	Various Manufacturers	spray	xylometazoline hydrochloride 0.1%
Demo-Cineol Suppositories Adults	Sandoz	suppository	
Demo-Cineol Suppositories Children	Sandoz	suppository	
Dequadin Lozenge Cherry/ Orange	Wellspring	lozenge	
Dimetapp	Pfizer Consumer Healthcare	liquid	phenylephrine hydrochloride 1 mg/mL
Dimetapp Chewables for Kids	Pfizer Consumer Healthcare	tablet, chewable	phenylephrine hydrochloride 2.5 mg
Dimetapp DM Cough & Cold	Pfizer Consumer Healthcare	liquid	phenylephrine hydrochloride 1 mg/mL
Dimetapp Extra Strength	Pfizer Consumer Healthcare	liquid	phenylephrine hydrochloride 10 mg
Dimetapp Extra Strength DM Cough and Cold	Pfizer Consumer Healthcare	liquid	phenylephrine hydrochloride 2 mg/mL
DM Children's Cough Syrup	Various Manufacturers	syrup	
DM Cough Syrup	Various Manufacturers	syrup	
DM Decongestant	Various Manufacturers	syrup	pseudoephedrine hydrochloride 6 mg/mL
DM Decongestant-Expectorant	Various Manufacturers	syrup	pseudoephedrine hydrochloride 6 mg/mL
DM Decongestant-Expectorant Extra Strength	Various Manufacturers	syrup	pseudoephedrine hydrochloride 6 mg/mL
DM Decongestant-Expectorant-Analgesic	Various Manufacturers	syrup	pseudoephedrine hydrochloride 2 mg/mL
DM Expectorant	Various Manufacturers	syrup	
DM Expectorant Cough Syrup	Various Manufacturers	syrup	
DM Expectorant Extra Strength	Various Manufacturers	syrup	
DM Plus Cough Syrup	Various Manufacturers	syrup	
DM Plus Decongestant Cough Syrup	Various Manufacturers	syrup	pseudoephedrine hydrochloride 6 mg/mL
DM Plus Decongestant Expectorant Cough Syrup	Various Manufacturers	syrup	pseudoephedrine hydrochloride 6 mg/mL
DM Plus Decongestant Expectorant Extra Strength Cough Syrup	Various Manufacturers	syrup	pseudoephedrine hydrochloride 6 mg/mL
DM Plus Expectorant Syrup	Various Manufacturers	syrup	
DM sans Sucre	Various Manufacturers	liquid	
DM-D Expectorant Cough & Cold Syrup	Various Manufacturers	liquid	pseudoephedrine hydrochloride 6 mg/mL
Dristan Extra Strength	Pfizer Consumer Healthcare	caplet	phenylephrine hydrochloride 5 mg
Dristan Long Lasting Mentholated Nasal Spray	Pfizer Consumer Healthcare	spray	oxymetazoline hydrochloride 0.05%
Dristan Long Lasting Nasal Mist	Pfizer Consumer Healthcare	spray	oxymetazoline hydrochloride 0.05%
Dristan Nasal Mist	Pfizer Consumer Healthcare	spray	phenylephrine hydrochloride 0.5%
Dristan Tablets	Pfizer Consumer Healthcare	tablet	phenylephrine hydrochloride 5 mg
Drixoral Cold & Sinus	Schering-Plough	tablet, sustained release	pseudoephedrine sulfate 120 mg
Drixoral Decongestant Nasal Spray	Schering-Plough	spray	oxymetazoline hydrochloride 0.05%
Drixoral No Drip Nasal Spray	Schering-Plough	spray	oxymetazoline hydrochloride 0.05%

Antihistamine	Antitussive	Expectorant	Other Active Ingredients
			acetaminophen 325 mg
		guaiacol 360 mg	camphor 40 mg eucalyptol 370 mg
		guaiacol 180 mg	camphor 20 mg eucalyptol 185 mg
			dequalinium chloride 0.25mg
brompheniramine maleate 0.4 mg/mL			
brompheniramine maleate 1 mg			
brompheniramine maleate 0.4 mg/mL	dextromethorphan hydrobromide 2 mg/mL		
brompheniramine maleate 4 mg			
brompheniramine maleate 0.8 mg/mL	dextromethorphan hydrobromide 4 mg/mL		
	dextromethorphan hydrobromide 1.5 mg/mL		
	dextromethorphan hydrobromide 3 mg/mL		
	dextromethorphan hydrobromide 3 mg/mL		
	dextromethorphan hydrobromide 3 mg/mL	guaifenesin 20 mg/mL	
	dextromethorphan hydrobromide 3 mg/mL	guaifenesin 40 mg/mL	
	dextromethorphan hydrobromide 1 mg/mL	guaifenesin 6.7 mg/mL	acetaminophen 21.7 mg/mL
	dextromethorphan hydrobromide 3 mg/mL	guaifenesin 20 mg/mL	
	dextromethorphan hydrobromide 3 mg/mL	guaifenesin 20 mg/mL	
	dextromethorphan hydrobromide 3 mg/mL	guaifenesin 40 mg/mL	
diphenhydramine hydrochloride 2.5 mg/mL	dextromethorphan hydrobromide 3 mg/mL	ammonium chloride 25 mg/mL	
	dextromethorphan hydrobromide 3 mg/mL		
	dextromethorphan hydrobromide 3 mg/mL	guaifenesin 20 mg/mL	
	dextromethorphan hydrobromide 3 mg/mL	guaifenesin 40 mg/mL	
	dextromethorphan hydrobromide 3 mg/mL	guaifenesin 20 mg/mL	
	dextromethorphan hydrobromide 3 mg/mL		
	dextromethorphan hydrobromide 3 mg/mL	guaifenesin 40 mg/mL	
chlorpheniramine maleate 2 mg			acetaminophen 500 mg
pheniramine maleate 0.2%			
chlorpheniramine maleate 2 mg			acetaminophen 325 mg
dexbrompheniramine maleate 6 mg			

Product	Manufacturer	Dosage Form	Decongestant
Echinacea	Jamp	capsule	
Echinacea	Jamieson	capsule	
Echinacea Herb Tincture	WN Pharmaceuticals	liquid tincture	
Echinacea Lozenges Cherry/ Orange	Swiss Herbal	lozenge	
Echinacea Purpurea	Holista	capsule	
Echinacea Tincture	Holista	liquid tincture	
Echinacea Tincture Alcohol Free Wild Cherry	Holista	liquid tincture	
EchinaMax Echinacea & Goldenseal Tincture	WN Pharmaceuticals	liquid tincture	
Eltor 120	sanofi-aventis	tablet, sustained release	pseudoephedrine hydrochloride 120 mg
Entex LA	Purdue Pharma	tablet, sustained release	pseudoephedrine hydrochloride 120 mg
Euro Cyproheptadine Syrup	Euro-Pharm	syrup	
Euro Cyproheptadine Tablets	Euro-Pharm	tablet	
Expectorant Cough Formula	Tanta	syrup	
Expectorant Cough Syrup	Various Manufacturers	syrup	
Expectorant Syrup (sucrose Free)	Various Manufacturers	syrup	
Guaifenesin Expectorant Syrup	Various Manufacturers	liquid	
Fisherman's Friend Milder Sucrose-Free Mint	Lofthouse	lozenge	
Fisherman's Friend Original Extra Strong	Lofthouse	lozenge	
Fisherman's Friend Regular Strength	Lofthouse	lozenge	
Fisherman's Friend Sucrose-Free Apple Cinnamon	Lofthouse	lozenge	
Fisherman's Friend Sucrose-Free Cherry	Lofthouse	lozenge	
Fisherman's Friend Sucrose-Free Lemon	Lofthouse	lozenge	
Halls Centres Cherry	Adams	lozenge	
Halls Centres Honey-Lemon	Adams	lozenge	
Halls Cherry	Adams	lozenge	
Halls Coolmint	Adams	lozenge	
Halls Extra Strong	Adams	lozenge	
Halls Extra Strong Spearmint	Adams	lozenge	
Halls Honey-Lemon	Adams	lozenge	
Halls Lemon-Lime	Adams	lozenge	
Halls Regular	Adams	lozenge	
Halls Strawberry	Adams	lozenge	

Antihistamine	Antitussive	Expectorant	Other Active Ingredients
			echinacea purpurea 200 mg
			echinacea angustifolia 200 mg
			echinacea purpurea 1 mL
			echinacea angustifolia 750 mg
			echinacea purpurea 500 mg
			echinacea angustifolia 1 mL
			echinacea purpurea 1 mL
			echinacea purpurea 514 mg echinacea purpurea roots 229 mg goldenseal (hydrastis canadensis) 62.5 mg
		guaifenesin 600 mg	
cyproheptadine hydrochloride 0.4 mg/mL			
cyproheptadine hydrochloride 4 mg			
		guaifenesin 20 mg/mL	
		guaifenesin 20 mg/mL	
		guaifenesin 20 mg/mL	
		guaifenesin	
			menthol 0.29%
			eucalyptus oil 0.15% menthol 0.9%
			menthol 0.5%
			menthol 0.35%
			menthol 0.55%
			menthol 0.4%
			eucalyptus oil 6.5 mg menthol 7.5 mg
			eucalyptus oil 4 mg menthol 10 mg
			eucalyptus oil 1.7 mg menthol 7.6 mg
			eucalyptus oil 1.5 mg menthol 6 mg
			eucalyptus oil 9.8 mg menthol 19.7 mg
			eucalyptus oil 6.5 mg menthol 19.7 mg
			eucalyptus oil 2.3 mg menthol 8.7 mg
			eucalyptus oil 1 mg menthol 2.3 mg
			eucalyptus oil 6.4 mg menthol 9.8 mg
			eucalyptus oil 2.8 mg menthol 3.8 mg

Product	Manufacturer	Dosage Form	Decongestant
Halls Sucrose-Free Black-Cherry	Adams	lozenge	
Histantil 50 mg	Pendopharm	tablet	
Histenol II	Zee Medical	tablet	phenylephrine hydrochloride 5 mg
Honey Lemon Cough Lozenges	H.J. Sutton	lozenge	
Hot Lemon Relief	Apotex	powder for solution	phenylephrine hydrochloride 10 mg
Hot Lemon Relief Extra Strength	Apotex	powder for solution	phenylephrine hydrochloride 10 mg
Hydrasense Congestion Relief Spray	Schering-Plough	liquid	
Hydrasense Easy Dose	Schering-Plough	liquid	
Hydrasense Nasal Spray Gentle Mist	Schering-Plough	liquid	
Hydrasense Nasal Spray Maximum	Schering-Plough	liquid	
Hydrasense Nasal Spray Medium Stream	Schering-Plough	liquid	
Jack & Jill Bedtime	W.K. Buckley	liquid	
Jack & Jill Cough & Cold Liquid	W.K. Buckley	liquid	pseudoephedrine hydrochloride 3 mg/mL
Jack & Jill Cough Liquid with DM	W.K. Buckley	liquid	
Jack & Jill Expectorant	W.K. Buckley	liquid	
Koffex DM	Teva	syrup	
Koffex DM Sucrose free	Teva	liquid	
Menthol Cough Lozenges	H.J. Sutton	lozenge	
Mentholatum Ointment	Mentholatum	ointment	
Neo Citran Cold & Flu	Novartis Consumer Health	powder for solution	phenylephrine hydrochloride 10 mg
Neo Citran Cough and Cold DM	Novartis Consumer Health	powder for solution	phenylephrine hydrochloride 10 mg
Neo Citran Extra Strength Total plus Mucous Relief	Novartis Consumer Health	powder for solution	pseudoephedrine hydrochloride 60 mg
Neo Citran Extra Strength Cold & Flu	Novartis Consumer Health	powder for solution	phenylephrine hydrochloride 10 mg
Neo Citran Extra Strength Cough, Cold & Flu/Total Nighttime	Novartis Consumer Health	powder for solution	pseudoephedrine hydrochloride 60 mg
Neo Citran Extra Strength Cold & Sinus	Novartis Consumer Health	powder for solution	phenylephrine hydrochloride 10 mg
Neo Citran Extra Strength Total Daytime	Novartis Consumer Health	powder for solution	phenylephrine hydrochloride 10 mg
Neo Citran Extra Strength Total Sugar Free	Novartis Consumer Health	powder for solution	phenylephrine hydrochloride 10 mg
Neo Citran Ultra Strength Total Flu	Novartis Consumer Health	powder for solution	pseudoephedrine hydrochloride 60 mg
Neo Citran Warming Extra Strength Chest Congestion, Cold & Mucous Relief	Novartis Consumer Health	syrup	phenylephrine hydrochloride 0.33 mg/mL
Neo Citran Warming Extra Strength Total Cold/Flu Daytime	Novartis Consumer Health	syrup	phenylephrine hydrochloride 0.33 mg/mL
Neo Citran Warming Extra Strength Total Cold/Flu Nighttime	Novartis Consumer Health	syrup	phenylephrine hydrochloride 0.33 mg/mL
Neo-Laryngobis	Teva	suppository	

Antihistamine	Antitussive	Expectorant	Other Active Ingredients
			eucalyptus oil 3.2 mg menthol 5.8 mg
promethazine hydrochloride 50 mg			
	dextromethorphan hydrobromide 15 mg	guaifenesin 200 mg	acetaminophen 325 mg
			menthol 8.6 mg
pheniramine maleate 20 mg			acetaminophen 325 mg ascorbic acid 50 mg
pheniramine maleate 20 mg			acetaminophen 500 mg ascorbic acid 50 mg
			natural source sea water 100%
			natural source sea water 100%
			natural source sea water 100%
			natural source sea water 100%
			natural source sea water 100%
diphenhydramine hydrochloride 1.25 mg/mL			
chlorpheniramine maleate 0.2 mg/mL	dextromethorphan hydrobromide 1.5 mg/mL		
chlorpheniramine maleate 0.4 mg/mL	dextromethorphan hydrobromide 1.5 mg/mL		
		guaifenesin 10 mg/mL	
	dextromethorphan hydrobromide 3 mg/mL		
	dextromethorphan hydrobromide 3 mg/mL		
			menthol 6.1 mg
			camphor 9% menthol 1.35%
pheniramine maleate 20 mg			acetaminophen 325 mg
pheniramine maleate 20 mg	dextromethorphan hydrobromide 30 mg		
	dextromethorphan hydrobromide 30 mg	guaifenesin 400 mg	acetaminophen 1000 mg
pheniramine maleate 20 mg			acetaminophen 650 mg
chlorpheniramine maleate 4 mg	dextromethorphan hydrobromide 20 mg		acetaminophen 650 mg
			acetaminophen 650 mg
	dextromethorphan hydrobromide 20 mg		acetaminophen 650 mg
diphenhydramine hydrochloride 25 mg			acetaminophen 650 mg
chlorpheniramine maleate 4 mg	dextromethorphan hydrobromide 30 mg		acetaminophen 1000 mg
		guaifenesin 13.33 mg/mL	acetaminophen 21.7 mg/mL
	dextromethorphan hydrobromide 0.67 mg/mL		acetaminophen 21.7 mg/mL
diphenhydramine hydrochloride 0.83 mg/mL			acetaminophen 21.7 mg/mL
			bismuth dipropylacetate 135 mg

Product	Manufacturer	Dosage Form	Decongestant
Nin Jiom Herbal Cough Syrup	Nin Jiom	liquid	
NyQuil Cold & Flu Multi-Symptom Relief Liquid	Procter & Gamble	liquid	
NyQuil Cold & Flu Multi-symptom Relief Liquicaps	Procter & Gamble	capsule	
NyQuil Cough	Procter & Gamble	liquid	
NyQuil Sinus Liquicaps	Procter & Gamble	capsule	phenylephrine hydrochloride 5 mg
Otrivin Cold & Allergy Nose Drops	Novartis Consumer Health	drops	xylometazoline hydrochloride 0.1%
Otrivin Measured Dose Pump	Novartis Consumer Health	liquid	xylometazoline hydrochloride 0.1%
Otrivin Nasal Solution	Novartis Consumer Health	drops	xylometazoline hydrochloride 0.1%
Otrivin Nasal Spray	Novartis Consumer Health	spray	xylometazoline hydrochloride 0.1%
Otrivin Saline Pediatric Nose Drops	Novartis Consumer Health	drops	
Otrivin Saline Sea Water & Aloe	Novartis Consumer Health	liquid	
Otrivin Saline with Moisturizers Measured Dose Pump	Novartis Consumer Health	spray	
Otrivin with Moisturizers Nasal Spray	Novartis Consumer Health	spray	xylometazoline hydrochloride 0.1%
PMS Cyproheptadine	Pendopharm	tablet	
Pseudofrin Syrup	Trianon	syrup	pseudoephedrine hydrochloride 6 mg/mL
Pseudofrin Tablets	Trianon	tablet	pseudoephedrine hydrochloride 60 mg
Reactine 5 mg	Pfizer Consumer Healthcare	tablet	
Reactine 10 mg	Pfizer Consumer Healthcare	tablet	
Reactine Allergy & Sinus	Pfizer Consumer Healthcare	tablet	pseudoephedrine hydrochloride 120 mg
Reactine Syrup	Pfizer Consumer Healthcare	syrup	
Rhinaris CS Anti-allergic	Pendopharm	metered-dose spray	
Rhinaris Lubricating Nasal Gel	Pendopharm	gel	
Rhinaris Lubricating Nasal Mist	Pendopharm	metered-dose spray	
Rhinaris Nozoil	Pendopharm	spray	
Rhinaris Saline Rinse	Pendopharm	liquid	
Rhinaris Saline Solution	Pendopharm	spray	
Rhinaris Sinomarin	Pendopharm	spray	
Rhinedrine Moisturizing Nasal Mist	Jamieson	liquid	
Ricola Green Tea & Echinacea Throat Drops	Ricola	lozenge	

Antihistamine	Antitussive	Expectorant	Other Active Ingredients
			ioquat 1.215 mg/mL dandelion 1.015 mg/mL peking spurge 0.473 mg/mL chinese licorice 0.4 mg/mL mandarin orange 0.34 mg/mL coltsfoot 0.34 mg/mL senega 0.34 mg/mL honey extract
doxylamine succinate 0.42 mg/mL	dextromethorphan hydrobromide 1 mg/mL		acetaminophen 21.7 mg/mL
doxylamine succinate 6.25 mg	dextromethorphan hydrobromide 15 mg		acetaminophen 325 mg
doxylamine succinate 0.42 mg/mL	dextromethorphan hydrobromide 1 mg/mL		
doxylamine succinate 6.25 mg			acetaminophen 325 mg
			sodium chloride 0.7%
			purified water sea water
			sodium chloride 0.7%
cyproheptadine hydrochloride 4 mg			
cetirizine hydrochloride 5 mg			
cetirizine hydrochloride 10 mg			
cetirizine hydrochloride 5 mg			
cetirizine hydrochloride 1 mg/mL			
			sodium cromoglycate 2%
			polyethylene glycol 15% propylene glycol 20%
			polyethylene glycol 15% propylene glycol 5%
			sesame oil 100%
			sodium chloride
			sodium chloride 0.9%
			natural source sea water 100%
			glycerin 3% propylene glycol 4.36%
			echinacea purpurea 205.2 mg mallow 0.864 mg red sage 11.64 mg thyme 3.2 mg

Product	Manufacturer	Dosage Form	Decongestant
Ricola Original Herb Cough Drops (No-sugar added)	Ricola	lozenge	
Ricola Swiss Herb Cough Drops	Ricola	lozenge	
Ricola Swiss Herb Cough Drops Cherry-Honey	Ricola	lozenge	
Ricola Swiss Herb Cough Drops Lemon-Mint	Ricola	lozenge	
Ricola Swiss Herb Cough Drops Orange-Mint	Ricola	lozenge	
Robitussin Children's Cough & Cold	Pfizer Consumer Healthcare	syrup	pseudoephedrine hydrochloride 3 mg/mL
Robitussin Cough & Cold	Pfizer Consumer Healthcare	syrup	pseudoephedrine hydrochloride 6 mg/mL

Antihistamine	Antitussive	Expectorant	Other Active Ingredients
			achillea millefolium 21.6 mg althea 28.08 mg cowslip 2.16 mg horehound 2.16 mg mallow 10.8 mg peppermint oil 28.08 mg pimpinella major 15.12 mg plantago lanceolata 34.56 mg salvia 21.6 mg sambucus nigra 6.48 mg thyme 3.2 mg veronica officinalis 3.2 mg
			althea 3.2 mg burnet 3.2 mg horehound 3.2 mg mallow 3.2 mg menthol 2 mg parsley piert 3.2 mg peppermint oil 2 mg plantago cordata 3.2 mg thyme 3.2 mg veronica officinalis 3.2 mg
			althea 0.8 mg ascorbic acid 10 mg burnet 0.8 mg horehound 0.8 mg mallow 0.8 mg menthol 1.5 mg parsley piert 0.8 mg peppermint oil 0.9 mg plantago cordata 0.8 mg thyme 0.8 mg veronica officinalis 0.8 mg
			althea 0.9 mg ascorbic acid 10 mg burnet 0.9 mg horehound 0.9 mg mallow 0.9 mg menthol 0.5 mg parsley piert 0.9 mg peppermint oil 1 mg plantago cordata 0.9 mg thyme 0.9 mg veronica officinalis 0.9 mg
			althea 0.5 mg ascorbic acid 25 mg burnet 0.5 mg horehound 0.5 mg mallow 0.5 mg menthol 0.5 mg parsley piert 0.5 mg peppermint oil 0.7 mg plantago cordata 0.5 mg thyme 0.5 mg veronica officinalis 0.5 mg
	dextromethorphan hydrobromide 1.5 mg/mL		
	dextromethorphan hydrobromide 3 mg/mL	guaifenesin 20 mg/mL	

Product	Manufacturer	Dosage Form	Decongestant
Robitussin Cough & Cold Extra Strength	Pfizer Consumer Healthcare	liquid	pseudoephedrine hydrochloride 6 mg/mL
Robitussin Cough Control	Pfizer Consumer Healthcare	liquid	
Robitussin Cough Control for People with Diabetes	Pfizer Consumer Healthcare	liquid	
Robitussin DM CoughGels	Pfizer Consumer Healthcare	capsule	
Robitussin Cough Control Extra Strength	Pfizer Consumer Healthcare	liquid	
Robitussin Chest Congestion	Pfizer Consumer Healthcare	liquid	
Robitussin Chest Congestion Extra Strength	Pfizer Consumer Healthcare	liquid	
Robitussin Total Cough, Cold & Flu	Pfizer Consumer Healthcare	liquid	pseudoephedrine hydrochloride 1 mg/mL
Robitussin Total Cough, Cold & Flu Extra Strength Nighttime	Pfizer Consumer Healthcare	liquid	pseudoephedrine hydrochloride 2 mg/mL
Rophelin Syrup	M. Vachon Group	syrup	
Salinex Nasal Drops	Sandoz	liquid	
Salinex Nasal Lubricant Gel	Sandoz	gel	
Salinex Nasal Lubricant Solution	Sandoz	liquid	
Salinex Nasal Mist	Sandoz	liquid	
Salinex Nasal Spray Adult	Sandoz	liquid	
Salinex Nasal Spray Children	Sandoz	liquid	
Secaris	Pendopharm	gel	
Sedatuss DM	Trianon	syrup	
Sinutab Extra Strength Daytime/Nightime Combo	Pfizer Consumer Healthcare	caplet	pseudoephedrine hydrochloride 30 mg (day) pseudoephedrine hydrochloride 30 mg (night)
Sinutab Nightime Extra Strength	Pfizer Consumer Healthcare	tablet	pseudoephedrine hydrochloride 30 mg
Sinutab Sinus & Allergy Extra Strength	Pfizer Consumer Healthcare	caplet	pseudoephedrine hydrochloride 30 mg
Sinutab Sinus & Allergy Regular	Pfizer Consumer Healthcare	caplet	pseudoephedrine hydrochloride 30 mg
Sinutab Sinus (Daytime) Non Drowsy Extra Strength	Pfizer Consumer Healthcare	tablet	pseudoephedrine hydrochloride 30 mg
Sinutab Sinus Non Drowsy	Pfizer Consumer Healthcare	tablet	pseudoephedrine hydrochloride 30 mg

Antihistamine	Antitussive	Expectorant	Other Active Ingredients
	dextromethorphan hydrobromide 3 mg/mL	guaifenesin 40 mg/mL	
	dextromethorphan hydrobromide 3 mg/mL	guaifenesin 20 mg/mL	
	dextromethorphan hydrobromide 2 mg/mL	guaifenesin 20 mg/mL	
	dextromethorphan hydrobromide 15 mg		
	dextromethorphan hydrobromide 3 mg/mL	guaifenesin 40 mg/mL	
		guaifenesin 20 mg/mL	
		guaifenesin 40 mg/mL	
	dextromethorphan hydrobromide 1 mg/mL		acetaminophen 21.6 mg/mL
chlorpheniramine maleate 0.13 mg/ml	dextromethorphan hydrobromide 1 mg/mL		acetaminophen 33.3 mg/mL
		ammonium chloride 5.8 mg/mL	
			sodium chloride 0.9%
			polyethylene glycol 15.2% propylene glycol 20% sodium chloride 0.9%
			polyethylene glycol 16% propylene glycol 5% sodium chloride 0.9%
			sodium chloride 0.9%
			sodium chloride 0.9%
			sodium chloride 0.9%
			polyethylene glycol 15% propylene glycol 20%
	dextromethorphan hydrobromide 3 mg/mL		
diphenhydramine hydrochloride 25 mg (night)			acetaminophen 500 mg (day) acetaminophen 500 mg (night)
diphenhydramine hydrochloride 25 mg			acetaminophen 500 mg
chlorpheniramine maleate 2 mg			acetaminophen 500 mg
chlorpheniramine maleate 2 mg			acetaminophen 325 mg
			acetaminophen 500 mg
			acetaminophen 325 mg

▶

Product	Manufacturer	Dosage Form	Decongestant
Slippery Elm Lozenges	Trophic	lozenge	
Soothe Aid Lozenge	Zee Medical	lozenge	
Sore Throat Lozenges Cherry/Menthol	H.J. Sutton	lozenge	
Strepsils Anesthetic Formula	Reckitt Benckiser	lozenge	
Strepsils Cherry	Reckitt Benckiser	lozenge	
Strepsils Sore Throat & Blocked Nose	Reckitt Benckiser	lozenge	
Strepsils Various Flavours	Reckitt Benckiser	lozenge	
Sucrets Complete Various Flavours	Insight	lozenge	
Sucrets Cough Control	Insight	lozenge	
Sucrets Cough Control Extra Strength	Insight	lozenge	
Sucrets DM Cough Suppresant Honey-Lemon	Insight	lozenge	
Sucrets Extra Strength	Insight	lozenge	
Sucrets for Kids	Insight	lozenge	
Sucrets Vapor Black Cherry	Insight	lozenge	
Sudafed Decongestant 12 Hour	McNeil Consumer Healthcare	caplet	pseudoephedrine hydrochloride 120 mg
Sudafed Head Cold & Sinus Extra Strength	McNeil Consumer Healthcare	caplet	pseudoephedrine hydrochloride 60 mg
Sudafed PE Decongestant	McNeil Consumer Healthcare	tablet	phenylephrine hydrochloride 10 mg
Sudafed Sinus Advance	McNeil Consumer Healthcare	tablet	pseudoephedrine hydrochloride 30 mg
Sunkist Lozenge Zinc & Vitamin C	WN Pharmaceuticals	lozenge	
Tantafed Decongestant	Tanta	tablet	pseudoephedrine hydrochloride 60 mg
Teva-Pheniram	Teva	tablet	
Triaminic Chest & Nasal Congestion	Novartis Consumer Health	liquid	phenylephrine hydrochloride 0.5 mg/mL
Triaminic Cold & Cough	Novartis Consumer Health	syrup	pseudoephedrine hydrochloride 3 mg/mL

Antihistamine	Antitussive	Expectorant	Other Active Ingredients
			slippery elm powder 600 mg fenugreek seed powder 10 mg
			hexylresorcinol 2.4 mg
			benzocaine 6 mg menthol 10 mg
			hexylresorcinol 2.4 mg
			amylmetacresol 0.6 mg dichlorobenzyl alcohol 1.2 mg menthol 5.0 mg
			amylmetacresol 0.6 mg dichlorobenzyl alcohol 1.2 mg menthol 8.0 mg
			amylmetacresol 0.6 mg dichlorobenzyl alcohol 1.2 mg
			dyclonine hydrochloride 3 mg menthol 6 mg
	dextromethorphan hydrobromide 5 mg		
	dextromethorphan hydrobromide 15 mg		
	dextromethorphan hydrobromide 10 mg		
			4-hexylresorcinol 3.5 mg
			dyclonine hydrochloride 1.2 mg
			dyclonine hydrochloride 3 mg
			acetaminophen 500 mg
			ibuprofen 200 mg
			vitamin C (sodium ascorbate) 50 mg zinc (citrate, gluconate) 5 mg
chlorpheniramine maleate 4 mg			
		guaifenesin 10 mg/mL	
chlorpheniramine maleate 0.2 mg/mL	dextromethorphan hydrobromide 1 mg/mL		

Product	Manufacturer	Dosage Form	Decongestant
Triaminic Cold & Nightime Cough	Novartis Consumer Health	syrup	pseudoephedrine hydrochloride 3 mg/mL
Triaminic Cold, Cough & Fever	Novartis Consumer Health	liquid	pseudoephedrine hydrochloride 3 mg/mL
Triaminic Cough	Novartis Consumer Health	syrup	pseudoephedrine hydrochloride 3 mg/mL
Triaminic Cough & Sore Throat	Novartis Consumer Health	syrup	pseudoephedrine hydrochloride 3 mg/mL
Triaminic Cough Long Acting	Novartis Consumer Health	syrup	
Triaminic Daytime Cough & Cold	Novartis Consumer Health	liquid	phenylephrine hydrochloride 0.5 mg/mL
Triaminic Thin Strips Cough	Novartis Consumer Health	strip	
Triaminic Thin Strips Cough & Congestion	Novartis Consumer Health	strip	phenylephrine hydrochloride 2.5 mg
Triaminic Thin Strips Nasal Congestion	Novartis Consumer Health	strip	phenylephrine hydrochloride 2.5 mg
Triaminic Thin Strips Nighttime Cough & Runny Nose	Novartis Consumer Health	strip	
Tylenol Allergy Extra Strength	McNeil Consumer Healthcare	tablet	phenylephrine hydrochloride 5 mg
Tylenol Children's Cold & Stuffy Nose	McNeil Consumer Healthcare	liquid	pseudoephedrine hydrochloride 3 mg/mL
Tylenol Children's Cold	McNeil Consumer Healthcare	liquid	pseudoephedrine hydrochloride 3 mg/mL
Tylenol Children's Cold & Cough	McNeil Consumer Healthcare	liquid	pseudoephedrine hydrochloride 3 mg/mL
Tylenol Children's Cold & Cough Nighttime	McNeil Consumer Healthcare	liquid	
Tylenol Children's Cough & Runny Nose	McNeil Consumer Healthcare	liquid	
Tylenol Cold Extra Strength Daytime	McNeil Consumer Healthcare	tablet	phenylephrine hydrochloride 5 mg
Tylenol Cold Extra Strength Nighttime	McNeil Consumer Healthcare	caplet	phenylephrine hydrochloride 5 mg
Tylenol Cold Regular Strength Daytime	McNeil Consumer Healthcare	caplet	phenylephrine hydrochloride 5 mg
Tylenol Cold Regular Strength Nighttime	McNeil Consumer Healthcare	caplet	phenylephrine hydrochloride 5 mg
Tylenol Cold & Sinus Extra Strength Daytime	McNeil Consumer Healthcare	caplet	pseudoephedrine hydrochloride 30 mg
Tylenol Cold & Sinus Extra Strength Nighttime	McNeil Consumer Healthcare	caplet	pseudoephedrine hydrochloride 30 mg
Tylenol Cough Medication	McNeil Consumer Healthcare	caplet	
Tylenol Extra Strength Nighttime	McNeil Consumer Healthcare	caplet	

Antihistamine	Antitussive	Expectorant	Other Active Ingredients
chlorpheniramine maleate 0.2 mg/mL	dextromethorphan hydrobromide 1.5 mg/mL		
chlorpheniramine maleate 0.2 mg/mL	dextromethorphan hydrobromide 1.5 mg/mL		acetaminophen 32 mg/mL
	dextromethorphan hydrobromide 1 mg/mL		
	dextromethorphan hydrobromide 1.5 mg/mL		acetaminophen 32 mg/mL
	dextromethorphan hydrobromide 1.5 mg/mL		
	dextromethorphan hydrobromide 1 mg/mL		
	dextromethorphan hydrobromide 7.5 mg		
	dextromethorphan hydrobromide 5 mg		
diphenhydramine hydrochloride 12.5 mg			
chlorpheniramine maleate 2 mg			acetaminophen 500 mg
			acetaminophen 32 mg/mL
chlorpheniramine maleate 0.2 mg/mL			acetaminophen 32 mg/mL
chlorpheniramine maleate 0.2 mg/mL	dextromethorphan hydrobromide 1.5 mg/mL		acetaminophen 32 mg/mL
diphenhydramine hydrochloride 1.25 mg/mL	dextromethorphan hydrobromide 1 mg/mL		acetaminophen 32 mg/mL
chlorpheniramine maleate 0.2 mg/mL	dextromethorphan hydrobromide 1 mg/mL		acetaminophen 32 mg/mL
	dextromethorphan hydrobromide 10 mg		acetaminophen 500 mg
chlorpheniramine maleate 2 mg	dextromethorphan hydrobromide 10 mg		acetaminophen 500 mg
	dextromethorphan hydrobromide 10 mg		acetaminophen 325 mg
chlorpheniramine maleate 2 mg	dextromethorphan hydrobromide 10 mg		acetaminophen 325 mg
			acetaminophen 500 mg
chlorpheniramine maleate 2 mg			acetaminophen 500 mg
	dextromethorphan hydrobromide 15 mg		acetaminophen 500 mg
diphenhydramine hydrochloride 25 mg			acetaminophen 500 mg

Product	Manufacturer	Dosage Form	Decongestant
Tylenol Flu Extra Strength Daytime	McNeil Consumer Healthcare	tablet	phenylephrine hydrochloride 5 mg
Tylenol Flu Extra Strength Nighttime	McNeil Consumer Healthcare	tablet	phenylephrine hydrochloride 5 mg
Tylenol Junior Strength Complete Cold, Cough & Fever	McNeil Consumer Healthcare	tablet, chewable	pseudoephedrine hydrochloride 15 mg
Tylenol Junior Strength Cold & Cough	McNeil Consumer Healthcare	tablet, chewable	pseudoephedrine hydrochloride 15 mg
Tylenol Sinus Extra Strength Daytime	McNeil Consumer Healthcare	caplet	phenylephrine hydrochloride 5 mg
Tylenol Sinus Extra Strength Nighttime	McNeil Consumer Healthcare	tablet	phenylephrine hydrochloride 5 mg
Tylenol Sinus Regular Strength Daytime	McNeil Consumer Healthcare	caplet	phenylephrine hydrochloride 5 mg
Vaporizing Colds Rub	Scott Chemical	ointment	
Vicks Cherry Throat Drops	Procter & Gamble	lozenge	
Vicks Chest Congestion Relief	Procter & Gamble	syrup	
Vicks Custom Care Chest Congestion & Cough	Procter & Gamble	liquid	
Vicks Custom Care Dry Cough	Procter & Gamble	liquid	
Vicks Custom Care Nasal Congestion & Cough	Procter & Gamble	liquid	pseudoephedrine hydrochloride 0.66 mg/ mL
Vicks Inhaler	Procter & Gamble	stick	
Vicks Lemon Throat Drops	Procter & Gamble	lozenge	
Vicks Menthol Throat Drops	Procter & Gamble	lozenge	
Vicks Vaporub Lotion	Procter & Gamble	lotion	
Vicks Vaporub Ointment	Procter & Gamble	ointment	
Zinc & Vitamin C	Nature's Sunshine	lozenge	
Zinc & Vitamin C	Quest	lozenge	
Zinc Lozenges with Vitamin C	Nutricorp	lozenge	
Zinc Lozenges with Vitamin C	General Nutrition Canada	lozenge	
Zinc Lozenges with Vitamin C	Jamieson	lozenge	
Zinc Lozenges with Vitamin C	WN Pharmaceuticals	lozenge	

Antihistamine	Antitussive	Expectorant	Other Active Ingredients
	dextromethorphan hydrobromide 10 mg		acetaminophen 500 mg
chlorpheniramine maleate 2 mg	dextromethorphan hydrobromide 10 mg		acetaminophen 500 mg
chlorpheniramine maleate 1 mg	dextromethorphan hydrobromide 7.5 mg		acetaminophen 160 mg
chlorpheniramine maleate 1 mg	dextromethorphan hydrobromide 7.5 mg		acetaminophen 160 mg
			acetaminophen 500 mg
chlorpheniramine maleate 2 mg			acetaminophen 500 mg
			acetaminophen 325 mg
			camphor 4.7% eucalyptus oil 1.2% menthol 2.6%
			menthol 0.0834%
		guaifenesin 13.3 mg/mL	
	dextromethorphan hydrobromide 1.33 mg/mL	guaifenesin 13.33 mg/mL	
	dextromethorphan hydrobromide 2 mg/mL		
	dextromethorphan hydrobromide 1.33 mg/mL		
			camphor 41.53% menthol 41.53%
			menthol 0.064%
			menthol 0.163%
			camphor 4.73% eucalyptus oil 1.2% menthol 2.6%
			camphor 4.73% eucalyptus oil 1.2% menthol 2.6%
			vitamin C 95 mg zinc (as acetate) 5 mg
			ascorbic acid 100 mg zinc 10 mg (as gluconate)
			ascorbic acid 25 mg zinc (zinc gluconate) 5 mg
			ascorbic acid 100 mg zinc 10 mg
			ascorbic acid 50 mg zinc 5 mg (as citrate)
			sodium ascorbate 50 mg zinc 5 mg (as citrate, gluconate)

Product	Manufacturer	Dosage Form	Decongestant
Zinc Lozenges with Vitamin C and non-medicinal Echinacea	Holista	lozenge	
Zinc Plus	Swiss Herbal	lozenge	
ZN-C Loz	Douglas	lozenge	

Antihistamine	Antitussive	Expectorant	Other Active Ingredients
			ascorbic acid 50 mg zinc 5 mg (as citrate)
			ascorbic acid 100 mg zinc 10 mg (as proteinate and gluconate)
			vitamin C (calcium ascorbate) 45 mg zinc (as gluconate, HVP chelate) 15 mg

Product	Manufacturer	Fluoride	Other Active Ingredients
Aim Gel	Church & Dwight	sodium fluoride 0.11%	
Aquafresh Advanced	GlaxoSmithKline Consumer Healthcare	sodium fluoride 0.243%	
Aquafresh Cavity Protection +	GlaxoSmithKline Consumer Healthcare	sodium monofluorophosphate 0.8%	
Aquafresh Extreme Clean Empowermint	GlaxoSmithKline Consumer Healthcare	sodium fluoride 0.243%	
Aquafresh Extreme Clean Original	GlaxoSmithKline Consumer Healthcare	sodium fluoride 0.243%	
Aquafresh Extreme Clean Powerwhite	GlaxoSmithKline Consumer Healthcare	sodium fluoride 0.243%	
Aquafresh Kids Toothpaste	GlaxoSmithKline Consumer Healthcare	sodium monofluorophosphate 0.8%	
Aquafresh Kidzmint Toothpaste	GlaxoSmithKline Consumer Healthcare	sodium monofluorophosphate 0.8%	
Aquafresh Sensitive Toothpaste	GlaxoSmithKline Consumer Healthcare	sodium fluoride 0.24%	potassium nitrate 5%
Aquafresh Ultimate White	GlaxoSmithKline Consumer Healthcare	sodium fluoride 0.243%	
Aquafresh White & Shine	GlaxoSmithKline Consumer Healthcare	sodium fluoride 0.11%	
Arm & Hammer Advance Care Gel	Church & Dwight	sodium fluoride 0.243%	
Arm & Hammer Complete Care Gel	Church & Dwight	sodium fluoride 0.243%	
Arm & Hammer Enamel Care Advanced Cleaning	Church & Dwight	sodium fluoride 0.11%	
Arm & Hammer Extra Whitening	Church & Dwight	sodium fluoride 0.243%	
Arm & Hammer Sensitive Gel	Church & Dwight	sodium fluoride 0.243%	potassium nitrate 5%
Arm & Hammer Sensitive Paste	Church & Dwight	sodium fluoride 0.243%	potassium nitrate 5%
Arm & Hammer Supreme Fresh Gel	Church & Dwight	sodium fluoride 0.243%	
Close-Up Gel	Church & Dwight	sodium fluoride 0.11%	
Colgate 2 in 1 Kids	Colgate-Palmolive	sodium fluoride 0.11%	
Colgate 2 in 1 Whitening	Colgate-Palmolive	sodium fluoride 0.11%	
Colgate Cavity Protection Gel	Colgate-Palmolive	sodium fluoride 0.243%	
Colgate Cavity Protection Regular	Colgate-Palmolive	sodium monofluorophosphate 0.76%	
Colgate Fluoride Toothpaste Winterfresh	Colgate-Palmolive	sodium monofluorophosphate 0.76%	
Colgate For Kids	Colgate-Palmolive	sodium fluoride 0.243%	
Colgate Maxfresh	Colgate-Palmolive	sodium fluoride 0.11%	
Colgate Maxfresh Liquid	Colgate-Palmolive	sodium fluoride 0.11%	
Colgate Optic White	Colgate-Palmolive	sodium monofluorophosphate 0.76%	
Colgate Platinum Whitening Toothpaste with Fluoride	Colgate-Palmolive	sodium monofluorophosphate 0.76%	
Colgate Sensitive	Colgate-Palmolive	sodium fluoride 0.11%	potassium nitrate 5%
Colgate Sensitive Whitening	Colgate-Palmolive	sodium fluoride 0.11%	potassium nitrate 5%
Colgate Tartar Control Mint	Colgate-Palmolive	sodium fluoride 0.243%	tetrapotassium pyrophosphate 6.2%
Colgate Tartar Control Mint Gel	Colgate-Palmolive	sodium fluoride 0.243%	tetrapotassium pyrophosphate 6.2%
Colgate Total	Colgate-Palmolive	sodium fluoride 0.243%	triclosan 0.3%
Colgate Total Advanced Health	Colgate-Palmolive	sodium fluoride 0.243%	triclosan 0.3%
Crest Complete	Procter & Gamble	sodium fluoride 0.243%	sodium acid pyrophosphate 1.65% tetrapotassium pyrophosphate 4.42% tetrasodium pyrophosphate 2.16%
Crest Cool Mint	Procter & Gamble	sodium fluoride 0.243%	
Crest Extra Whitening	Procter & Gamble	sodium fluoride 0.243%	tetrapotassium pyrophosphate 5.05%
Crest for Kids Toothpaste	Procter & Gamble	sodium fluoride 0.243%	
Crest Icy Clean Toothpaste	Procter & Gamble	sodium fluoride 0.243%	

Product	Manufacturer	Fluoride	Other Active Ingredients
Crest Multicare Toothpaste	Procter & Gamble	sodium fluoride 0.243%	tetrapotassium pyrophosphate 5.05%
Crest Pro-Health	Procter & Gamble	stannous fluoride 0.454%	sodium hexametaphosphate 13%
Crest Pro-Health Whitening	Procter & Gamble	stannous fluoride 0.454%	sodium hexametaphosphate 13%
Crest Regular Toothpaste	Procter & Gamble	sodium fluoride 0.243%	
Crest Sensitivity Protection Toothpaste	Procter & Gamble	sodium fluoride 0.243%	potassium nitrate 5%
Crest Spiderman Liquid Gel	Procter & Gamble	sodium fluoride 0.243%	
Crest Tartar Protection	Procter & Gamble	sodium fluoride 0.243%	sodium acid pyrophosphate 2.1% tetrapotassium pyrophosphate 3.82% tetrasodium pyrophosphate 2.05%
Crest Vivid White	Procter & Gamble	sodium fluoride 0.243%	sodium hexametaphosphate 7.326%
Crest Vivid White Night	Procter & Gamble	sodium fluoride 0.243%	
Natural Anticavity Fluoride Toothpaste	Tom's of Maine	sodium monofluorophosphate 0.76%	
Natural Whole Care Fluoride Gel	Tom's of Maine	sodium flouride 0.11% zinc 0.31%	
Oral-B Stages Toothpaste	Procter & Gamble	sodium fluoride 0.243%	
Pearl Drops Triple Power Whitening	Church & Dwight	sodium fluoride 0.11%	
Plus White Xtra Whitening	Farleyco	sodium monofluorophosphate 0.9%	
PreviDent 5000 Plus	Colgate-Palmolive	sodium fluoride 1.1 %	
PreviDent Sensitive	Colgate-Palmolive	sodium fluoride 1.1 %	potassium nitrate 5%
Rembrandt Complete	Johnson & Johnson	sodium monofluorophosphate 0.88%	
Rembrandt Intense Stain	Johnson & Johnson	sodium monofluorophosphate 0.88%	
Rembrandt Plus	Johnson & Johnson	sodium monofluorophosphate 0.88%	
Sensodyne Original	GlaxoSmithKline Consumer Healthcare		strontium chloride 10%
Sensodyne Baking Soda Clean with Fluoride	GlaxoSmithKline Consumer Healthcare	sodium fluoride 0.243%	potassium nitrate 5%
Sensodyne-F iso-active	GlaxoSmithKline Consumer Healthcare	sodium fluoride 0.254%	potassium nitrate 5%
Sensodyne with Fluoride (Various Flavours)	GlaxoSmithKline Consumer Healthcare	sodium fluoride 0.243%	potassium nitrate 5%
Sensodyne Pronamel	GlaxoSmithKline Consumer Healthcare	sodium fluoride 0.254%	potassium nitrate 5%
Sensodyne Pronamel for Children	GlaxoSmithKline Consumer Healthcare	sodium fluoride 0.254%	
Sensodyne Whitening / Brilliant Whitening	GlaxoSmithKline Consumer Healthcare	sodium fluoride 0.243%	potassium nitrate 5%
TheraBreath Fresh Breath Toothpaste	Dr. Harold Katz	sodium fluoride 0.24%	
TheraBreath Oxygenating Toothpaste with Aloe Vera	Dr. Harold Katz	sodium fluoride 0.24%	
Topol Professional	Nicene Brands	sodium monofluorophosphate 0.83%	

Product	Manufacturer	Dosage Form	Fluoride	Other Active Ingredients
Fluor-A-Day 0.56 mg	Pendopharm	tablet, chewable	sodium fluoride 0.56 mg	
Fluor-A-Day 1.1 mg	Pendopharm	tablet, chewable	sodium fluoride 1.1 mg	
Fluor-A-Day 2.21 mg	Pendopharm	tablet, chewable	sodium fluoride 2.21 mg	
Fluor-A-Day Drops	Pendopharm	drops	sodium fluoride 5.56 mg/mL	
Listerine Platinum	Johnson & Johnson	rinse	sodium fluoride 0.22%	eucalyptus oil 0.092% thymol 0.064% menthol 0.042%
Neutragel Neutral Gel	Germiphene	gel	sodium fluoride 1.1%	
PreviDent 5000 Plus	Colgate Oral Pharmaceuticals	paste	sodium fluoride 1.1%	
PediaFluor	Euro-Pharm	liquid	sodium fluoride 5.56 mg/mL	
PediaVit Minimum Oral Solution	Euro-Pharm	liquid	potassium fluoride 0.25 mg/mL	ascorbic acid 30 mg/mL vitamin A 1500 IU/mL vitamin D 400 IU/mL
PediaVit Plus Oral Solution	Euro-Pharm	liquid	potassium fluoride 0.50 mg/mL	ascorbic acid 30 mg/mL vitamin A 1500 IU/mL vitamin D 400 IU/mL

Dental Products: Topical Analgesics for Teething

Product	Manufacturer	Dosage Form	Active Ingredients
Anbesol Baby Gel	Wyeth Consumer Healthcare	gel	benzocaine 7.5%
Anbesol Baby Grape Gel	Wyeth Consumer Healthcare	gel	benzocaine 7.5%
Baby Orajel	Church & Dwight	gel	benzocaine 7.5%
Baby Orajel Night time Cherry	Church & Dwight	gel	benzocaine 10%
Baby Orajel Teething Swabs	Church & Dwight	swab	benzocaine 7.5%

Product	Manufacturer	Dosage Form	Active Ingredients
Anbesol Gel	Wyeth Consumer Healthcare	gel	benzocaine 10%
Anbesol Extra Strength Gel	Wyeth Consumer Healthcare	gel	benzocaine 20%
Anbesol Extra Strength Liquid	Wyeth Consumer Healthcare	liquid	benzocaine 20% camphor 0.25% menthol 0.25% phenol 0.45%
Orajel Denture Plus	Church & Dwight	gel	benzocaine 15% menthol 2%
Orajel Maximum Strength	Church & Dwight	gel	benzocaine 20%
Orajel Maximum Strength Liquid	Church & Dwight	liquid	benzocaine 20%
Orajel Maximum Strength PM	Church & Dwight	paste	benzocaine 20%
Orajel Maximum Strength Swabs	Church & Dwight	swab	benzocaine 20%
Orajel Regular Strength	Church & Dwight	gel	benzocaine 10%

Product	Manufacturer	Test Strips	Time to Read Result	Calibration (Coding)	Dimensions (L xW x H)	Weight	Memory Capacity
Accu-Chek Aviva	Roche Diagnostics	Accu-Chek Aviva	5 sec.	Lot specific Program strip with each new vial of test strips	94 x 53 x 22 mm	60 g (with battery)	500 results with time and date, average, highest and lowest value for 7, 14 and 30 days
Accu-Chek Aviva Nano	Roche Diagnostics	Accu-Chek Aviva	5 sec.	Lot specific Program strip with each new vial of test strips	69 x 43 x 20 mm	40 g (with batteries)	500 results with time and date, average, highest and lowest value for 7, 14, 30 and 90 days
Accu-Chek Compact Plus	Roche Diagnostics	Accu-Chek Compact Test Strip Drum	5 sec.	Fully automatic calibration and safety checks	125 x 64 x 32 mm (with lancing device)	147 g (with batteries, lancing device and test strip drum)	500 results with time and date average, highest and lowest value for 7, 14 and 30 days
Accu-Chek Mobile	Roche Diagnostics	Accu-Chek Mobile	5 sec.	No coding	123 x 66 x 28 mm	150 g (with batteries, test cassette and lancet drum)	500 results with time and date average, highest and lowest value for 7, 14 and 30 days
Accu-Chek Voicemate Plus(to be used with Accu-Chek Compact Plus)	Roche Diagnostics				113 x 49 x 30 mm	130 g (with batteries)	5000 results
Accutrend GC	Roche Diagnostics	Accutrend Glucose	12 sec.	Lot specific Program strip with each new vial of test strips	150 x 62 x 19 mm	100 g	50 values with date and time
BG Star	sanofi-aventis	BG Star test strips	6 sec.	No coding	86 x 46 x 16 mm	48 g	1800 most recent results, average, high and low results for 7,14, 30 and 90 days
Bionime Rightest GM100	Bionime	Bionime GS100	8 sec.	No coding	95 x 44 x 13 mm	43 g	150 most recent results, average, high and low results for 7,14, 30 and 90 days
Breeze 2	Bayer Healthcare	Breeze 2 Strip Disc	5 sec.	No coding	104 x 63 x 25 mm	46 g	420 results
Contour	Bayer Healthcare	Contour	5 sec.	No coding	77 x 57 x 19 mm	47.5 g	480 most recent results, average, high and low results for 7 and 14 days
Contour Link	Bayer Healthcare	Contour	5 sec.	No coding	77 x 57 x 19 mm	47.5 g	480 most recent results, average, high and low results for 7 and 14 days

Size of Blood Sample	Warranty	Battery	Measurement Range	Computer Data Systems	Special Features	Lancing Device
0.6 µL	Lifetime warranty	1 x 3-volt lithium battery (CR 2032)	0.6-33.3 mmol/L	Data transferable to computer through wireless infrared data port or cable		Softclix
0.6 µL	Lifetime warranty	2 x 3-volt lithium batteries (CR 2032)	0.6-33.3 mmol/L	Data transferable to computer through wireless infrared data port or cable	Can add meal markers Post meal alarms and logbook results	Softclix
1.5 µL	Lifetime warranty	2 x AAA batteries	0.6-33.3 mmol/L	Data transferable to computer through wireless infrared data port	All-in-one system No strip handling Automatic calibration Discreet look	Softclix
0.3 µL	Lifetime warranty	Main Battery: 2 x AAA batteries. Back-up battery: 1 x 3-volt lithium (CR 1025)	0.6-33.3 mmol/L		Pre-loaded cassette of test strips	Fastclix Mobile
	Lifetime warranty	2 x AAA batteries		Data transferable to computer and to Accu-Chek Compact Plus meter through wireless infrared data port or cable	Talking system to be used with Accu-Chek Compact Plus Has electronic diary that can store results as well as comments about them	
	Lifetime warranty	2 x AAA batteries	1.1-33.3 mmol/L (20-600 mg/dL) glucose 3.88-7.75 mmol/L cholesterol		Measures also Blood Cholesterol levels with appropriate strips Back up visual blood glucose reading Measures whole blood only	Softclix
0.5 µ46 x 16 mmL	Lifetime warranty	2 x 3-volt lithium battery (CR 2032)	1.1-33.3 mmol/L	BG Star Diabetes Management Software		BG Star Ultra Thin
1.4 µL	Lifetime warranty	1 x 3-volt lithium battery (CR 2032)	1.1-33.3 mmol/L			Rightest Lancing Device
1 µL	Lifetime warranty	1 x 3-volt lithium battery (CR 2032)	0.6-33.3 mmol/L	Diabetes Management Software - Glucofacts Deluxe data transferable to computer through cable	No strip handling Available as a disc	Microlet Lancing Device
0.6 µL	Lifetime warranty	2 x 3-volt lithium batteries (CR 2032)	0.6-33.3 mmol/L	Diabetes Management Software - Glucofacts Deluxe	Can add meal markers, post meal alarms and logbook results	Microlet Lancing Device
0.6 µL	Lifetime warranty	2 x 3-volt lithium batteries (CR 2032)	0.6-33.3 mmol/L	Diabetes Management Software - Glucofacts Deluxe or Medtronic CareLink Therapy Management Software	Can connect wirelessly with Medtronic insulin pumps and can automatically calibrate Guardian REAL-time continuous glucose monitoring system once a reading has been done Can add meal markers, post meal alarms and logbook results	Microlet Lancing Device

Product	Manufacturer	Test Strips	Time to Read Result	Calibration (Coding)	Dimensions (L xW x H)	Weight	Memory Capacity
Contour USB	Bayer Healthcare	Contour	5 sec.	No coding	97 x 30 x 16 mm	43 g	2000 most recent results, also 500 MB flash-drive
Didget Kid's Glucometer	Bayer Healthcare	Contour	5 sec.	No coding	95 x 77 x 21 mm	76 g	480 most recent results
EZ Health Oracle Talking Meter	Tremblay Harrison	EZ Health Oracle	6 sec.	No coding	96 x 46 x 20 mm	70 g	450 results with date and time, average of 7, 14, 21, 30, 60 and 90 days
FreeStyle Freedom Lite	Abbott Diabetes Care	Freestyle	5 sec.	Lot specific Program strip with each new vial of test strips	83 x 55 x 16	44 g	400 results with date and time
FreeStyle InsuLinx	Abbott Diabetes Care	Freestyle	5 sec				
FreeStyle Lite	Abbott Diabetes Care	Freestyle	5 sec.	Lot specific Program strip with each new vial of test strips	74 x 40 x 17	40 g	400 results with date and time
iBG Star	sanofi-aventis	BG Star Test Strips	6 sec.	No coding	55 x 24 x 10 mm		300 results with time, date, average of 14, 30, 90 days
iTest	Auto Control Medical	iTest	4 sec.	Lot specific Program strip with each new vial of test strips	77 x 44 x 16 mm	44 g	300 results with time, date, average of 14, 30, 90 days
Nova Max	Nova Biomedical	NovaMax	5 sec.	No coding	91 x 58 x 23 mm	75 g	400 results
OneTouch Ultra 2	Lifescan	OneTouch Ultra	5 sec.	Lot specific Program strip with each new vial of test strips	79 x 57 x 23 mm	42.5 g (with batteries)	500 results
OneTouch Ultra Smart	Lifescan	One Touch Ultra	5 sec.	Lot specific Program strip with each new vial of test strips	94 x 58 x 21 mm	79 g (with battery)	3,000 results

Size of Blood Sample	Warranty	Battery	Measurement Range	Computer Data Systems	Special Features	Lancing Device
0.6 µL	5 years	Rechargeable battery from the wall or from computer USB port	1.1-33.3 mmol/L	Diabetes Management Software - Glucofacts Deluxe	Plug & Play technology with built-in Glucofacts Deluxe for instant access to patterns and trends 500 MB of memory available as a flash drive	Microlet Lancing Device
0.6 µL	Lifetime warranty	1 x 3-volt lithium battery (CR 2032) approx. 1000 tests)	1.1-33.3 mmol/L	Diabetes Management Software - Glucofacts Deluxe	Comes with games and plugs into a Nintendo DS or Nintendo DS Lite system Has two testing levels to grow with child's ability and testing routine	Microlet Lancing Device
0.6 µL	5 years	2 x AAA batteries	1.1-33.3 mmol/L	Data transferable to computer via USB cable (not included) Data can be viewed using Oracle DMS (diabetes management software)	Talking Function in either English or French; can be turned off Ketone Warning when result is above 13.3 mmol/L	Oracle Lancing Device
0.3 µL	Lifetime warranty	1 x 3-volt lithium battery (CR 2032) approx. 1000 tests	1.1-33.3 mmol/L	Data transferable to computer through cable Uses Co-Pilot Management system software		FreeStyle Lancing Device
				Uses FreeStyle Auto-Assist data management software	Plug & Play reports via FreeStyle Auto-Assist Software. Touchscreen	FreeStyle Lancing Device
0.3 µL	Lifetime warranty	1 x 3-volt lithium battery (CR 2032) approx. 500 tests	1.1-33.3 mmol/L	Data transferable to computer through cable Uses Co-Pilot Management system software		FreeStyle Lancing Device
0.5 µL	Lifetime warranty		1.1-33.3 mmol/L	BG Star Diabetes Management Software	Designed to be used with iPhone & iPod Touch Requires App to be downloaded	BG Star Ultra Thin
0.5 µL	Lifetime warranty	2 x 3-volt lithium batteries (CR 2032)	1.1-33.3 mmol/L			iTest Lancing Device
0.3 µL	Lifetime warranty		1.1-33.3 mmol/L			Nova Sureflex Lancing device
1 µL	Lifetime warranty	2 x 3-volt lithium batteries (CR 2032)	1.1-33.3 mmol/L	Data transferable to computer via USB cable Data can be viewed using OneTouch DMS (diabetes management software)	Can review past results and averages Can add meal flags or comments to a result Computer software can be used to store your results and to analyze patterns for planning meals, exercise and medication Puts information into charts and graphs	One Touch Lancing Device
1 µL	Lifetime warranty	2 x AAA batteries	1.1-33.3 mmol/L	Data transferable to computer via USB cable Data can be viewed using OneTouch DMS (diabetes management software)	Meter and electronic logbook Automatically captures and organizes results Entries displayed in 12 different charts and graphs at the push of a button Gives you the option to track exercise, health, medication and food to see patterns and trends	One Touch Lancing Device

Product	Manufacturer	Test Strips	Time to Read Result	Calibration (Coding)	Dimensions (L xW x H)	Weight	Memory Capacity
OneTouch UltraMini	Lifescan	One Touch Ultra	5 sec.	Lot specific Program strip with each new vial of test strips	108 x 32 x 17 mm	40 g	500 results
One Touch Verio IQ	Lifescan	One Touch Verio Gold	5 sec.	No coding	88 x 47 x 12 mm	47 g	750 most recent results
Precision Xtra	MediSense	Precision Xtra	5 sec.	By lot with calibrator in each box of strips	75 x 53 x 43 x 16	41.5 g (with battery)	450 values with date and time and 1, 2 and 4 week averaging
Sidekick	Home Diagnostics	Sidekick	10 sec.	No coding	36 x 13 mm	40 g (with strips)	50 results
TrueTrack	Home Diagnostics	True Track	5 sec.	Lot specific Program strip with each new vial of test strips	89 x 55 x 17 mm	47 g	365 results

Size of Blood Sample	Warranty	Battery	Measurement Range	Computer Data Systems	Special Features	Lancing Device
1 µL	Lifetime warranty	1 x 3-volt lithium battery (CR 2032)	1.1-33.3 mmol/L	Data transferable to computer via USB cable Data can be viewed using OneTouch DMS (diabetes management software)	Computer software can be used to store your results and to analyze patterns for planning meals, exercise and medication Puts information into charts and graphs	One Touch Lancing Device
0.4 µL	3 years	Rechargeable battery from the wall or from computer USB port	1.1-33.3 mmol/L	Data transferable to computer via USB cable Data can be viewed using OneTouch DMS (diabetes management software)		One Touch Delica
0.6 µL	4 years	1 x 3-volt lithium battery (CR 2032)	1.1-27.8 mmol/L	Data transferable to computer through cable Uses Co-Pilot Management system software	Ability to test blood ketones, strip to finger, finger to strip ease of application, top-fill or end-fill, fill trigger removes errors, strips waste & finger sticks	Precision Autolancet
1 µL	Lifetime warranty		1.1-33.3 mmol/L		All-in-one disposable blood glucose testing Meter built into the cap of bottle of test strips New monitor with every bottle of test strips Alternate site testing	Gentle Draw Lancing Device
1 µL	Lifetime warranty	1 x 3-volt lithium battery (CR 2032)	1.1-33.3 mmol/L	TrueTrack Diabetes Management Software Data transferable to computer via USB cable		Gentle Draw Lancing Device

Product	Manufacturer	Dosage Form	Active Ingredients	Comments
DEX-4	AMG Medical	tablet	glucose 4 g	Variety of flavours
DEX-4 Glucose Gel	AMG Medical	gel	dextrose 15 g	Incremental 5 g dosing with gel level indicator Re-sealable container
DEX-4 Liquiblast	AMG Medical	liquid	dextrose 15 g	Drinkable Liquid Variety of flavours
Insta-Glucose	Valeant	gel	glucose 30 g	

Type	Product	Manufacturer	Dosage Form	Source
Rapid-Acting	Humalog	Lilly	10 mL vial 3 mL cartridge 3 mL prefilled pen	lispro
	NovoRapid Penfill	Novo Nordisk	10 mL vial 3 mL cartridge	aspart
	Apidra	Sanofi Aventis	10 mL vial 3 mL cartridge	glulisine
	Apidra SoloSTAR	Sanofi Aventis	3 mL prefilled pen	glulisine
Regular	Humulin R	Lilly	10 mL vial 3 mL penfill cartridge	BHI[a]
	Novolin ge Toronto	Novo Nordisk	10 mL vial 3 mL penfill cartridge	BHI[a]
	Hypurin Regular	Wockhardt UK	10 mL vial	pork
Intermediate	Humulin N	Lilly	10 mL vial 3 mL penfill cartridge	BHI[a]
	Novolin ge NPH	Novo Nordisk	10 mL vial 3 mL penfill cartridge	BHI[a]
	Hypurin NPH Isophane	Wockhardt UK	10 mL vial	pork
Long-Acting	Levemir	Novo Nordisk	10 mL vial	detemir
	Lantus	Sanofi Aventis	10 mL vial 3 mL penfill cartridge	glargine
	Lantus SoloSTAR	Sanofi Aventis	3 mL prefilled pen	glargine
Mixtures	Humalog Mix25 (25% lispro/75% lispro protamine)	Lilly	3 mL cartridge 3 mL prefilled pen	lispro
	Humalog Mix50 (50% lispro/50% lispro protamine)	Lilly	3 mL cartridge	lispro
	Humulin 30/70 (30% reg/70% NPH)	Lilly	10 mL vial 3 mL cartridge	BHI[a]
	Novolin ge 30/70 (30% reg/70% NPH)	Novo Nordisk	10 mL vial 3 mL cartridge	BHI[a]
	Novolin ge 40/60 (40% reg/60% NPH)	Novo Nordisk	3 mL cartridge	BHI[a]
	Novolin ge 50/50 (50% reg/50% NPH)	Novo Nordisk	3 mL cartridge	BHI[a]
	NovoMix 30 (30% aspart/70% aspart protamine)	Novo Nordisk	3 mL cartridge	aspart

Abbreviations:
[a] BHI: biosynthetic human insulin (rDNA-recombinant DNA technology)

Product	Manufacturer	Insulin	Needle
Apidra SoloSTAR	sanofi-aventis	Apidra Pre-filled pen injector	Most needles
Autopen 24	Owen Mumford	Lantus 3 mL cartridges	Most needles
Blue ClickSTAR	sanofi-aventis	Apidra Pre-filled pen injector	Most needles
ClickSTAR	sanofi-aventis	Lantus 3 mL cartridges	Most needles
Humalog KwikPen	Lilly	Humalog 3 mL cartridges Humalog Mix25 3 mL cartridges Humalog Mix50 3 mL cartridges	Most needles
HumaPen Luxura	Lilly	Humalog 3 mL cartridges Humulin 3 mL cartridges	B-D Ultra-Fine III 29G (12 mm) B-D Ultra-Fine III 31 G (5 mm, 8 mm)
HumaPen Memoir (Digital Pen with Memory Feature)	Becton-Dickinson	Humalog 3 mL cartridges Humulin 3 mL cartridges	B-D Ultra-Fine III 29G (12 mm) B-D Ultra-Fine III 31 G (5 mm, 8 mm)
Lantus SoloSTAR	sanofi-aventis	Lantus Pre-filled pen injector	Most needles
Novolin-Pen 4	Novo Nordisk	Novolin ge Penfill 3 mL cartridges NovoRapid 3 mL cartridges Levemir 3 mL cartridges	NovoFine 28G (12 mm) NovoFine 30G (6 mm, 8 mm) NovoFine 32G (6 mm) ETW
Novolin-Pen Junior	Novo Nordisk	Novolin ge Penfill 3 mL cartridges NovoRapid 3 mL cartridges Levemir 3 mL cartridges	NovoFine 32G (6 mm) ETW

Test	Product	Manufacturer	Also detects:
Glucose	Diastix	Bayer Healthcare	
Glucose	Chemstrip GP	Roche Diagnostics	protein
Glucose	Chemstrip 5	Roche Diagnostics	protein blood nitrite leukocytes
Glucose and Ketones	Chemstrip uG/K	Roche Diagnostics	
Glucose and Ketones	Keto-Diastix	Bayer Healthcare	
Glucose and Ketones	Chemstrip 7	Roche Diagnostics	protein blood nitrite leukocytes pH
Glucose and Ketones	Chemstrip 9	Roche Diagnostics	protein blood nitrite leukocytes pH urobilinogen bilirubin
Glucose and Ketones	Chemstrip 10	Roche Diagnostics	protein blood nitrite leukocytes pH urobilinogen bilirubin specific gravity
Ketones	Acetest Tablets	Bayer Healthcare	
Ketones	Ketostix	Bayer Healthcare	

Product	Manufacturer	Dosage Form	Size	Active Ingredients
CanesOral	Bayer Consumer	oral tablet	1 oral tablet	fluconazole 150 mg
CanesOral Combi-Pak	Bayer Consumer	oral tablet/cream	1 oral tablet/10 g cream	fluconazole 150 mg (oral tablet) clotrimazole 1% (cream)
Canesten 1 Cream	Bayer Consumer	cream	1 prefilled vaginal applicator	clotrimazole 10%
Canesten 1 Cream Combi-Pak	Bayer Consumer	cream/cream	1 prefilled vaginal applicator/ 10 g cream	clotrimazole 10% (vaginal cream) clotrimazole 1% (vulvar cream)
Canesten 1 Insert Combi-Pak	Bayer Consumer	tablet/cream	1 vaginal tablet/10 g cream	clotrimazole 500 mg (vaginal tablet) clotrimazole 1% (cream)
Canesten 3 Cream	Bayer Consumer	cream	25 g tube with 3 applicators	clotrimazole 2%
Canesten 3 Insert Combi-Pak	Bayer Consumer	tablet/cream	3 vaginal tablets/10 g cream	clotrimazole 200 mg (vaginal tablet) clotrimazole 1% (cream)
Canesten 6 Cream	Bayer Consumer	cream	50 g tube with 6 applicators	clotrimazole 1%
Clotrimaderm Vaginal Cream 1%	Taro	cream	50 g tube with 6 applicators	clotrimazole 1%
Clotrimaderm Vaginal Cream 2%	Taro	cream	25 g with 3 applicators	clotrimazole 2%
Clotrimazole Vaginal Cream 1%	Various Manufacturers	cream	50 g tube with 6 applicators	clotrimazole 1%
Clotrimazole Vaginal Cream 2%	Various Manufacturers	cream	25 g with 3 applicators	clotrimazole 2%
Clotrimazole Vaginal Cream	Various Manufacturers	cream	various	clotrimazole 2%
Diflucan One	Pfizer	oral tablet	1 oral tablet	fluconazole 150 mg
Fluconazole 150 mg	Various Manufacturers	oral tablet	1 oral tablet	fluconazole 150 mg
Miconazole Vaginal Cream	Taro	cream	45 g	miconazole nitrate 2%
Monistat 1 Combination Pack	McNeil Consumer Healthcare	ovule/cream	1 ovule/9 g cream	miconazole nitrate 1200 mg (ovule) miconazole nitrate 2% (cream)
Monistat 1 Vaginal Ovule	McNeil Consumer Healthcare	ovule	1 ovule	miconazole nitrate 1200 mg
Monistat 3 Dual-Pak	McNeil Consumer Healthcare	ovules/cream	3 ovules/9 g cream	miconazole nitrate 400 mg (ovule) miconazole nitrate 2% (cream)
Monistat 3 Vaginal Cream	McNeil Consumer Healthcare	cream	3 prefilled applicators	miconazole nitrate 4%
Monistat 3 Vaginal Ovules	McNeil Consumer Healthcare	ovule	3 ovules	miconazole nitrate 400 mg
Monistat 7 Cream	McNeil Consumer Healthcare	cream	7 prefilled applicators	miconazole nitrate 2%
Monistat 7 Dual-Pak	McNeil Consumer Healthcare	suppository/cream	7 vaginal suppositories/9 g cream	miconazole nitrate 100 mg (suppository) miconazole nitrate 2% (cream)
Nystatin Cream	Various Manufacturers	cream		nystatin 100,000 units/g
PS Miconazole 3 Days Ovules +Cream	Pendopharm	ovules/cream	3 ovules/9 g cream	miconazole nitrate 400 mg (ovule) miconazole nitrate 2% (cream)
ratio-Nystatin cream	Teva	cream	75 g	nystatin 100,000 units/g

Product	Manufacturer	Dosage Form	Active Ingredients
Advil Caplets	Pfizer Consumer Healthcare	caplet	ibuprofen 200 mg
Advil Extra Strength Caplets	Pfizer Consumer Healthcare	caplet	ibuprofen 400 mg
Advil Gel Caplet	Pfizer Consumer Healthcare	gelatin caplet	ibuprofen 200 mg
Advil Liqui-Gels	Pfizer Consumer Healthcare	capsule	ibuprofen 200 mg
Advil Liqui-Gels Extra Strength	Pfizer Consumer Healthcare	capsule	ibuprofen 400 mg
Advil Tablets	Pfizer Consumer Healthcare	tablet	ibuprofen 200 mg
Aleve Caplets	Bayer Consumer	caplet	naproxen sodium 220 mg
Aleve Liqui-Gels	Bayer Consumer	capsule	naproxen sodium 220 mg
Aleve Tablets	Bayer Consumer	tablet	naproxen sodium 220 mg
Ibuprofen Caplets 200 mg	Various Manufacturers	caplet	ibuprofen 200 mg
Ibuprofen Caplets 400 mg	Various Manufacturers	caplet	ibuprofen 400 mg
Ibuprofen Tablets 200 mg	Various Manufacturers	tablet	ibuprofen 200 mg
Ibuprofen Tablets 400 mg	Various Manufacturers	tablet	ibuprofen 400 mg
Maxidol Liquid Gels	Bayer Consumer	capsule	naproxen sodium 220 mg
Midol Extra Strength Caplets	Bayer Consumer	caplet	acetaminophen 500 mg caffeine 60 mg pyrilamine maleate 15 mg
Midol PMS Extra Strength	Bayer Consumer	caplet	acetaminophen 500 mg pamabrom 25 mg pyrilamine maleate 15 mg
Midol Teen Complete	Bayer Consumer	caplet	acetaminophen 325 mg caffeine 60 mg pyrilamine maleate 15 mg
Motrin IB Caplets	McNeil Consumer Healthcare	caplet	ibuprofen 200 mg
Motrin IB Extra Strength	McNeil Consumer Healthcare	tablet	ibuprofen 300 mg
Motrin IB Liquid Gels	McNeil Consumer Healthcare	gelcap	ibuprofen 200 mg
Motrin IB Super Strength	McNeil Consumer Healthcare	tablet	ibuprofen 400 mg
Motrin IB Tablets	McNeil Consumer Healthcare	tablet	ibuprofen 200 mg
Pamprin Extra Strength Caplets	Chattem	caplet	acetaminophen 500 mg pamabrom 25 mg pyrilamine maleate 15 mg
Pamprin PMS	Chattem	caplet	acetaminophen 500 mg pamabrom 25 mg pyrilamine maleate 15 mg
Relievol PMS Extra Strength	Tanta	tablet	acetaminophen 500 mg pamabrom 25 mg pyrilamine maleate 15 mg
Tylenol Menstrual Extra Strength	McNeil Consumer Healthcare	tablet	acetaminophen 500 mg pamabrom 25 mg pyrilamine maleate 15 mg

Product	Manufacturer	Dosage Form	Active Ingredients
Massengil	GlaxoSmithKline	liquid	vinegar water
Fermalac Vaginal	Rougier	capsule, vaginal	lactobacillus bulgaricus lactobacillus rhamnosus streptococcus thermophilus
Summer's Eve Cleansing Cloths (16)	CB Fleet	wipe	aloe barbadensis water
Summer's Eve Cleansing Cloths (32)	CB Fleet	wipe	aloe barbadensis lanolin water
Summer's Eve Douche	CB Fleet	liquid	vinegar water
Summer's Eve Feminine Deodorant Spray	CB Fleet	spray	corn starch isopropyl myristate mineral oil sodium bicarbonate tocopherol
Tucks Feminine Cleansing Wipes	Pfizer Consumer Healthcare	pad	hamamelis water 50% glycerin 10%
Vagisil	Combe	cream	benzocaine 5% resorcinol 2%
Vagisil Extra Strength	Combe	cream	benzocaine 20% resorcinol 3%
Vagisil Wipes	Combe	wipe	hamamelis water

Product	Manufacturer	Dosage Form	Ingredients
Astroglide	Biofilm	gel	water soluble lubricant
ContraGel Green	DeltaMed GmbH	gel	lactic acid (milk acid) methylcellulose sodium lactate sorbic acid water
Durex Play Lubricants	Durex Canada	gel	water soluble lubricant
Gyne-Moistrin	Schering-Plough	gel	polyglyceryl methacrylate propylene glycol
K-Y Jelly Personal Lubricant	Johnson & Johnson	gel	water soluble lubricant
K-Y Liquibeads	Johnson & Johnson	ovule	water soluble lubricant
K-Y Silk E Vaginal Moisturizer	Johnson & Johnson	liquid	vitamin E water soluble lubricant
K-Y Yours and Mine Couple Lubricant	Johnson & Johnson	gel	aloe vitamin E water soluble lubricant
Muko Lubricating Jelly	Source Medical	gel	water soluble lubricant
O'My Natural Lubricant	O'My Products	gel	water soluble lubricant
Pre-seed	INGfertility	gel	arabinogalactan carbomer hydroxyethylcellulose sodium chloride sodium hydroxide sodium phosphate methylparaben pluronic potassium phosphate water
Replens Moisturizer	WellSpring	gel	polycarbophil water
Splash Lubricant	Medisca	gel	hyaluronic acid
Taro Lubricating Gel	Taro	jelly	carbomer glycerin propylene glycol sodium hydroxide
Zestica	Burdica	gel	hyaluronic acid

Product	Manufacturer	Dosage Form	Active Ingredients
Canesten Topical	Bayer Consumer	cream	clotrimazole 1%
Clotrimazole Cream	Various Manufacturers	cream	clotrimazole 1%
Dr. Scholl's Athlete's Foot Powder	Schering-Plough	powder	tolnaftate 1%
Dr. Scholl's Athlete's Foot Spray Powder	Schering-Plough	aerosol	tolnaftate 1%
Flexitol Antifungal Liquid	LaCorium	liquid	undecylenic acid 25%
Footworks Antifungal Foot Spray	Avon	liquid	tolnaftate 1%
Fungicure Gel	Alva-Amco Pharmacal	gel	tolnaftate 1%
Fungicure Liquid	Alva-Amco Pharmacal	liquid	undecylenic acid 10%
Fungicure Professional Formula	Alva-Amco Pharmacal	liquid	undecylenic acid 12.5%
Micatin Cream	Wellspring Pharmaceutical	cream	miconazole nitrate 2%
Micatin Spray	Wellspring Pharmaceutical	aerosol	miconazole nitrate 2%
Odor-Eaters Athlete's Foot & Sneaker Spray Powder	Combe	aerosol	tolnaftate 1%
Proclearz Antifungal Liquid	Profoot	liquid	tolnaftate 1%
Tinactin Aerosol Powder	Schering-Plough	aerosol	tolnaftate 1%
Tinactin Cream	Schering-Plough	cream	tolnaftate 1%
Tinactin Powder	Schering-Plough	powder	tolnaftate 1%
Tinactin Pump Spray	Schering-Plough	spray	tolnaftate 1%
Thursday Plantation Anti-fungal Gel	Abundace Naturally	gel	tea tree oil 5%

Product	Manufacturer	Dosage Form	Active Ingredients
Canthacur	Paladin	liquid	cantharidin 0.7%
Canthacur-PS	Paladin	liquid	cantharidin 1% podophyllin 5% salicylic acid 30%
Cantharone	Dormer	liquid	cantharidin 0.7%
Cantharone Plus	Dormer	liquid	cantharidin 1% podophyllin 2% salicylic acid 30%
Compound W Dual Power Pads	Medtech	pad	salicylic acid 40%
Compound W Freeze Off Wart Removal System	Medtech	liquid	cryotherapy mixture: dimethyl ether and propane (DMEP)
Compound W Gel	Medtech	gel	salicylic acid 17%
Compound W Liquid	Medtech	liquid	salicylic acid 20%
Compound W One Step Pads	Medtech	pad	salicylic acid 40%
Compound W Pads for Kids	Medtech	pad	salicylic acid 40%
Compound W Plantar Pads	Medtech	pad	salicylic acid 40%
Compound W Plus	Medtech	liquid	salicylic acid 30%
Freezone Liquid	Medtech	liquid	salicylic acid 17.6%
Freezone One Step Corn & Callus Remover	Medtech	pad	salicylic acid 40%
Scholl 2-Drop Corn & Callus Remedy	Schering-Plough	liquid	salicylic acid 17%
Scholl Clear Away Liquid Wart Remover	Schering-Plough	liquid	salicylic acid 17%
Scholl Clear Away One Step Wart Remover	Schering-Plough	gel	salicylic acid 17%
Scholl Clear Away Plantar Wart Remover	Schering-Plough	plaster	salicylic acid 40%
Scholl Clear Away Wart Remover	Schering-Plough	plaster	salicylic acid 40%
Scholl Freeze Away	Schering-Plough	liquid	cryotherapy mixture: dimethyl ether and propane (DMEP)
Scholl Freeze Away Dual Action	Schering-Plough	liquid	cryotherapy mixture: dimethyl ether and propane (DMEP)
Scholl One Step Callus Remover	Schering-Plough	plaster	salicylic acid 40%
Scholl One Step Corn Remover	Schering-Plough	plaster	salicylic acid 40%
Scholl One Step Plantar Wart Remover	Schering-Plough	pad	salicylic acid 40%
Scholl One Step Wart Remover	Schering-Plough	plaster	salicylic acid 40%
Scholl Ultra Thin Corn Removers	Schering-Plough	plaster	salicylic acid 40%
Scholl Zino Callus Remover	Schering-Plough	plaster	salicylic acid 40%
Scholl Zino Corn Remover	Schering-Plough	plaster	salicylic acid 40%
Soluver	Dermtek	liquid	salicylic acid 20%
Soluver Plus	Dermtek	liquid	salicylic acid 27%
Wart Removal Gel	Various Manufacturers	liquid	salicylic acid 17%
Wart Remover	Various Manufacturers	liquid	cryotherapy mixture: dimethyl ether and propane (DMEP)
WartFreeze Hands & Feet	Aurium	liquid	cryotherapy mixture: dimethyl ether and propane (DMEP)
Wartner for Kids	Aurium	liquid	cryotherapy mixture: dimethyl ether and propane (DMEP)
Wartner Original	Aurium	liquid	cryotherapy mixture: dimethyl ether and propane (DMEP)
Wartner Plantar Warts	Aurium	liquid	cryotherapy mixture: dimethyl ether and propane (DMEP)

Product	Manufacturer	Dosage Form	Comments
Dr. Scholl's Foot Deodorant Pump Spray	Schering-Plough	spray pump	
Dr. Scholl's Foot Powder Spray	Schering-Plough	aerosol	
Dr. Scholl's Odor Destroyers Shoe Powder with Zinoxol	Schering-Plough	powder	
Dr. Scholl's Odor Destroyers with Zinoxol Deodorant Foot Powder/Spray	Schering-Plough	powder/spray	
Dr. Scholl's Odor Destroyers All Day Powder	Schering-Plough	powder	Contains cornstarch
Dr. Scholl's Sneaker Treater Deodorizer	Schering-Plough	aerosol	
Gold Bond Extra Strength Foot Powder	Chattem	powder	Contains menthol
Gold Bond Foot Powder	Chattem	powder	Contains menthol
Johnson's Foot Soap	Combe	bar	
Odor Eaters Foot Powder	Combe	powder	Contains baking soda
Odor Eaters Foot Spray	Combe	spray pump	
PediFresh Gel	Aurium Pharma	gel	
PediFresh Spray	Aurium Pharma	spray pump	

Product	Manufacturer	Size (shoe size)	Form	Comments
Airplus Coolmax EveryDay Insoles	Implus	women 6-11 men 7-12	insole	Breathable insoles
Airplus Gel Ball-of-Foot Cushion	Implus	women 6-11	insert	
Airplus Gel Cushion	Implus	men 7-12	insole	Foam insole with gel insert in heel
Airplus Gel Heel Cup	Implus	women 6-11	insert	
Airplus Gel Heel Savers	Implus	women 6-11	insert	
Airplus Gel Cell Insole	Implus	women 6-11 men 7-12	insole	Made up of over 100 cushion cells
Airplus Gellies Gel Insole	Implus		insole	Made up of over 100 cushion cells
Airplus Hug my Heels Gel Cushion	Implus	women 6-11	insert	
Airplus My Arch	Implus	women 6-11 men 7-12		
Airplus Save My Soles Gel	Implus	women 6-11	insole	
Airplus Sport & Work Gel Insoles	Implus	men 7-12	insole	
Airplus Steppies Gel Insert	Implus	women 6-11	insert	
Airplus Ultra Arch Gel Insoles	Implus	women 6-11	insole	
Dr. Scholl's Active Series Insoles	Schering-Plough	women 5 ½ -11 men 7 ½ -13	insole	Designed for Athletes Reinforced Arch Designed to help prevent pain from shin splints, runner's knee and plantar fasciitis
Dr. Scholl's Air Pillo Insoles	Schering-Plough	women 5-10 men 7-13	insole	
Dr. Scholl's Air Pillo Ultra Insoles	Schering-Plough	women 6-10 men 8-12	insole	
Dr. Scholl's Diabetes Foot Health Insoles	Schering-Plough	women 6-10 men 8-12	insole	
Dr. Scholl's for Her Heel Gel Cushions	Schering-Plough	women 1 size	insert	
Dr. Scholl's for Her Hidden Arch Support	Schering-Plough	women 1 size	insert	
Dr. Scholl's for Her High Heel Insoles	Schering-Plough	women 6-10	insert	
Dr. Scholl's for Her Open Shoe Insoles	Schering-Plough	women 6-10	insert	
Dr. Scholl's Gel Ball of Foot Cushion	Schering-Plough	1 size	insert	Contains soft polymer gel
Dr. Scholl's Heel Liners	Schering-Plough	women 1 size	insert	Helps prevent heels from slipping and rubbing
Dr. Scholl's Heel Spur	Schering-Plough	women 1 size men 1 size	insert	
Dr. Scholl's Knee Pain Relief	Schering-Plough	women 6-10 men 8-12	insole	
Dr. Scholl's Massaging Gel Arch Support	Schering-Plough	women 6-10 men 8-12	insert	
Dr. Scholl's Massaging Gel Ball of Foot Cushion	Schering-Plough	1 size	insert	
Dr. Scholl's Massaging Gel -Dual Gel Insoles	Schering-Plough	women 6-10 men 8-12	insole	Dual Gel design to provide cushion and absorb shock
Dr. Scholl's Massaging Gel Heel Cup	Schering-Plough	1 size	insert	Lightweight, gel construction
Dr. Scholl's Massaging Gel Heel Cushion	Schering-Plough	1 size	insert	
Dr. Scholl's Massaging Gel Slimsole Insoles	Schering-Plough	men 8-13	insert	Ideal for men's dress shoes

▶

Product	Manufacturer	Size (shoe size)	Form	Comments
Dr. Scholl's Massaging Gel Sport Replacement Insoles	Schering-Plough	women 6-10 men 8-12	insole	Ideal for sport shoes
Dr. Scholl's Memory Fit Plus Insoles	Schering-Plough	women 1 size men 1 size	insole	
Dr. Scholl's Memory Fit Work Insoles	Schering-Plough	men 1 size	insole	
Dr. Scholl's Tri Comfort Insert	Schering-Plough	women 6-10 men 8-12	insert	
Dr.Scholl's Sheep Wool Fleece Winter Insoles	Schering-Plough	1 size	insert	
ProFoot 2 oz. Miracle Custom Molding	ProFoot	women 6-10 men 8-13	insole	Memory foam that molds to foot and arch
ProFoot Aero-3 Insoles	ProFoot	women 6-10 men 8-13	insole	Air-cell cushioning, memory foam
ProFoot Bottom of the Foot Cushion	ProFoot	1 size	insert	Helps relieve knee, leg and back pain
ProFoot Gel Toe Bed	ProFoot	1 size	insert	Cradles toes Cushions ball of foot to prevent fatigue and callus formation
ProFoot Smart Arch Support	ProFoot	women 1 size men 1 size	insert	Good for supporting high or low arches
ProFoot Super Sport Arch Support	ProFoot	women 1 size men 1 size	insert	Supports for heel and arch
ProFoot Triad Orthotic Insoles	ProFoot	women 1 size men 1 size	insole	Designed to relieve knee, leg and back pain
ProFoot Ultra Gel Energizing Insoles	ProFoot	men 8-13	insole	2 Layers of gel

Condition	Product	Manufacturer	Form	Comments
Blisters	Dr. Scholl's Blister Treatment	Schering-Plough	cushion	Water-resistant Can be used on open blisters
Blisters	Dr. Scholl's Moleskin Cushion	Schering-Plough	sheet	Soft latex foam Beige
Blisters	Dr. Scholl's Moleskin Kurotex	Schering-Plough	sheet, roll	Cut to size required 100% cotton flannel backed by self-stick
Blisters	Profoot Velvetex Moleskin	Profoot	sheets	Latex-free Breathable material
Bunions	Dr. Scholl's Bunion Cushions-Foam Ease	Schering-Plough	cushion	Ring of foam Self-stick Waterproof adhesive
Bunions	Dr. Scholl's Bunion Felt Cushions	Schering-Plough	cushion	Made of felt
Calluses	Profoot Velvetex Callus Cushions	Profoot	cushion	Latex-free Breathable material
Calluses	Dr. Scholl's Callus Cushions	Schering-Plough	cushion	Waterproof adhesive
Corns	Profoot Velvetex Corn Cushions	Profoot	cushion	Latex-free Breathable material
Corns	Profoot Vita-Gel Corn Wraps	Profoot	wraps	Full wrap around toes
Corns	Dr. Scholl's Corn Cushions	Schering-Plough	cushion	Waterproof adhesive
Toe Bandages	Profoot Toe Bandages	Profoot	bandages	Trim to fit Wraps toe Protects and soothes toes Can be used instead of corn cushions
Toe Beds	Profoot Gel Toe Beds	Profoot	cushion	Cushions ball-of-foot Prevents corns and calluses Promotes proper toe placement
Toe Protector	Profoot Vita-Gel Toe Protector	Profoot	cap	Covers entire toe Gel cap contains mineral oil Relieves corns, hammer toes and toe tips
Toe Relief	Profoot Vita-Gel Toe Relief Pad	Profoot	cushion	Corrects hammer and bent toes Relieves pressure and friction which causes corn and soreness
Toe Spacer	Profoot Vita-Gel Toe Spacer	Profoot	spacers	Separates and cushions toes Relieves pressure on bunion joint Straightens problem toes

Product	Manufacturer	Dosage Form	Aluminum	Magnesium	Calcium	Other Antacids	Histamine H2-Receptor Antagonist	Other Active Ingredients
Alka-Seltzer	Bayer Consumer	tablet, effervescent				sodium bicarbonate 1916 mg		acetylsalicylic acid 325 mg citric acid 1000 mg
Alka-Seltzer Flavored	Bayer Consumer	tablet, effervescent				sodium bicarbonate 1700 mg		acetylsalicylic acid 325 mg citric acid 1000 mg
Almagel 200	Atlas	suspension	aluminum hydroxide 40 mg/mL	magnesium hydroxide 40 mg/mL				
Almagel Plus	Atlas	suspension	aluminum hydroxide 40 mg/mL	magnesium hydroxide 40 mg/mL				simethicone 5 mg/mL
Alugel	Atlas	liquid	aluminum hydroxide 60 mg/mL					
Amphojel Suspension	Axcan	liquid	aluminum hydroxide 64 mg/mL					
Amphojel Tablets	Axcan	tablet	aluminum hydroxide 600 mg					
Antacid Plus Antiflatulent	Various Manufacturers	suspension	aluminum hydroxide 40 mg/mL	magnesium hydroxide 40 mg/mL				simethicone 5 mg/mL
Antacid Suspension	Various Manufacturers	suspension	aluminum hydroxide 40 mg/mL	magnesium hydroxide 40 mg/mL				
Antacid Tablet	Swiss Herbal	tablet		magnesium hydroxide 172.2 mg	calcium carbonate 327.8 mg			
Axia3 ProDigestive Antacid	Axia Canada	tablet			calcium carbonate 145 mg	sodium bicarbonate 50 mg		
Beano Tablets	GlaxoSmithKline Consumer Healthcare	tablet						alpha-D-galactosidase 150 GalU (galactose units)
Bismuth Subsalicylate Suspension	Various Manufacturers	suspension						bismuth subsalicylate 17.6 mg/mL
Bismuth Subsalicylate Extra Strength Suspension	Various Manufacturers	suspension						bismuth subsalicylate 35.2 mg/mL
Bismuth Subsalicylate Tablets	Various Manufacturers	tablet						bismuth subsalicylate 262 mg
Diovol Caplets	Church & Dwight	caplet	dried aluminum hydroxide gel 165 mg	magnesium hydroxide 200 mg				
Diovol Extra Strength Suspension	Church & Dwight	suspension	aluminum hydroxide gel 120 mg/mL	magnesium hydroxide 60 mg/mL				

Product	Manufacturer	Dosage Form	Aluminum	Magnesium	Calcium	Other Antacids	Histamine H2-Receptor Antagonist	Other Active Ingredients
Diovol Plus AF Suspension	Church & Dwight	suspension		magnesium hydroxide 40 mg/mL	calcium carbonate 40 mg/mL			simethicone 5 mg/mL
Diovol Plus AF Tablets	Church & Dwight	tablet		magnesium hydroxide 200 mg	calcium carbonate 200 mg			simethicone 25 mg
Diovol Plus Suspension	Church & Dwight	suspension	aluminum hydroxide gel 33 mg/mL	magnesium hydroxide 40 mg/mL				simethicone 5 mg/mL
Diovol Plus Tablets	Church & Dwight	tablet		magnesium hydroxide 100 mg		aluminum hydroxide/ magnesium carbonate co-dried gel 300 mg		simethicone 25 mg
Diovol Suspension	Church & Dwight	liquid	dried aluminum hydroxide gel 40 mg/mL	magnesium hydroxide 40 mg/mL				
ENO	GlaxoSmithKline Consumer Healthcare	powder						sodium citrate 536 mg/g
Famotidine Tablets	Various Manufacturers	tablet					famotidine 10 mg	
Famotidine Tablets	Various Manufacturers	tablet					famotidine 20 mg	
Gastrifom	Tanta	tablet	aluminum hydroxide 80 mg					alginic acid 200 mg
Gas-X	Novartis Consumer Health	tablet						simethicone 80 mg
Gas-X Extra Strength	Novartis Consumer Health	tablet						simethicone 125 mg
Gas-X Thin Strips	Novartis Consumer Health	lozenge						simethicone 62.5 mg
Gas-X Ultra Strength	Novartis Consumer Health	capsule						simethicone 180 mg
Gaviscon Heartburn Relief Extra Strength Chewable	GlaxoSmithKline Consumer Healthcare	tablet, chewable		magnesium carbonate 40 mg				alginic acid 200 mg
Gaviscon Heartburn & Acid Reflux Relief Tablets	GlaxoSmithKline Consumer Healthcare	tablet		magnesium carbonate 40 mg				alginic acid 200 mg
Gaviscon Heartburn & Acid Reflux Relief Extra Strength	GlaxoSmithKline Consumer Healthcare	tablet		magnesium carbonate 63 mg				alginic acid 313 mg

Product	Manufacturer	Dosage Form	Aluminum	Magnesium	Calcium	Other Antacids	Histamine H2-Receptor Antagonist	Other Active Ingredients
Gaviscon Liquid	GlaxoSmithKline Consumer Healthcare	liquid	aluminum hydroxide 20 mg/mL					sodium alginate 50 mg/mL
Gaviscon MaxRelief Heartburn & Acid Reflux Relief	GlaxoSmithKline Consumer Healthcare	tablet		magnesium carbonate 72 mg				alginic acid 360 mg
Gaz Away	Swiss Herbal	tablet						alpha-D-galactosidase 150 GalU
Gelusil Tablets	Pfizer Consumer Healthcare	tablet	aluminum hydroxide 200 mg	magnesium hydroxide 200 mg				
Little Tummys Gas Relief Drops	Prestige Brands	liquid						simethicone 66 mg/mL
Maalox Antacid Extra Strength with Anti-Gas	Novartis Consumer Health	suspension	aluminum hydroxide 80 mg/mL	magnesium hydroxide 80 mg/mL				simethicone 8 mg/mL
Maalox Anti-Gas Suspension	Novartis Consumer Health	suspension	aluminum hydroxide 40 mg/mL	magnesium hydroxide 40 mg/mL				simethicone 4 mg/mL
Maalox Multi Action	Novartis Consumer Health	suspension						bismuth subsalicylate 35 mg/mL
Maalox Nighttime Suspension	Novartis Consumer Health	suspension		magnesium carbonate 25 mg/mL	calcium carbonate 60 mg/mL			sodium alginate 55 mg/mL
Maalox Nighttime Tablets	Novartis Consumer Health	tablet			calcium carbonate 500 mg			alginic acid 200 mg
Maalox Quick Dissolve	Novartis Consumer Health	tablet, chewable			calcium carbonate 600 mg			
Maalox Quick Dissolve Anti-Gas Extra Strength	Novartis Consumer Health	tablet, chewable			calcium carbonate 1000 mg			simethicone 60 mg
Maalox Quick Dissolve Extra Strength	Novartis Consumer Health	tablet, chewable			calcium carbonate 1000 mg			
Milk of Magnesia	Various Manufacturers	liquid		magnesium hydroxide 70 to 88 mg/mL				
Mucaine - Sus	Aurium	suspension	aluminum hydroxide 60 mg/mL	magnesium hydroxide 20 mg/mL				oxetacaine 2 mg/mL
Neutra Seltzer	Teva Canada	tablet, effervescent				sodium bicarbonate 1916 mg		acetylsalicylic acid 325 mg citric acid 1000 mg
Ovol Drops	Church & Dwight	liquid						simethicone 40 mg/mL
Ovol Ultra Strength	Church & Dwight	tablet						simethicone 180 mg
Ovol Ultra Strength Softgels	Church & Dwight	capsule						simethicone 180 mg

Product	Manufacturer	Dosage Form	Aluminum	Magnesium	Calcium	Other Antacids	Histamine H2-Receptor Antagonist	Other Active Ingredients
Ovol-80	Church & Dwight	tablet, chewable						simethicone 80 mg
Pediacol	Euro-Pharm	liquid						simethicone 40 mg/mL
Pepcid AC	Johnson & Johnson Merck	tablet					famotidine 10 mg	
Pepcid AC Maximum Strength	Johnson & Johnson Merck	tablet					famotidine 20 mg	
Pepcid Complete	Johnson & Johnson Merck	tablet, chewable		magnesium hydroxide 165 mg	calcium carbonate 800 mg		famotidine 10 mg	
Pepto-Bismol Caplets	Procter & Gamble	caplet						bismuth subsalicylate 262 mg
Pepto-Bismol Liquid	Procter & Gamble	liquid						bismuth subsalicylate 17.6 mg/mL
Pepto-Bismol Liquid Extra Strength	Procter & Gamble	liquid						bismuth subsalicylate 35.2 mg/mL
Pepto-Bismol Tablets	Procter & Gamble	tablet, chewable			calcium carbonate 350 mg			bismuth subsalicylate 262 mg
Phazyme-125	GlaxoSmithKline Consumer Healthcare	softgel						simethicone 125 mg
Phazyme-180 Softgels	GlaxoSmithKline Consumer Healthcare	capsule						simethicone 180 mg
Phillips' Milk of Magnesia Liquid Plain/Cherry/Mint	Bayer Consumer	liquid		magnesium hydroxide 80 mg/mL				
Phillips' Milk of Magnesia Tablets	Bayer Consumer	tablet		magnesium hydroxide 311 mg				
Ranitidine 150 mg Tablets	Various Manufacturers	tablet					ranitidine hydrochloride 150 mg	
Ranitidine 75 mg Tablets	Various Manufacturers	tablet					ranitidine hydrochloride 75 mg	
Rolaids Extra Strength	Pfizer Consumer Healthcare	tablet		magnesium hydroxide 135 mg	calcium carbonate 750 mg			
Rolaids Extra Strength Multi-Symptom	Pfizer Consumer Healthcare	tablet		magnesium hydroxide 135 mg	calcium carbonate 750 mg			simethicone 60 mg
Rolaids Regular	Pfizer Consumer Healthcare	tablet		magnesium hydroxide 110 mg	calcium carbonate 550 mg			
Sodium Bicarbonate	Various Manufacturers	powder / tablets				sodium bicarbonate		
Sodium Bicarbonate Powder	Atlas	powder				sodium bicarbonate 300 mg/g		

Product	Manufacturer	Dosage Form	Aluminum	Magnesium	Calcium	Other Antacids	Histamine H2-Receptor Antagonist	Other Active Ingredients
Sodium Bicarbonate Tablets	Xenex	tablet				sodium bicarbonate 325 mg		
Sodium Bicarbonate Tablets	Sandoz	tablet				sodium bicarbonate 500 mg		
Tums Extra Strength	GlaxoSmithKline Consumer Healthcare	tablet			calcium carbonate 750 mg			
Tums Extra Strength Smoothies	GlaxoSmithKline Consumer Healthcare	tablet			calcium carbonate 750 mg			
Tums Regular	GlaxoSmithKline Consumer Healthcare	tablet			calcium carbonate 500 mg			
Tums Ultra Strength	GlaxoSmithKline Consumer Healthcare	tablet			calcium carbonate 1000 mg			
Zantac 75	Pfizer Consumer Healthcare	tablet					ranitidine hydrochloride 75 mg	
Zantac Extra Strength 150 mg	Pfizer Consumer Healthcare	tablet					ranitidine hydrochloride 150 mg	
Zantac Maximum Strength 150 mg	Pfizer Consumer Healthcare	tablet					ranitidine hydrochloride 150 mg	

Product	Manufacturer	Dosage Form	Active Ingredients
Bacid	Erfa	capsule	lactobacillus rhamnosus 1 billion units
Bismuth Subsalicylate Suspension	Various Manufacturers	suspension	bismuth subsalicylate 17.6 mg/mL
Bismuth Subsalicylate Extra Strength Suspension	Various Manufacturers	suspension	bismuth subsalicylate 35.2 mg/mL
Bismuth Subsalicylate Tablets	Various Manufacturers	suspension	bismuth subsalicylate 262 mg
Culturelle	Locin Industries	capsule	lactobacillus rhamnosus GG 10 billion units
Diarr-eze Caplet	Pharmascience	caplet	loperamide hydrochloride 2 mg
Diarr-eze Liquid	Pharmascience	liquid	loperamide hydrochloride 0.2 mg/mL
Florastor	Medical Futures	capsule	saccharomyces boulardii lyo 5 billion units (250 mg)
Fowler's Oral Suspension	Columbia	suspension	attapulgite (activated) 60 mg/mL
Fowler's Tablet	Columbia	tablet	attapulgite (activated) 630 mg
Imodium Advanced	McNeil Consumer Healthcare	tablet, chewable	loperamide hydrochloride 2 mg simethicone 125 mg
Imodium Caplets	McNeil Consumer Healthcare	caplet	loperamide hydrochloride 2 mg
Imodium Liquid	McNeil Consumer Healthcare	liquid	loperamide hydrochloride 0.13 mg/mL
Imodium Quick Dissolve	McNeil Consumer Healthcare	tablet	loperamide hydrochloride 2 mg
Kaopectate Children's Suspension	Johnson & Johnson Merck	suspension	attapulgite (activated) 40 mg/mL
Kaopectate Extra Strength Suspension	Johnson & Johnson Merck	suspension	attapulgite (activated) 50 mg/mL
Kaopectate Regular Strength Suspension	Johnson & Johnson Merck	liquid	attapulgite (activated) 40 mg/mL
Lacidofil Probiotic	Institut Rosell	tablet	lactobacillus rhamnosus 1.9 billion units lactobacillus acidophilus 0.1 billion units
Loperamide	Various Manufacturers	tablet	loperamide hydrochloride 2 mg
Metamucil Powder Original	Procter & Gamble	powder	psyllium hydrophilic mucilloid 0.5 g/g
Metamucil Powder Smooth Orange	Procter & Gamble	powder	psyllium hydrophilic mucilloid 0.3 g/g
Metamucil Powder Smooth Sugar-Free	Procter & Gamble	powder	psyllium hydrophilic mucilloid 0.6 g/g
Mucillium Powder	Pendopharm	powder	psyllium hydrophilic mucilloid 0.5 g/g
Pepto-Bismol Caplets	Procter & Gamble	caplet	bismuth subsalicylate 262 mg
Pepto-Bismol Liquid	Procter & Gamble	liquid	bismuth subsalicylate 17.6 mg/mL
Pepto-Bismol Liquid Extra Strength	Procter & Gamble	liquid	bismuth subsalicylate 35.2 mg/mL
Pepto-Bismol Tablets	Procter & Gamble	tablet, chewable	bismuth subsalicylate 262 mg calcium carbonate 350 mg
Riva - Loperamide	Riva Laboratories	tablet	loperamide hydrochloride 2 mg
VSL #3	Ferring	powder	bifidobacterium breve bifidobacterium longum bifidobacterium infantis lactobacillus acidophilus lactobacillus plantarum lactobacillus paracasei lactobacillus bulgaricus streptococcus thermophilus 450 billion units (combined count)

Product	Manufacturer	Dosage Form	Dimenhydrinate	Other Active Ingredients
Benadryl	McNeil Consumer Healtcare	capsule		diphenhydramine 25 mg
Benadryl Children's Liquid	McNeil Consumer Healtcare	liquid		diphenhydramine 1.25 mg/mL
Benadryl Elixir	McNeil Consumer Healtcare	liquid		diphenhydramine 2.5 mg/mL
Bismuth Subsalicylate	Various Manufacturers	liquid		bismuth subsalicylate 17.6 mg/mL
Bismuth Subsalicylate Extra Strength	Various Manufacturers	liquid		bismuth subsalicylate 35.2 mg/mL
Bismuth Subsalicylate Tablets	Various Manufacturers	tablet		bismuth subsalicylate 262 mg
Children's Motion Sickness Liquid	Tanta	liquid	3 mg/mL	
Dimenhydrinate 50 mg	Various Manufacturers	tablet	50 mg	
Dimenhydrinate 100 mg Suppositories	Various Manufacturers	suppository	100 mg	
Diphenhydramine 25 mg	Various Manufacturers	capsule		diphenhydramine 25 mg
Diphenhydramine 50 mg	Various Manufacturers	capsule		diphenhydramine 50 mg
Gravol Chewable Tablets for Adults	Church & Dwight	tablet, chewable	50 mg	
Gravol Chewable Tablets for Children	Church & Dwight	tablet, chewable	15 mg	
Gravol Filmkote Tablets 50 mg	Church & Dwight	tablet	50 mg	
Gravol Liquid	Church & Dwight	syrup	3 mg/mL	
Gravol Long Action Dual Relief Tablets	Church & Dwight	tablet (combined long acting & short acting)	25 mg immediate release 75 mg sustained release	
Gravol Natural Source	Church & Dwight	tablet		ginger 500 mg
Gravol Soft chew Ginger	Church & Dwight	tablet		ginger 500 mg
Gravol Softgel	Church & Dwight	capsule	50 mg	
Gravol Suppositories Adult	Church & Dwight	suppository	100 mg	
Gravol Suppositories Children	Church & Dwight	suppository	25 mg	
Histantil 50 mg	Pharmascience	tablet		promethazine hydrochloride 50 mg
Pepto-Bismol Caplet	Procter & Gamble	caplet		bismuth subsalicylate 262 mg
Pepto-Bismol Liquid	Procter & Gamble	liquid		bismuth subsalicylate 17.6 mg/mL
Pepto-Bismol Tablets	Procter & Gamble	tablet, chewable		bismuth subsalicylate 262 mg calcium carbonate 350 mg
Transderm-V	Pharmascience	patch, sustained-release		scopolamine 1.5 mg

Product	Manufacturer	Dosage Form	Active Ingredients
Bi-Peglyte	PendoPharm	powder for solution (sachet) + tablets	bisacodyl (tablets) 5 mg/tab polyethylene glycol 3350 59.55 g potassium chloride 760 mg sodium bicarbonate 1.69 g sodium chloride 1.46 g sodium sulfate 5.74 g
Colyte	GlaxoSmithKline Consumer Healthcare	powder for solution	polyethylene glycol 3350 240 g potassium chloride 2.98 g sodium bicarbonate 6.72 g sodium chloride 5.84 g sodium sulfate 22.72 g
GoLytely Gastrointestinal Lavage Solution	Braintree Labs	powder for solution	polyethylene glycol 3350 236 g potassium chloride 2.97 g sodium bicarbonate 6.74 g sodium chloride 5.86 g sodium sulfate 22.72 g
Klean-Prep	Helix Biopharma	powder for solution	polyethylene glycol 3350 59 g potassium chloride 740 mg sodium bicarbonate 1.68 g sodium chloride 1.46 g sodium sulfate 5.68 g
Peglyte Powder	PendoPharm	powder for solution	polyethylene glycol 3350 238.18 g potassium chloride 3.05 g sodium bicarbonate 6.76 g sodium chloride 5.85 g sodium sulfate 22.96 g
Peglyte Powder Sachet	PendoPharm	powder for solution (sachet)	polyethylene glycol 3350 59.55 g potassium chloride 760 mg sodium bicarbonate 1.69 g sodium chloride 1.46 g sodium sulfate 5.74 g
Pico-Salax	Ferring	powder for solution	citric acid 12 g magnesium oxide 3.5 g sodium picosulfate 10 mg
Purg-Odan	Odan	powder for solution	citric acid 12 g magnesium oxide 3.5 g sodium picosulfate 10 mg

Product	Manufacturer	Dosage Form	Active Ingredients
Anurex Hemorrhoidal Kit	Anurex	kit	Cryotherapy device No active ingredients Made of surgical plastic To be inserted in the rectum for 6-10 minutes Freeze for 2 hours prior to use
Anusol Ointment	McNeil Consumer Healthcare	ointment	zinc sulfate monohydrate 0.5%
Anusol Plus Ointment	McNeil Consumer Healthcare	ointment	pramoxine hydrochloride 1% zinc sulfate monohydrate 0.5%
Anusol Plus Suppositories	McNeil Consumer Healthcare	suppository	pramoxine hydrochloride 20 mg zinc sulfate monohydrate 10 mg
Anusol Suppositories	McNeil Consumer Healthcare	suppository	zinc sulfate monohydrate 10 mg
Anuzinc Ointment	Sandoz	ointment	zinc sulfate 0.5%
Anuzinc Suppositories	Sandoz	suppository	zinc sulfate 10 mg
Hemoclin Gel	YouMedical	gel	aloe barbadensis 40%
Hemorrhoid Ointment	Various Manufacturers	ointment	pramoxine hydrochloride 1% zinc sulfate 0.5%
Hemorrhoidal Pads	Various Manufacturers	pad	glycerin 10% hamamelis 50%
Nupercainal Ointment	Novartis Consumer Health	ointment	dibucaine 1%
Preparation H PE Gel	Pfizer Consumer Healthcare	gel	hamamelis 50% phenylephrine hydrochloride 0.25%
Preparation H Cream	Pfizer Consumer Healthcare	cream	shark liver oil 3% yeast 1%
Preparation H Ointment	Pfizer Consumer Healthcare	ointment	shark liver oil 3% yeast 1%
Preparation H Suppositories	Pfizer Consumer Healthcare	suppository	shark liver oil 66 mg yeast 22 mg
Tucks Cleansing Wipes	Johnson & Johnson	pad	glycerin 10% hamamelis 50%

Product	Manufacturer	Dosage Form	Bulk Forming	Osmotic	Stimulant	Emollient	Other Active Ingredients
ABCO Enema	Unico Holdings	enema		sodium phosphate (dibasic) 59 mg/mL sodium phosphate (monobasic) 161 mg/mL			
Agarol Plain	Numark	emulsion				glycerin 160 mg/mL mineral oil 0.32 mL/mL	
Benefibre Powder	Novartis Consumer Health	powder	guar gum 100%				
Benefibre Tablets	Novartis Consumer Health	chewable tablets	partially hydrolyzed guar gum 1.3 g				
Biolax	M. Vachon Group	liquid			cascara sagrada 2.73 mg/mL		
Bisacodyl Suppositories 10 mg	Various Manufacturers	suppository			bisacodyl 10 mg		
Bisacodyl Tablets	Various Manufacturers	tablet, enteric coated			bisacodyl 5 mg		
Carters Little Pills	Church & Dwight	tablet			bisacodyl 5 mg		
Cas-Mag Suspension	Omega	liquid		magnesium hydroxide 50 mg/mL	cascara sagrada 0.33 mg/mL		
Cascara Aromatique	Atlas	liquid			cascara sagrada 15%	glycerin 4.4%	caraway 0.026% orange 0.15% licorice 1.2% anise 0.023%
Cascara Sagrada Capsules	Various Manufacturers	capsule			cascara sagrada 320 to 450 mg		
Cascara Sagrada Tablets	Various Manufacturers	tablet			cascara sagrada 325 to 487.5 mg		
Castor Oil	Various Manufacturers	liquid			castor oil		
Cholasyn II	M. Vachon Group	tablet			cascara sagrada 3.34 mg sennosides 12 mg	bile salts 65 mg	
Citrodan	Odan	liquid		magnesium citrate 50 mg/mL			
Citro-Mag	Rougier	liquid		magnesium citrate 50 mg/mL			
Colace Capsules	WellSpring	capsule				docusate sodium 100 mg	
Colace Drops	WellSpring	drops				docusate sodium 10 mg/mL	
Colace Syrup	WellSpring	syrup				docusate sodium 4 mg/mL	
Docusate Calcium Capsules	Various Manufacturers	capsule				docusate calcium 240 mg	
Docusate Sodium Capsules	Various Manufacturers	capsule				docusate sodium 100 mg	

▶

Product	Manufacturer	Dosage Form	Bulk Forming	Osmotic	Stimulant	Emollient	Other Active Ingredients
Docusate Sodium Drops	Various Manufacturers	drops				docusate sodium 10 mg/mL	
Docusate Sodium Syrup	Various Manufacturers	syrup				docusate sodium 4 mg/mL	
Dulcolax	Boehringer Ingelheim Consumer Health Care	tablet, enteric coated			bisacodyl 5 mg		
Dulcolax Suppositories 10 mg	Boehringer Ingelheim Consumer Health Care	suppository			bisacodyl 10 mg		
Dulcolax Suppositories 5 mg	Boehringer Ingelheim Consumer Health Care	suppository			bisacodyl 5 mg		
Enemol	Pendopharm	enema		sodium acid phosphate 160 mg/mL sodium phosphate 60 mg/mL			
Epsom Salts	Various Manufacturers	powder for solution		magnesium sulfate 100%			
Ex-Lax Chocolate Pieces	Novartis Consumer Health	tablet			sennosides 15 mg		
Ex-Lax Extra Strength	Novartis Consumer Health	tablet			sennosides 25 mg		
Ex-Lax Sugar-Coated	Novartis Consumer Health	tablet			sennosides 15 mg		
Fleet Enema Regular (130 mL)	Johnson & Johnson Merck	liquid		sodium phosphate (dibasic) 60 mg/mL sodium phosphate (monobasic) 160 mg/mL			
Fleet Enema Mineral Oil	Johnson & Johnson Merck	enema				mineral oil 100%	
Fleet Enema Pediatric (65 mL)	Johnson & Johnson Merck	enema		sodium phosphate (dibasic) 60 mg/mL sodium phosphate (monobasic) 160 mg/mL			
Garilax-2X	Gerbex	liquid		magnesium sulfate 176 mg/mL	cascara sagrada 26.4 mg/mL		
Gerbelax	Gerbex	liquid			cascara sagrada 35.1 mg/mL		
Glycerin Suppositories Adult	Various Manufacturers	suppository		glycerin			
Glycerin Suppositories Adult	Teva Canada	suppository		glycerin 2.4 g			
Glycerin Suppositories Infant/Child	Teva Canada	suppository		glycerin 1.62 g			
Glycerin Suppositories Infants & Children	Various Manufacturers	suppository		glycerin			

Product	Manufacturer	Dosage Form	Bulk Forming	Osmotic	Stimulant	Emollient	Other Active Ingredients
Herbal Laxative	Swiss Herbal	tablet			cascara sagrada 150 mg rhubarb 8 mg senna 240 mg	gentian 8 mg	
Herbal Laxative	Trophic	tablet			buchu 5 mg cascara sagrada 150 mg licorice 50 mg senna 250 mg	fennel 50 mg gentian 10 mg juniper berries 5 mg leptandra 10 mg	
Herbal Tea #1 Laxative	Robert et fils	tea bags					fennel 150 mg peppermint 135 mg
Herbalax	Sante Naturelle	tablet			cascara sagrada 70 mg frangula 100 mg rhubarb 25 mg senna 20 mg	bile salts 50 mg	
Herborex Capsule	Rolmex	capsule			cascara sagrada 81 mg yellow dock 81 mg		
Herborex Forte Liquid	Rolmex	liquid			cascara sagrada 15.1 mg/mL yellow dock 10.83 mg/mL		
Herborex Liquid	Rolmex	liquid			cascara sagrada 10.83 mg/mL yellow dock 10.83 mg/mL		
Lactulose	Various Manufacturers	syrup		lactulose 667 mg/mL			
Lansoyl	Axcan Pharma	jelly				mineral oil 78%	
Lansoyl Sugar Free	Axcan Pharma	jelly				mineral oil 78%	
Lax A Day	Pendopharm	powder		polyethylene glycol (PEG) 3350			
Laxaco Herbal Laxative	Jamieson	capsule			cascara sagrada 150 mg senna 240 mg		
Laxative	Lab Lalco	tablet			aloe 60 mg cascara sagrada 100 mg	bile salts 60 mg	
Laxcodyl	Tanta	tablet			bisacodyl 5 mg		
Magnolax	Pendopharm	emulsion		magnesium hydroxide 60 mg/mL		mineral oil 0.25 mL/mL	
Metamucil Fibre Therapy Capsules	Procter & Gamble	capsules	psyllium seed husks 550 mg				
Metamucil Powder Original Texture, Unflavoured	Procter & Gamble	powder for solution	psyllium hydrophilic mucilloid 0.5 g/g				

Product	Manufacturer	Dosage Form	Bulk Forming	Osmotic	Stimulant	Emollient	Other Active Ingredients
Metamucil Powder Smooth Texture Orange	Procter & Gamble	powder for solution	psyllium hydrophilic mucilloid 0.3 g/g				
Metamucil Powder Smooth Texture Orange Sugar-Free	Procter & Gamble	powder for solution	psyllium hydrophilic mucilloid 0.6 g/g				
Metamucil Powder Smooth Texture Unflavoured Sugar-Free	Procter & Gamble	powder for solution	psyllium hydrophilic mucilloid 0.6 g/g				
Metamucil Wafers	Procter & Gamble	wafer	psyllium hydrophilic mucilloid 3.4 g				
Microlax Micro Enema	McNeil Consumer Healthcare			sodium citrate 90 mg/mL			sodium lauryl sulfoacetate 9 mg/mL sorbitol 625 mg/mL
Milk of Magnesia	Various Manufacturers	liquid		magnesium hydroxide 70 to 88 mg/mL			
Milk of Magnesia Mineral Oil Emulsion	Various Manufacturers	liquid		magnesium hydroxide 64 to 80 mg/mL		mineral oil 0.2 to 0.25 mL/mL	
Milk of Magnesia Tablets	Various Manufacturers	tablet		magnesium hydroxide 300 to 385 mg			
Mineral Oil	Various Manufacturers	liquid				petrolatum liquid	
Mucillium Powder	Pharmascience	powder	psyllium hydrophilic mucilloid 0.5 g/g				
Nature's Remedy	GlaxoSmithKline Consumer Healthcare	tablet			sennosides 8.6 mg		
Normacol	Helix Biopharma	powder	sterculia urens 62%				
Novo-Fibre-Tab	Novopharm	tablet	fibre (grain & citrus) 469 mg				
PegaLAX	Medical Futures	powder		polyethylene glycol (PEG) 3350			
Peri-Colace	WellSpring	capsule			casanthranol 30 mg	docusate sodium 100 mg	
Phillips' Milk of Magnesia Liquid Plain/Cherry/Mint	Bayer Consumer	liquid		magnesium hydroxide 80 mg/mL			
Phosphates Solution	Various Manufacturers	enema		sodium phosphate (dibasic) 180 mg/mL sodium phosphate (monobasic) 480 mg/mL			

Product	Manufacturer	Dosage Form	Bulk Forming	Osmotic	Stimulant	Emollient	Other Active Ingredients
Prodiem Bulk Fibre Therapy	Novartis Consumer Health	tablet	polycarbophil calcium 625 mg				
Prodiem Overnight Relief Therapy	Novartis Consumer Health	tablet			sennosides 15 mg		
Psyllium Seed Bulk-Forming Laxative	Nature's Way	powder for solution	plantago ovata 610 mg				
Relaxa	Red Leaf Medical	powder		polyethylene glycol (PEG) 3350			
RestoraLax	Schering-Plough	powder		polyethylene glycol (PEG) 3350			
Selax Capsules 100 mg	Odan	capsule				docusate sodium 100 mg	
Selax Syrup	Odan	syrup				docusate sodium 4 mg/mL	
Senna 12 mg Tablets	Various Manufacturers	tablet			sennosides 12 mg/g		
Senna Tablets	Various Manufacturers	tablet			sennosides 8.6 mg		
Senokot S	Purdue Pharma	tablet			sennosides 8.6 mg	docusate sodium 50 mg	
Senokot Syrup	Purdue Pharma	syrup			sennosides 1.7 mg/mL		
Senokot Tablets	Purdue Pharma	tablet			sennosides 8.6 mg		
Sodium Phosphates Enema	Various Manufacturers			sodium phosphate (dibasic) 60 mg/mL sodium phosphate (monobasic) 160 mg/mL			
Soflax Capsules	Pharmascience	capsule				docusate sodium 100 mg	
Soflax 200 mg Capsules	Pharmascience	capsule				docusate sodium 200 mg	
Soflax Pediatric Drops	Pharmascience	drops				docusate sodium 10 g/mL	
Soflax Syrup	Pharmascience	syrup				docusate sodium 4 mg/mL	
Stomach Ease Herbal Laxative	Nature's Harmony (Purity Life)	tablet					gentian 8 mg peppermint extract 0.2 mL
Tri-Lax Bulk	Trophic	powder	psyllium husks 18.57 g	lactose 11.43 g	bentonite 2.5 g dolomite 5.71 g whey powder 41.14 g dextrose 16.8 g		
Vitality Herbelax	Vitality	tablet			cascara sagrada 64.8 mg licorice 32.4 mg rhubarb 48.6 mg senna 194.4 mL	anise 32.4 mg	

Product	Manufacturer	Dosage Form	Ingredients	Standardization
Aloelax 530 mg	Nature's Way	capsule	aloe vera 250 mg fennel seed 280 mg	
Chondroitin and Glucosamine Sulfate	Quest	capsule	chondroitin sulfate 200 mg glucosamine sulfate 300 mg	
CoQ$_{10}$ with Omega-3	Jamieson	capsule	coenzyme Q$_{10}$ 100 mg fish oil 850 mg	docosahexaenoic acid 150 mg eicosapentaenoic acid 300 mg
Double Strength Glucosamine and Chondroitin	Holista	capsule	chondroitin sulfate 450 mg glucosamine sulfate 500 mg	>95% chondroitin sulfate A
Echinacea and Goldenseal	Jamieson	capsule	echinacea purpurea raw herb extract (1:4) 185 mg goldenseal raw herb extract (1:2) 45 mg	
Echinacea with Garlic and Ginger	Jamieson	capsule	echinacea purpurea raw herb extract (1:3) 100 mg garlic 300 mg ginger raw herb extract (1:6) 50 mg	
Efalex	Efamol	gelatin capsule	arachidonic acid 5.25 mg docosahexaenoic acid 60 mg gamma-linolenic acid 12 mg linoleic acid 100 mg thyme oil 1 mg vitamin E 15 IU	
Efalex Liquid	Efamol	liquid	arachidonic acid 2.5 mg/mL docosahexaenoic acid 28 mg/mL eicosapentaenoic acid 6.4 mg/mL	
Estrosoy	Nature's Way	capsule	red clover 200 mg soy extract 335 mg	6% isoflavones
Estrosoy Plus	Nature's Way	capsule	black cohosh 20 mg red clover 200 mg soy extract 335 mg	2.5% triterpene glycosides 6% isoflavones
Feminex Meno	Santé Naturelle	capsule	black cohosh 40 mg FOS (fructooligosaccharides) 75 mg kudzu root 40 mg red clover 50 mg sage leaves 20 mg	2.5% triterpenes glycosides 40% isoflavones 8% isoflavones
Feminex Post-Meno	Santé Naturelle	capsule	kudzu root 65 mg red clover 125 mg soy extract 25 mg	40% isoflavones 8% isoflavones 40% isoflavones
Feminex Pre-Meno	Santé Naturelle	capsule	kudzu root 75 mg red clover 75 mg	40% isoflavones 8% isoflavones
Focus with Omega-3 Fatty Acids	Swiss Herbal	softgel capsule	evening primrose oil 155 mg tuna oil 255 mg vitamin E 20 IU	docosahexaenoic acid 63.75 mg eicosapentaenoic acid 12.75 mg
Glucosamine & Chondroitin	Holista	capsule	chondroitin sulfate 200 mg glucosamine sulfate 250 mg	>95% chondroitin sulfate A
Glucosamine and Chondroitin	Nutravite	gelatin capsule	chondroitin sulfate 500 mg glucosamine sulfate 500 mg	
Glucosamine and Chondroitin	Nutravite	gelatin capsule	chondroitin sulfate 250 mg glucosamine sulfate 250 mg	
Glucosamine/Chondroitin Complex	Jamieson	capsule	chondroitin sulfate 200 mg glucosamine hydrochloride 250 mg	
Glucosamine Joint and Muscle Cream with MSM	Nutravite	cream	evening primrose oil glucosamine sulfate 5% grape seed oil methylsulfonylmethane (MSM) 4.95%	

Product	Manufacturer	Dosage Form	Ingredients	Standardization
Green Tea Phytosome Complex	Quest	capsule	green tea phytosome complex : greenselect tea leaf extract 33 mg green tea 40 mg phosphatidylcholine 67 mg	
Herbal Diuretic	Nature's Harmony	tablet	buchu leaf 100 mg celery seed 75 mg juniper berries 100 mg parsley leaf 75 mg uva ursi 100 mg	buchu leaf 25 mg (4:1) juniper berries 25 mg (4:1) uva ursi 33.3 mg (3:1)
Herbal Diuretic Maximum Strength	Swiss Herbal	tablet	buchu leaves 100 mg celery seed powder 75 mg juniper berries 100 mg parsley leaf 75 mg uva ursi 100 mg	
Herbal Insomnia Formula	Nature's Harmony	tablet	chamomile flower 80 mg hops flower 50 mg mistletoe herb 50 mg passion flower 80 mg valerian root 200 mg wild lettuce leaf 40 mg	chamomile flower 15 mg (4:1) valerian root 50 mg (4:1)
Herbal Laxative	Swiss Herbal	tablet	cascara sagrada 150 mg gentian root 8 mg rhubarb root 8 mg senna leaves 240 mg	
Herbal Laxative	Trophic	tablet	buchu 5 mg cascara sagrada 150 mg fennel 50 mg gentian 10 mg juniper 5 mg leptandra 10 mg licorice 50 mg senna 250 mg yoghurt 10 mg	
Herbal Nerve	Nature's Harmony	tablet	hops flower 50 mg skullcap herb 100 mg valerian root 200 mg	valerian root 50 mg (4:1)
Herbal Sleepwell	Swiss Herbal	tablet	hops 200 mg lemon balm herb 10 mg linden flower 10 mg passion flower 400 mg valerian root 400 mg	hops 50 mg (4:1) passion flower 100 mg (4:1) valerian root 100 mg (4:1)
Kyolic 104	Wakunaga	capsule	aged garlic extract 300 mg lecithin 190 mg	S-allyl cysteine
Kyolic 108	Wakunaga	capsule	aged garlic extract 250 mg folic acid 300 µg l-arginine 100 mg vitamin B_6 12.5 mg vitamin B_{12} 100 µg	
Kyolic Omega 3	Wakunaga	capsule	aged garlic extract 120 mg docosahexaenoic acid 120 mg eicosapentaenoic acid 280 mg vitamin E 5 IU	S-allyl cysteine
Meno Caps	Genuine Health	capsule	black cohosh 480 mg chastetree 1250 mg dandelion 250 mg dong quai 1250 mg	2.5% triterpene glycosides 0.5% agnuside 1% ligustilide

Product	Manufacturer	Dosage Form	Ingredients	Standardization
Milk Thistle Extract Formula	Quest	caplet	burdock root 155 mg dandelion root 155 mg licorice root 40 mg milk thistle seed extract (1:8) 60 mg wild yam root 10 mg	6.0% diosgenin 80% silymarin
MSM and Glucosamine Sulfate	Quest	tablet	glucosamine sulfate 300 mg methylsulfonylmethane 200 mg	
Natural HRT Nightime Herbal Relief Therapy	Swiss Herbal	capsule	black cohosh 100 mg lemon balm 300 mg passion flower 150 mg	
Omega 3-6-9	Jamieson	capsule	borage oil 400 mg fish oil 400 mg flax seed oil 400 mg vitamin E 10 IU	alpha linolenic acid 212 mg eicosapentaenoic acid 72 mg docosahexaenoic acid 48 mg gamma-linolenic acid 76 mg linoleic acid 207 mg oleic acid 173 mg
Omega 3-6-9 Hi-Potency	WN Pharmaceuticals	softgel capsule	borage oil 400 mg fish oil 400 mg flax seed oil 400 mg	alpha linolenic acid 200 mg eicosapentaenoic acid 120 mg docosahexaenoic acid 80 mg gamma-linolenic acid 75 mg
Phyto Cold	Sisu	gelatin capsule	ginger 100 mg kalmegh - andrographis paniculata 300 mg	5% gingenosides 10% andrographolides
Phytovision	Sisu	gelatin capsule	bilberry extract (100:1) 25 mg ginkgo biloba extract 30 mg grape seed extract (100:1) 25 mg lutein 2 mg multi anthocyanadins 25 mg	25% anthocyanadins 24% flavone glycosides 85-95% proanthocyanadins 6% terpene lactones
Phytovision Plus	Sisu	gelatin capsule	bilberry extract (100:1) 25 mg ginkgo biloba extract 30 mg grape seed extract (100:1) 25 mg lutein 4 mg multi anthocyanadins 25 mg	24% flavone glycosides 85-95% proanthocyanadins 6% terpene lactones
Prosta Ease	Swiss Herbal	capsule	flax seed oil 125 mg pumpkin seed oil 125 mg pygeum extract 15 mg saw palmetto extract 80 mg	13% beta-sitosterols 85%-95% fatty acids
Prostate Formula	Sisu	capsule	phytosterols 45 mg rye pollen extract 190 mg saw palmetto extract 160 mg vitamin E 50 IU	40-58% beta-sitosterols 45% free fatty acids
Prostate Formula	Holista	softgel capsule	flax seed oil 130 mg pumpkin seed oil 130 mg pygeum bark 20 mg saw palmetto berry oil 80 mg	85%-95% free fatty acids, esters & sterols 13% sterols
Prostease Saw Palmetto Complex	Jamieson	capsule	cranberry extract (1:25) 10 mg pumpkin seed oil 130 mg pygeum bark extract 1(150) 50 mg saw palmetto berry extract (1:4) 50 mg	80% fatty acids

Product	Manufacturer	Dosage Form	Ingredients	Standardization
Restorativ Glucosamine Muscle & Joint Cream	Holista	cream	borage oil boswellia/frankincense camphor oil cetylmyristoleate devil's claw evening primrose oil glucosamine sulfate grape seed oil peppermint oil rosemary oil	
Saw Palmetto Complex	Sisu	gelatin capsule	pumpkin seed extract (5:1) 50 mg pygeum bark extract (30:1) 25 mg saw palmetto fruit extract (4:1) 125 mg stinging nettle (10:1) 75 mg uva ursi (4:1) 15 mg	pumpkin seed 25% fatty acids saw palmetto 25% fatty acids uva ursi 10% arbutin
Slippery Elm Lozenges	Trophic	lozenges	fenugreek seed powder 10 mg slippery elm powder 600 mg	
Stomach Ease	Nature's Harmony	tablet	buchu 4 mg cascara sagrada 150 mg gentian 8 m g juniper 8 mg licorice 30 mg peppermint extract 0.2 mg rhubarb 4 mg senna 240 mg	
Tri Lax Colon Cleanser	Trophic	powder	bentonite 2.5 g dextrose 16.8 g dolomite 5.71 g kelp 1.07 g lactose 11.43 g psyllium husk 18.57 g slippery elm bark whey powder 41.14 g yoghurt 0.71 g	

Common Name	Product	Manufacturer	Dosage Form	Strength	Standardization
alfalfa	Alfalfa Leaf	Nature's Harmony	capsule	alfalfa leaf 500 mg	
bilberry	Bilberry Extract	Various Manufacturers	capsule	bilberry extract 40 mg	25% anthocyanidins
black cohosh	Black Cohosh	Various Manufacturers	capsule	black cohosh extract 40 mg	2.5% triterpene glycosides
	Black Cohosh	Jamieson	caplet	black cohosh raw herb extract (1:2) 20 mg	2.5% triterpene glycosides
	Black Cohosh	Sisu	gelatin capsule	black cohosh root extract 150 mg	2.5% triterpene glycosides
burdock	Burdock Root	Nature's Harmony	capsule	burdock root 430 mg	
butterbur	Petadolex	Sisu	gelatin capsule	butterbur root 50 mg	15% petasin and isopetasin
cascara sagrada	Cascara Sagrada Bark	Nature's Harmony	capsule	cascara sagrada 450 mg	7% hydroxyanthracene derivatives (HAD)
cayenne	Cayenne Extract	WN Pharmaceuticals	capsule	cayenne extract 470 mg	42,000 heat units
chasteberry	Chasteberry	Various Manufacturers	capsule	chasteberry 100 mg	
	Vitex	Nature's Way	capsule	chasteberry 400 mg	
chlorophyll	Chlorofresh	Nature's Way	gelatin capsule	chlorophyllin copper complex 50 mg	
	Chlorofresh Liquid	Nature's Way	liquid	chlorophyllin copper complex 3.33 mg/mL	
cinnamon	Cinnamon Extract	WN Pharmaceuticals	capsule	cinnamon extract (20:1) 150 mg	
coenzyme Q_{10}	CoEnzyme Q_{10} 30 mg	Various Manufacturers	capsule	coenzyme Q_{10} 30 mg	
	CoEnzyme Q_{10} 60 mg	Various Manufacturers	capsule	coenzyme Q_{10} 60 mg	
	CoEnzyme Q_{10} 100 mg	Various Manufacturers	capsule	coenzyme Q_{10} 100 mg	
	Q-Sorb CoEnzyme Q_{10}	Vita-Health	capsule	coenzyme Q_{10} 200 mg	
cranberry	Completely Cranberry	Nature's Harmony	capsule	cranberry extract (1:35) 500 mg	
	Cranberry Capsules	Various Manufacturers	capsule	cranberry extract 250 mg	
	Cranberry Capsules	Various Manufacturers	capsule	cranberry extract 500 mg	
	Cran-C	Holista	gelatin capsule	cranberry extract (1:25) 45.3 mg vitamin C 100 mg	
dandelion	Dandelion Root	Nature's Way	capsule	dandelion root 540 mg	
devil's claw	Devil's Claw	Holista	tablet	devil's claw 500 mg	3% harpagoside
	Devil's Claw	Jamieson	capsule	devil's claw raw herb extract (1:3) 400 mg	3.5% harpagoside
	Devil's Claw	Nutravite	gelatin capsule	devil's claw 200 mg	5% harpagoside
	Devil's Claw Secondary Root	Nature's Way	capsule	devil's claw 480 mg	
	Triple Strength Devil's Claw	Swiss Herbal	soft gelatin capsule	devil's claw 1230 mg	5% harpagoside (12.3 mg)
echinacea	Cold-A-Tak Echinilin	WN Pharmaceuticals	softgel	echinacea purpurea standardized extract 2.4:1 250 mg	
	Echinacea 1000 mg	Jamieson	capsule	echinacea angustifolia raw herb extract (1:5) 200 mg	4% echinacosides
	Echinacea Extract	WN Pharmaceuticals	capsule	echinacea purpurea 500 mg	
	Echinacea 4% Standardized	Nutravite	gelatin capsule	echinacea extract (1:4) 125 mg (from 500 mg of fresh herb)	4% phenolic compounds

Common Name	Product	Manufacturer	Dosage Form	Strength	Standardization
echinacea	Echinacea Liquid	Holista	liquid	echinacea angustifolia dried root 200 mg/mL	4% echinacosides
	Echinacea Standardized to 4% Phenolic Compounds	Holista	gelatin capsule	echinacea purpurea extract (1:3) 167 mg	4% phenolic compounds
	Echinacea Tincture	Various Manufacturers	liquid	echinacea angustifolia raw root extract (1:2) 500 mg/2 mL	
	Premium Echinacea	Holista	gelatin capsule	echinacea angustifolia extract (1:4) 125 mg	4% echinacosides
	Standard Echinacea Angustifolia	Swiss Herbal	gelatin capsule	echinacea angustifolia extract (1:7) 500 mg	4% echinacosides (2.6 mg)
	Triple Blend Echinacea Time Release	Swiss Herbal	caplet	echinacea 1000 mg (E. angustifolia, E. purpurea, E. pallida)	4% echinacosides 4% phenolics
evening primrose	Efamol 500 mg	Efamol	gelatin capsule	gamma-linolenic acid 60 mg linoleic acid 350 mg vitamin E 13.6 IU 12% gamma-linolenic acid	
	Efamol 1000 mg	Efamol	gelatin capsule	gamma-linolenic acid 120 mg linoleic acid 700 mg vitamin E 27.2 IU 12% gamma-linolenic acid	
	Evening Primrose Oil 500 mg	Various Manufacturers	capsule	gamma-linolenic acid 50 mg linoleic acid 350 mg 10% gamma-linolenic acid	
	Evening Primrose Oil 1000 mg	Various Manufacturers	capsule	gamma-linolenic acid 100 mg linoleic acid 650 mg	
	Evening Primrose Oil 1300 mg	Quest	softgel capsule	gamma-linolenic acid 130 mg linoleic acid 936 mg	
	Focus	Swiss Herbal	capsule	gamma-linolenic acid 14 mg linoleic acid 111 mg vitamin E 20 IU	
	Women's Evening Primrose Oil 500 mg	General Nutrition Products	capsule	gamma-linolenic acid 45 mg linoleic acid 350 mg	
	Women's Evening Primrose Oil 1300 mg	General Nutrition Products	capsule	gamma-linolenic acid 130 mg linoleic acid 940 mg	
feverfew	Feverfew 125	Various Manufacturers	capsule	feverfew 125 mg	0.2% parthenolide (250 µg)
	Feverfew Tincture	Various Manufacturers	liquid	feverfew extract 200 mg/mL	
fish oil	Omega-3 Capsules 500 mg	Various Manufacturers	softgel capsule	fish oils 500 mg	
	Omega-3 Capsules 1000 mg	Various Manufacturers	softgel capsule	fish oils 1000 mg	
	Omega-3 Super Concentrate	WN Pharmaceuticals	softgel capsule	fish oils 1000 mg	400 mg eicosapentaenoic acid 200 mg docosahexaenoic acid 30 mg other omega-3 fatty acids
	Triameg Omega-3	Nicar	capsule	fish oils 500 mg	60% eicosapentaenoic acid 30% docosahexaenoic acid
flax	Flax Seed Oil	Various Manufacturers	gelatin capsule	flax seed oil (certified organic) 1000 mg	

Common Name	Product	Manufacturer	Dosage Form	Strength	Standardization
flax	Flax Seed Oil	WN Pharmaceuticals	liquid	flax seed oil (certified organic)	alpha-linolenic acid 0.46 g/mL gamma-linolenic acid 0.13 g/mL oleic acid 0.13 g/mL
	Ground Flaxseed	WN Pharmaceuticals	ground seeds	100% organic, cold-milled ground flaxseed	
garlic	Allicin Rich Garlic	Jamieson	capsule	garlic raw herb 500 mg	allicin 1000 µg
	Garlic	Sisu	enteric-coated tablet	garlic extract 250 mg	allicin 2.5 mg
garlic	Kwai Garlic Tablets	Hilary's Salesmaster	tablet	odourless garlic powder concentrate (LI 111) 100 mg	0.6% allicin
	Kyolic	Wakunaga	liquid	aged garlic extract 100%	S-allyl cysteine
	Kyolic 100 Capsules	Wakunaga	capsule	aged garlic extract 300 mg	S-allyl cysteine
	Kyolic Once A Day	Wakunaga	caplet	aged garlic extract 600 mg	S-allyl cysteine
	Odourless Garlic	Various Manufacturers	capsule	garlic powder 500 mg	
	Pur-Gar Garlic	Trophic	capsule	de-odorized garlic 500 mg	0.15% allicin
	Super Garlic Oil	Jamieson	capsule	fresh garlic 1500 mg	
	Triple Strength Odour Reduced Garlic	Holista	gelatin capsule	garlic oil 1500 mg	
ginger	Ginger	Jamieson	capsule	ginger root extract (1:10) 100 mg	20% actives
	Ginger Root	Various Manufacturers	gelatin capsule	ginger root 500 mg	
ginkgo	Ginkgo	Holista	gelatin capsule	ginkgo biloba 200 mg	24% flavoglycosides 6% terpene lactones
	Ginkgo Biloba	Nutravite	gelatin capsule	ginkgo biloba 60 mg	24% flavoglycosides 6% terpene lactones
	Ginkgo Biloba 40 mg	Swiss Herbal	capsule	ginkgo biloba 40 mg	flavoglycosides 9.6 mg terpene lactones 2.4 mg
	Ginkgo Biloba	Trophic	gelatin capsule	ginkgo biloba extract 60 mg	24% flavoglycosides 6% terpene lactones
	Ginkgo Biloba	WN Pharmaceuticals	gelatin capsule	ginkgo biloba extract 60 mg	24% flavoglycosides 6% terpene lactones
	Ginkgo Biloba Extract	Quest	caplet	ginkgo biloba extract (1:50) 60 mg 200 mg of hesperidin 24% ginkgosides hesperidin 50 mg	
	Ginkgo Max 120	Jamieson	caplet	ginkgo biloba leaf extract (1:50) 40 mg	24% flavoglycosides 10% quercetin
	Ginkgo Tincture	Jamieson	liquid	ginkgo leaf extract (1:2) 500 mg/mL	
ginseng	Canadian Ginseng	Jamieson	tablet	panax quinquefolius 250 mg	5% ginsenosides
	Nature Made Ginseng 500 mg (Chinese Red Panax)	Nature Made	softgel capsule	ginseng root (NM-1000 extract) 250 mg	2% ginsenosides (0.5 mg)
	Panax Ginseng (Korean Red Ginseng)	Various Manufacturers	gelatin capsule	panax ginseng 500 mg	7% ginsenosides
	Red Korean Ginseng	Jamieson	caplet	panax ginseng root 250 mg	6% ginsenosides

Common Name	Product	Manufacturer	Dosage Form	Strength	Standardization
ginseng	Siberian Ginseng	Various Manufacturers	capsule	siberian ginseng 500 mg	
grape seed extract	Grape Seed Extract	Quest	caplet	grape seed extract 2,500 mg	grape seed extract 25 mg (100:1) 90% proanthocyanadins
	Grape Seed Extract	Sisu	gelatin capsule	grape seed extract (100:1) 50 mg	85-95% proanthocyanadins
green tea	Green Tea Extract	WN Pharmaceuticals	capsule	green tea extract 200 mg	15% caffeine 25% epigallocatechin gallate (EGCG)
hawthorn	Hawthorn Berries	Various Manufacturers	capsule	hawthorn flower extract (1:5) 250 mg	1.8% vitexin (4.5 mg)
melatonin	Melatonin Easy Dissolve	WN Pharmaceuticals	tablet	melatonin 3 mg	
	Melatonin Easy Dissolve Extra Strength	WN Pharmaceuticals	tablet	melatonin 5 mg	
melatonin	Melatonin Sublingual Tablets	Jamieson	tablet	melatonin 3 mg	
	Quest Melatonin	Quest	capsule	melatonin 3 mg	
milk thistle	Milk Thistle	Various Manufacturers	capsule	milk thistle seed extract (1:30) 150 mg	80% silymarin
	Milk Thistle	Quest	tincture	milk thistle 350 mg/mL	
	Milk Thistle	Swiss Herbal	capsule	milk thistle 250 mg	80% silymarin (200 mg)
psyllium	Psyllium Seeds	Nature's Way	capsule	psyllium seeds 610 mg	
red clover	Herbal Select Red Clover	Puresource	capsule	red clover 450 mg	
s-adenosyl L-methionine	SAMe	Various Manufacturers	tablet	s-adenosyl-L-methionine (SAMe) 200 mg	
saw palmetto	Nature Made Saw Palmetto	Various Manufacturers	softgel capsule	saw palmetto berry extract (1:10) 160 mg	85-95% free fatty acids
	Saw Palmetto	Nutravite	gelatin capsule	saw palmetto berries 500 mg	
	Saw Palmetto	Quest	tincture	saw palmetto 272 mg/mL	
	Super Saw Palmetto 800 mg	Swiss Herbal	gelatin capsule	saw palmetto 800 mg	96% fatty acids (76 mg)
senna	Senna Leaves	Nature's Way	capsule	senna leaves 450 mg	
St. John's Wort	Neurosome St. John's Wort	Jamieson	tablet	st. john's wort raw herb extract (1:5) 200 mg	0.3% hypericin 3% hyperforin
	St. John's Wort	Various Manufacturers	caplet	st. john's wort extract (1:5) 300 mg	0.3% hypericin
	St. John's Wort	Nutravite	gelatin capsule	st. john's wort extract (1:6) 500 mg	0.3% hypericin
	St. John's Wort Tincture	Jamieson	liquid	st. john's wort raw herb extract (1:2) 500 mg/mL	
	St. John's Wort Tincture	Quest	tincture	st. john's wort 233 mg/mL	
valerian	Valerian	Various Manufacturers	gelatin capsule	valerian root extract 500 mg	0.8% valerenic acid
	Valerian	Various Manufacturers	caplet	valerian extract (1:4) 100 mg	0.8% valerenic acid
white willow	White Willow	Various Manufacturers	capsule	salix alba 400 mg	

Product	Manufacturer	Test Strips	Memory	Power Options	Time to result (minutes)	Dimensions (LxWxH)	Weight	Measurement Range	Comments
Coaguchek XS	Roche Diagnostics	Coaguchek XS	100 results with time and date	4 X AAA	1	138 x 78 x 28 mm	127 g (without batteries)	INR: 0.8-8.0	Model for customers
Coaguchek XS Plus	Roche Diagnostics	Coaguchek XS	500 results with time and date, 60 code chip records	4 X AAA or rechargeable power pack or AC power adapter	1	185 x 98 x 42 mm	311 g (without batteries)	INR: 0.8-8.0	Model for health care practitioners with extra features
Coaguchek XS Pro	Roche Diagnostics	Coaguchek XS	Stores 1000 patients and 500 results; Data storage for 60 code chips	4 X AA or rechargeable power pack or AC power adapter	1	231 x 97 x 43 mm	350 g (without batteries)	INR: 0.8-8.0	Model for health care practitioners with extra features; Integrated barcode scanner.

Product	Manufacturer	Reaction Time	End Points			Contents	Comments
			Positive	**Negative**	**Control**		
Biocard Kit	2G Pharma (distributor)	10 min	1 line in control window and 1 line in test window	1 line in control window only	Yes, red line in control window	1 test and a dropper tip 1 sterile lancet 1 capillary tube (10 µL) 0.5 mL sample diluent 1 alcohol swab Instructions for use	Uses capillary blood sample Red line in control window ensures that test is done properly Test detects anti-tissue transglutaminase (anti-tTG) IgA antibodies from blood sample Patient must be consuming gluten for the test to work

Product	Manufacturer	Test Strips	Time to Read Result	Calibration (Coding)	Memory Capacity	Measurement Range	Special Features
Accutrend GC Digital Monitor	Roche Diagnostics	Accutrend Cholesterol Strips	3 min	Lot specific Barcode included with each new vial of test strips	15 results with time and date	3.88-7.76 mmol/L (150-300 mg/dL)	Also measures Blood Glucose levels with appropriate strips Can measure in mg/dL or in mmol/L
CardioChek Digital Monitor	Polymer Technology	CardioChek Total Cholesterol Strips CardioChek HDL Test Strips CardioChek Tryglycerides Test Strips	2 min	Lot specific MEMo Chip included with each new vial of test strips	30 results with time and date	Total cholesterol strips: 2.59-10.36 mmol/L (100-400 mg/dL) HDL strips: 0.65-2.20 mmol/L (25-85 mg/dL) Tryglyceride strips: 0.56-5.65 mmol/L (50-500 mg/dL)	6 languages: English, French, Spanish, German, Italian and Portuguese Can measure in mg/dL or in mmol/L

Product	Manufacturer	Model No	User Storage Capacity	Warranty	Memory	Battery	Dimensions without cuff (LxWxH)	Weight with cuff and batteries	Comments
Auto Inflation 3-Series Digital BP Monitor	Omron	BP710CAN	1 user	2 years	14 results	4 AAA	128 x 104 x 64 mm	295 g	One button operation Medium cuff only; large cuff available Detects and corrects for an irregular heartbeat Displays average reading
Auto Inflation 5-Series Digital BP Monitor	Omron	BP742CAN	2 users	2 years	30 results per user with time and date (60 total)	4 AA	141 x 123 x 85 mm	420 g	One button operation Medium cuff only; large cuff available Detects and corrects for an irregular heartbeat AC adapter (not included) Advanced averaging
Auto Inflation 7-Series Intellisense Monitor with ComFit Cuff	Omron	BP760CAN	1 user	2 years	60 results with time and date	4 AA	158 x 124 x 86 mm	520 g	One button operation Detects and corrects for an irregular heartbeat AC adapter included Advanced averaging
Auto Inflation 10-Series Intellisense Monitor with ComFit Cuff	Omron	BP785CAN	2 users	2 years	100 results per user with time and date (200 total)	4 AA	158 x 124 x 86 mm	520 g	One button operation Calibration Check System: automatically double check each reading TruRead feature that automatically takes three readings one minute apart, and displays average AM/PM averaging Detects and corrects for an irregular heartbeat AC adapter included Advanced averaging
Automatic BP Monitor	HoMedics	BPA-110-2CA	2 users	5 years	60 results per user with date and time(120 total)	4 AA	149 x 112 x 57 mm	420 g	One button operation AC adapter included Displays average reading
Automatic BP Monitor with Voice Assist	HoMedics	BP-A26-0ACA	2 users	5 years	60 results per user with date and time(120 total)	4 AA	143 x 109 x 63 mm	390 g	One button operation Detects and corrects for an irregular heartbeat AC adapter included Voice Assist Talking Function guides you through process
Automatic BP Monitor for Pregnancy	Microlife	BP 3BT0-A(2)	1 user	3 years	30 results with date and time	4 AA	115 x 182 x 76 mm	460 g	Medium and large cuffs included
Automatic BP Monitor with Arrythmia Detection	Microlife	BP 3AG1	1 user	3 years	Saves only previous reading	4 AA	140 x 120 x 70 mm	400 g	AC adapter (not included)

▶

Product	Manufacturer	Model No	User Storage Capacity	Warranty	Memory	Battery	Dimensions without cuff (LxWxH)	Weight with cuff and batteries	Comments
Automatic BP Monitor with Arrythmia Detection	Microlife	BP A100	1 user	5 years	30 results with date and time	4 AA	160 x 125 x 98 mm	610 g	Arrythmia detection AC adapter (not included) Washable cuff 2 alarm times
Automatic BP Monitor with Arrythmia Detection	Microlife	BP 3BT0-A	1 user	1 year	99 results with date and time	4 AA	115 x 182 x 76 mm	460 g	Arrythmia detection AC adapter (not included) Washable cuff
Automatic BP Monitor with Arrythmia Detection & Triple Measurement Feature	Microlife	BP A100 Plus	1 user	5 years	200 results with date and time	4 AA	160 x 140 x 98 mm	735 g	Arrythmia detection MAM Technology: Automatically takes 3 consecutive measurements and then displays average AC adapter (not included) Washable cuff 2 alarm times
Automatic BP Monitor with Arrythmia Detection & Triple Measurement Feature with PC Download	Microlife	BP 3AC1-PC	1 user	3 years	99 results with date and time	4 AA	118 x 177 x 77 mm	503 g	Arrythmia detection MAM technology: Automatically takes 3 consecutive measurements and then displays average AC adapter (not included) Washable cuff 2 alarm times Information can be downloaded to a PC using cable provided; software needed is included
Automatic BP Monitor with MAM Technology and Risk Factor Classification	Microlife	BP RM 100	1 user	3 years	NA	4 AA	155 x 127 x 45 mm	600 g	MAM Technology: Automatically takes 3 consecutive measurements and then displays average Gives a "Risk Factor" based on WHO blood pressure classification Washable cuff 2 alarm times
Easy One Step Auto Inflate	Lifesource	UA-631V		5 year	60 results	4 AA	130 x 144 x 55 mm	390 g	One button operation Medium cuff only; small or large cuff available AC adapter included Detects and corrects for an irregular heartbeat Displays average reading
EssentiA Blood Pressure Monitor	Physiologic	106-930	4 users	2 year	30 results per user with time and date (120 total)	4 AA	110 x 155 x 70 mm	490 g	One button operation Medium cuff AC adapter (not included)

Product	Manufacturer	Model No	User Storage Capacity	Warranty	Memory	Battery	Dimensions without cuff (LxWxH)	Weight with cuff and batteries	Comments
One Step Advanced/Deluxe Plus Memory	LifeSource	UA-767P	1 user	Lifetime	90 results	4 AA	110 x 147 x 64 mm	390 g	One button operation Medium cuff only; small or large cuff available AC adapter included Detects and corrects for an irregular heartbeat
Premium Automatic Blood Pressure Monitor	Lifesource	UA-853AC	1 user	Lifetime	90 results with date and time	4 AA	126 x 150 x 156 mm	440 g	One button operation AM/PM TimeWise tracking technology Detects and corrects for an irregular heartbeat 3 alarm times AC adapter included
PrismA Blood Pressure Monitor	Physiologic	106-950	1 user	2 years	60 results	4 AAA	200 x 60 x 56 mm	350 g	One button operation AC adapter (not included)
Quick Response BP Monitor with Easy Fit Cuff	LifeSource	UA-787 EJ	1 user	Lifetime	280 results with date and time	4 AA	112 x 163 x 62 mm	440 g	One button operation Semi-hard cuff Detects and corrects for an irregular heartbeat 3 alarm times AC adapter included

[a] All monitors listed in this table use the oscillometric method to measure blood pressure and are endorsed by Hypertension Canada.

			End Points				
Product	Manufacturer	Reaction Time	Positive	Negative	Control	Contents	Comments
MySet Test	2G Pharma (distributor)	10 min	Results line is same colour or darker than reference line	Results line is lighter than reference line, or it is absent	Reference line: 1 bar in control window	2 tests packs in sealed pouch Instruction sheet	Requires mid-stream urine sample

			End Points			
Product	**Manufacturer**	**Reaction Time (minutes)**	**Positive**	**Negative**	**Number of Tests/Kits**	**Comments**
ClearBlue Fertility Monitor	Procter & Gamble	5	Result indicated by number of bars to show days of low, high or peak fertility		10	Electronic monitor, keeps track of 2 hormones through the cycle to indicate most fertile days Can indicate the 2 days of peak fertility and up to 6 fertile days
ClearBlue Ovulation Test	Procter & Gamble	3	"Results" line is same colour or darker than "reference" line	"Results" line is lighter than "reference" line	7	Ignore results after 10 minutes
ClearBlue Ovulation Test Digital	Procter & Gamble	3	Happy face in display	Circle shape in display	7	
Clearplan Easy	Novartis Consumer Health	3	blue		5	Stick No urine collection Test urine same time each day
Conceive LH One-Step Ovulation Predictor	Pendopharm	3	"Results" line is same colour or darker than "reference" line	"Results" line is lighter than "reference" line	3	Ignore changes after 4 minutes
First Response	Church & Dwight	5	Purple	Light purple	5	Stick Direct in urine stream Test urine same time each day
Luna Fertility Kit	Luna products		Appearance of ferning phenomenon, when viewing dried saliva	No sign of ferning in dried saliva	reusable slide	Saliva test Dried sample of saliva on a slide is viewed through a microscope and checked for the presence of salt formations on the slide
Ovusee Ovulation Test	Mansfield	3	"Results" line is same colour or darker than "reference" line	"Results" line is lighter than "reference" line	5	
Ovu-Trac Ovulation Test	OvumOptics		Appearance of ferning phenomenon when viewing dried saliva	No sign of ferning in dried saliva	6 reusable slides	Saliva test Dried sample of saliva on a slide is viewed through a microscope and checked for the presence of salt formations on the slide

Product	Manufacturer	mIU hcg/mL urine: Ealiest Detection	Reaction Time (minutes)	End Points			
				Positive	Negative	Control	Comments
ClearBlue Easy	Procter & Gamble	50: up to 4 days before missed period	2	Symbol: +	Symbol: -	Yes, blue line in control window	1 step, stick, any urine Tip changes colour while test is being performed
ClearBlue Easy Digital	Procter & Gamble	50: up to 4 days before missed period	3	Word: Pregnant	Words: Not pregnant	NA	1 step, any urine Result will remain in the display for about 24 hours
ClearBlue Easy Digital with Conception Indicator	Procter & Gamble	50: up to 4 days before missed period	3	Word: Pregnant & displays how many weeks	Words: Not pregnant	NA	1 step, any urine Result will remain in the display for about 24 hours Displays how many weeks have passed since conception (gives number in the display)
Conceive 1 Step Pregnancy Test	Pendopharm	50: day of missed period	3	1 line in control window and 1 line in results window	1 line in control window only	Yes, coloured line in control window	1 step, any urine
Fact Plus One Step	Procter & Gamble	50: day of missed period	1	2 bars (II)	1 bar (I)	Yes, red colour in test window	1 step, any urine
First Response Early Result	Church & Dwight	50: up to 4 days before missed period	3	2 bars (II)	1 bar (I)	Yes, pink colour in test window	1 step, any urine
First Response Gold Early Result Digital	Church & Dwight	50: up to 4 days before missed period	3	Word: Yes	Word: No	NA	1 step, any urine
First Response Rapid Result	Church & Dwight	50: day of missed period	1	2 bars (II)	1 bar (I)	Yes, pink colour in test window	1 step, any urine
Pregnansee Test	Ethix	50: day of missed period	3	1 line in control window and 1 line in results window	1 line in control window only	Yes, red colour in test window	1 step, any urine
Result Pregnancy Test	Tanta	50: day of missed period	3	1 line in control window and 1 line in results window	1 line in control window only	Yes, red colour in test window	1 step, any urine

Product	Manufacturer	Model No.	Type	Warranty	Memory	Time to Result	Battery	Comments
Accuflex Flexible Thermometer	Physio Logic	016-637 (5-second model) 016-635 (10-second model)	Oral Rectal Underarm	Lifetime	5 readings	5 sec. or 10 sec. depending on model	1 x SR41 or 1 x LR41	Soft flexible tip for added comfort °C / °F convertible Storage case included Waterproof Available in 5-second or 10-second model
B-D Rapid Digital Thermometer	Becton Dickinson	524-952	Oral Rectal Underarm	Lifetime	Last reading	9 sec.	1 x SR41 or 1 x LR41	°C / °F convertible Battery/Storage case included Large night light display for easy reading
B-D Rapid Flex Digital Thermometer	Becton Dickinson	524-950	Oral Rectal Underarm	Lifetime	Last reading	9 sec.	1 x SR41 or 1 x LR41	Soft flexible tip for added comfort °C / °F convertible Battery/Storage case included Large night light display for easy reading
Bios Ear/ Forehead Thermometer	Microlife	BD-802	Ear Forehead	2 years	9 readings with time/ date	Instant	1 x CR2032	°C / °F convertible Large LCD display with time and date Does not require a probe cover for ear measurements Fever alarm
Digital Thermometer	PharmaSystems	PS-720 (flexible tip) PS-730 (rigid tip)	Oral Underarm	Lifetime	Last reading	10 sec.	1 x SR41 or 1 x LR41	Available with rigid tip or flexible tip Large LCD display °C / °F convertible
Digital Flex Tip Basal Thermometer	PharmaSystems	PS-740	Oral Rectal Vaginal	Lifetime	Last reading	10 sec.	1 x SR41 or 1 x LR41	2 decimal places of accuracy May be used for fertility awareness Soft flexible tip Large LCD display Celsius (°C) scale only
Dual Scale Digital Thermometer	Mansfield	DUODIG	Oral Rectal Underarm	Lifetime		20-30 sec.	1 x SR41 or 1 x LR41	Rigid tip °C / °F convertible
Dual Scale Mercury Thermometer	Mansfield	CFDO	Oral Rectal Underarm	Lifetime		60 sec.		Traditional design Dual °C and °F scale Available as either oral/ underarm or rectal thermometer
FeverBugz Stick-On Fever Indicators	Physio Logic	016-700	Chest Forehead Underarm	Disposable		Continuous monitoring		Sticker that provides continuous reading of temperature Quick at-a-glance visibility Easy to use Provides up to 48 hours of monitoring Can be worn while bathing
FeverTemp Forehead Strip Thermometer	Mansfield	FEVER	Forehead			30-60 sec.		Reusable strip for quick temperature check Dual °C and °F scale

Product	Manufacturer	Model No.	Type	Warranty	Memory	Time to Result	Battery	Comments
Flex-Tip Digital Thermometer	Lifesource	DT-611	Oral Rectal Underarm	Lifetime	Last reading	10 sec.	1 x SR41 or 1 x LR41	Soft flexible tip for added comfort °C / °F convertible Storage case included Large night light display for easy reading Water resistant
Forehead Digital Thermometer	Microlife	FR 1DM1	Forehead	2 years	12 readings	3 sec.	1 x CR 2032	°C / °F convertible Large LCD display Green backlight turns red if temperature above 37.5 °C (99.5 °F) Fever alarm sounds when temperature above 37.5 °C (99.5 °F)
Forehead Fever Strip	PharmaSystems	PS-700	Forehead			30-60 sec.		Reusable strip for quick temperature check Dual °C and °F scale
High Speed Digital Zoonometer Thermometer	PharmaSystems	327-05	Oral Underarm	Lifetime	Last reading	10 sec.	1 x SR41 or 1 x LR41	Child friendly with an animal top Soft flexible tip for added comfort °C / °F convertible Large night light display Storage case included
Insta-Therm Instant-Read Ear Thermometer	Physio Logic	016-640	Ear	1 year	Last reading	Instant	1 x CR 2032	Easy to read LCD display Celsius (°C) scale only Waterproof lens cleans up easily with a moist cloth or cotton swab No probe cover needed Fever alarm: Upset face L shows on display followed by two long beeps
Insta-Therm Quick Scan Ear/Forehead Thermometer	Physio Logic	016-670	Ear Forehead	1 year	10 readings	Instant	1 x CR 2032	°C / °F convertible Large LCD display Does not require a probe cover Colour coded display changes colour from green to orange if there is a fever
Lifesource Digital Thermometer	Lifesource	DT-607	Oral Rectal Underarm	Lifetime	Last reading	60 sec.	1 x SR41 or 1 x LR41	Rigid tip °C / °F convertible
Mercury Free Thermometer	Mansfield	GER-THERM	Oral	Lifetime		60 sec.		Uses Galinstan, an enviromentally safe alternative to mercury Dual °C and °F scale Includes storage case
Mercury Free Thermometer	PharmaSystems	PS-750	Oral	Lifetime		60 sec.		Uses Galinstan, an enviromentally safe alternative to mercury Dual °C and °F scale Includes storage case

Product	Manufacturer	Model No.	Type	Warranty	Memory	Time to Result	Battery	Comments
Omron 10-Second Digital Thermometer	Omron	MC-106	Oral Rectal Underarm	Lifetime	Last reading	Oral: 10 sec. Rectal: 10 sec. Underarm: 20-30 sec.	1 x SR41 or 1 x LR41	°C / °F convertible 5 Probe covers included Waterproof
Omron 10-Second Flexible Digital Thermometer	Omron	MC-206	Oral Rectal Underarm	Lifetime	Last reading	Oral: 10-20 sec. Rectal: 10 sec. Underarm: 20-30 sec.	1 x SR41 or 1 x LR41	Soft, Flexible tip for added comfort °C / °F convertible 5 Probe covers included
Omron Compact Digital Thermometer	Omron	MC-110	Oral Rectal Underarm	1 year		Oral: 60 sec. Rectal: 40 sec. Underarm: 90 sec.	non-replaceable	Available in °F only Waterproof Optional probe covers sold separately Non-replaceable battery; once depleted, themometer must be replaced
Omron Digital Basal Thermometer	Omron	MC-301N	Oral Rectal Vaginal	Lifetime	Last reading	60 sec.	1 x SR41 or 1 x LR41	Basal thermometer °C / °F convertible Includes 5 probe covers Beep confirms that you are using the thermometer correctly Includes ovulation tracking chart
Omron IntelliTemp Ear Thermometer	Omron	MC-514	Ear	5 years	Last reading	1 sec.	1 x CR 2032	With IntelliTemp Technology mode, which allows to scan temperature for 10 seconds and then displays the highest reading registered °C / °F convertible Probe covers sold separately
Ovu-Therm Basal Thermometer	Mansfield	OVU	Oral Rectal Vaginal	1 year		60 sec.		Basal thermometer Recording chart included Celsius (°C) scale only
Thermoflash Infrared Thermometer	ThermoFlash	LX-26	Forehead	2 years	32 readings	Instant	2 x AA	Infrared thermometer measures temperature without contact, from a distance of 5 cm Can be used to measure temperature of other objects as well °C / °F convertible
ThermoScan ExacTemp Ear Thermometer	Braun	IRT-4520	Ear	3 years	8 readings	Instant	2 x AA	°C / °F convertible Includes 20 probe covers Guidance system confirms that you are using the thermometer correctly Pre-warmed tip
Thermotalk Talking Digital Ear Thermometer	Tremblay Harrison	IRE-A1	Ear	1 year	30 readings	2 sec.	2 x AAA	Real time clock and calendar display (with auto-sleep mode) °C / °F convertible English only

Product	Manufacturer	Model No.	Type	Warranty	Memory	Time to Result	Battery	Comments
Vicks ComfortFlex Digital Thermometer with Fever InSight Feature	Vicks	V966F-CAN	Oral Rectal Underarm	Lifetime	Last reading	8 sec.	1 x SR41 or 1 x LR41	Soft ComfortFlex tip Fever InSight large backlit display changes colour (green, yellow, red) to indicate temperature level °C / °F convertible Waterproof
Vicks Digital Thermometer	Vicks	V901G-CAN	Oral Rectal Underarm	Lifetime	Last reading	30 sec.	1 x SR41 or 1 x LR41	°C / °F convertible Waterproof
Vicks Digital Plus Thermometer	Vicks	V906G-CAN	Oral Rectal Underarm	Lifetime	Last reading	30 sec.	1 x SR41 or 1 x LR41	Large LCD display, easy to read °C / °F convertible Waterproof for easy cleaning
Vicks Ear Thermometer	Vicks	V971CFN-CAN	Ear	1 year	12 readings	Instant	2 x AA	Gentle ComfortTouch soft sensor tip Audible fever alert indicates temperature over 37.5 °C (99.5 °F) °C / °F convertible Large, lighted LCD display Includes probe cover applicator and 20 probe covers
Vicks Forehead Thermometer	Vicks	V977N-CAN	Forehead	3 years	12 readings	3 sec.	2 x AAA	Fever InSight large backlit display changes colour (green, yellow, red) to indicate temperature level Beeps when temperature reading is complete °C / °F convertible
Vicks SpeedRead Digital Thermometer with Fever InSight Feature	Vicks	V912F-CAN	Oral Rectal Underarm	Lifetime	Last reading	8 sec.	1 x SR41 or 1 x LR41	Fever InSight large backlit display changes colour (green, yellow, red) to indicate temperature level °C / °F convertible Waterproof
Vicks Underarm Thermometer	Vicks	V932-CAN	Underarm	Lifetime	Last reading	30 sec.	1 x SR41 or 1 x LR41	Takes underarm measurements only Ideal for toddlers and older children Large LCD display Comfort disc shaped to fit under arm

Disease/Condition	Product	Manufacturer	Recommended Use	Dosage Form	Active Ingredients
Allergies	Allergies	Homeocan	Allergies	granules	allium cepa 6X aralia racemosa 6X arsenicum album 6X cuprum metallicum 8X euphrasia 6X nux vomica 8X sabadilla 6X sticta pulmonaria 6X
	Hay Fever	Homeocan	Hay fever	granules	allium cepa 6X apis mellifica 9CH aralia racemosa 6X cuprum metallicum 9X sabadilla 6X sticta pulmonaria 6X
	Hayfever	Hylands	Hay fever	tablet	allium cepa 3X ambrosia 3X euphrasia officinalis 3X sabadilla 3X
	Hives	Hylands	Hives	tablet	apis mellifica 3X arsenicum album 6X natrum muriaticum 6X urtica urens 3X
Anxiety	Calms Forté	Hylands	Nervous tension, sleeplessness	caplet	avena sativa 1X calcarea phosphorica 3X chamomilla 2X ferrum phosphorica 3X humulus lupulus 1X kali phosphoricum 3X magnesia phosphoricum 3X natrum phosphoricum 3X passiflora 1X
	Calms Forté 4 Kids	Hylands	Mental and physical restlessness in children ages 2 and up	tablet	aconitum nap. 6X calc. phos 12X chamomilla 6X cina 6X lycopodium 6X nat. mur. 6X pulsatilla 6X sulphur 6X
	Nerve Tonic	Hylands	Nervous tension, sleeplessness	caplet	calcarea phosphorica 3X ferrum phosphorica 3X kali phosphoricum 3X magnesia phosphoricum 3X natrum phosphoricum 3X
	Stress	Homeocan	Stress, anxiety, moodiness, fatigue	granules	argentum nitricum 9X asa foetida 3X avena sativa 3X ignatia amara 4X valeriana officinalis 3X
Baby Colic	Cocyntal	Boiron	Baby colic	liquid unidoses	carbo vegetabilis 5CH colocynthis 9CH cuprum metallicum 5CH
	Colic	Hylands	Baby colic	tablet	chamomilla 3X colocynthis 3X dioscorea 12X
	Kid's Colic	Homeocan	Intestinal gas, colic	pellets	chamomilla 6X colocynthis 6X dioscorea villosa 6X magnesia phosphorica 6X

Disease/Condition	Product	Manufacturer	Recommended Use	Dosage Form	Active Ingredients
Bumps and Bruises	Arnica	Homeocan	Pain due to bumps, bruises, strains, etc.	granules	arnica montana 10X, 30X, 100X
Bumps and Bruises	Arnica plus, Pain Relief Cream	Homeocan	Minor bruises, strains, sprains	topical	arnica montana 4X hypericum perforatum 4X symphytum officinalis 4X
	Arnicare Sport	Boiron	Bruises, muscle pain	tablet	arnica montana 9CH sarcolacticum acidum 3CH zincum oxydatum 3CH
	Bumps and Bruises	Hylands	Bumps and bruises	tablet	arnica 6X hypericum perforatum 6X bellis perennis 6X ruta graveolens 6X
Colds and Flu	Bronchial Cough	Hylands	Cough with mucus	tablet	kalium bichromium 3X rumex crispus 3X sanguinaria canadensis 3X
	Coryzalia	Boiron	Colds, runny nose, congestion	tablet	allium cepa 3CH belladonna 3CH gelsemium 3CH kalium bichromium 3CH pulsatilla 3CH sabadilla 3CH
	Coryzalia for Children	Boiron	Colds, runny nose, congestion	liquid unidoses	allium cepa 3CH belladonna 3CH gelsemium 3CH kalium bichromium 3CH pulsatilla 3CH sabadilla 3CH
	Cough & Cold	Homeocan	Cough, sore throat, runny nose, bronchitis	granules	belladonna 4X drosera 3X ipecacuanha 6X kali bichromicum 12X mercurius solubilis 30X pulsatilla 12X
	Cough	Hylands	Cough due to common cold	tablet	antimonium tartaricum 6X bryonia 3X causticum 3X hepar sulphuricum 3X
	C-Plus	Hylands	Runny nose, sneezing in children	tablet	eupatorium perfoliatum 2X euphrasia officinalis 2X gelsemium sempervirens 3X kali Iodatum 3X
	Echinacea	Homeocan	Immunity, sinusitis, repeated infections	granules	echinacea purpurea 6X echinacea purpurea12X zincum metallicum 10X
	Homeocoksinum	Homeocan	Flu symptoms, chills, aches and pains, fever	single dose tubes	anas barbariae hepatis et cordis extractum 200C
	Hylands Flu	Hylands	Fever, chills, body aches and pains	tablet	eupatorium perfoliatum 3X bryonia 3X gelsemium 3X euphrasia officinalis 3X kali iodatum 3X anas barbaria hepatis et cordis 200C
	Oscillococcinum	Boiron	Flu symptoms	single dose tubes	anas barbariae hepatis et cordis extractum 200C
	Oscillococcinum for Children	Boiron	Flu symptoms in children	single dose tubes	anas barbariae hepatis et cordis extractum 200C

Disease/Condition	Product	Manufacturer	Recommended Use	Dosage Form	Active Ingredients
Cold and Flu	Sinus	Hylands	Sinus congestion	tablet	calcarea carbonica 3X hydrastis canadensis 3X kali bichromicum 3X pulsatilla 3X
Constipation	Constipation L.106	Homeocan	Constipation, flatulence	drops	alumina 6X argentum met. 6X bryonia 6X magnesia oxyd. 8X plumbum acet. 6X valeriana officinalis 8X zincum metallicum 8X
Cough	Hylands Cough	Hylands	Cough	tablet	antimonium tartaricum 6X bryonia 3X causticum 3X hepar sulfuricum 3X
	Phytotux H	Homeocan	Cough, cold, bronchitis	syrup	arnica 3CH belladonna 3CH bryonia 3CH cetraria 1CH coccus cacti 3CH corallium rubrum 3CH drosera 1CH ipeca 3CH stannum metallicum 3CH
	Stodal Pellets	Boiron	Cough	pellets	anemone pulsatilla 3CH antimonium tartaricum 6CH bryonia dioica 3CH coccus cacti 3CH ipecacuahna 3CH rumex crispus 6CH spongia tosta 3CH sticta pulmonaria 3CH
	Stodal Syrup	Boiron	Cough	syrup	anemone pulsatilla 6CH antimonium tartaricum 6CH bryonia dioica 3CH coccus cacti 3CH drosera MT ipecacuanha 3CH rumex crispus 6CH spongia tosta 3CH sticta pulmonaria 3CH polygala syrup 19g tolu syrup 19g
	Stodal for Children	Boiron	Cough	syrup	anemone pulsatilla 6CH antimonium tartaricum 6CH bryonia dioica 3CH coccus cacti 3CH drosera 3CH ipecacuanha 3CH rumex crispus 6CH spongia tosta 3CH sticta pulmonaria 3CH
Dental	Camilia	Boiron	Baby teething	liquid unidoses	belladonna 5CH chamomilla 9CH ferrum phosphoricum 5CH
	Kids' Teething	Homeocan	Baby teething and irritability	pellets	arnica 5C borax 5C chamomilla 5C hypericum 5C

Disease/Condition	Product	Manufacturer	Recommended Use	Dosage Form	Active Ingredients
Dental	Orajel Homeopathic Remedy Teething Gel	Church & Dwight	Baby teething	gel	calcarea phosphorica 12X chamomilla 6X coffea cruda 6X
	Teething	Hylands	Restlessness and wakeful irritability	tablet	belladonna 3X calcarea phosphorica 3X chamomilla 3X coffee cruda 3X
	Teething Gel	Hylands	Restlessness and wakeful irritability	gel	belladonna 6X calcarea phosphorica 12X chamomilla 6X coffee cruda 6X
Dermatological	Acne	Homeocan	Acne, oily skin	granules	antimonium tartaricum 6X calcarea picrata 6K echinacea ang. 3K kalium bromatum 6K nux vomica 6K pulsatilla 6K selenium metallicum 3K sulfur iodatum 6K thuja occidentalis 6K viola tricolor 3K
	Calendula	Homeocan	Minor cuts, scrapes, burns	topical	calendula off. MT cantharis 3X echinacea ang. MT hypericum perf. 3X phytolacca decandra 3X sulfur 3X
	Calendula Gel	Boiron	Cuts, burns, sunburn	topical	calendula officinalis 7%
	Cold Sores	Hylands	Cold sores, cracked lips	tablet	antimonium crudum 3X baptisia tinctoria 3X borax 2X natrum muriaticum 3X
	Poison Ivy/Oak	Hylands	Itching, burning and crusting skin	tablet	croton tiglium 6X rhus toxicodendron 6X xerophyllum 6X
Dysmenorrhea/PMS	Hylands Menstrual Cramps	Hylands	Cramps	tablet	cimicifuga racemosa 12X colocynthis 12X magnesia phosphorica 12X pulsatilla 6X
	Hylands PMS	Hylands	Painful menstruation, cramping, irritability	tablet	caulophyllum 3X cocculus indicus 3X gelsemium sempervirens 3X viburnum opulus 2X
	P.M.S.	Homeocan	Menstrual cramping, irritability, fatigue, anxiety	granules	cimicifuga racemosa 4X hydrastis canadensis 4X hyoscyamus niger 4X lycopodium clavatum 4X mercurius corrosivus 4X nitricum acidum 9X sabina 8X secale cornutum 14X
Ears	Earache	Hylands	Earache symptoms, fever, pain, irritability and sleeplessness	liquid / tablet	belladonna 30C calcarea carbonica 30C chamomilla 30C lycopodium 30C pulsatilla 30C sulfur 30C

Disease/Condition	Product	Manufacturer	Recommended Use	Dosage Form	Active Ingredients
Ears	Earache Pain	Homeocan	Earache pain	granules	aurum met. 30K capsicum annuum 30K ferrum phosphoricum 30K kalium sulphuricum 6K mercurius vivus 6K pyrogenium 30K thuja occidentalis 30K
	Kids' Earache	Homeocan	Earache pain in children	pellets	belladonna 30K capsicum 30K ferrum phosphoricum 30K metallum album 30K pyrogenium 30K
Fatigue	Alfalfa Tonic	Boiron	Fatigue	syrup	alfalfa MT avena sativa MT cyclamen europaeum 6X eleutherococcus MT ginseng MT kalium phosphoricum 5CH menyanthes trifoliata 3X
	Alfalfa Tonic	Homeocan	Physical and intellectual fatigue	liquid	agnus castus 3X alfalfa MT avena sativa MT cinnamomum 1X ginseng MT kali arsenicosum 6X phosphoricum acidum 3X selenium metallicum 4X
	Magnesium +	Homeocan	Fatigue, cramps	tablet	ambra grisea 5X kalium phosphoricum 5X magnesii chloras. 1X magnesii phosphas 1X magnesii stereate 3X plumbum metallicum 8X
Gastrointestinal	Diarrex	Hylands	Acute diarrhea	tablet	arsenicum album 6X chamomilla 6X mercurius viv. 6X phosphorus 6X podophyllum peltatum 6X
	Digestion	Homeocan	Digestive discomfort, nausea, bloating	drops	carduus marianus 3X chelidonium majus 3X dolichos pruriens 3X leptandra 3X lycopodium 3X nux vomica 3X
	Hylands Gas	Hylands	Flatulence, belching, gas	tablet	asafoetida 3X ignatia 3X lycopodium 6X nux moschata 3X
	Hylands Upset Stomach	Hylands	Improper digestion and gastric upset	tablet	carbo vegetalis 3X nux vomica 3X
	Indigestion	Hylands	Hyperacidity	tablet	cinchona officinalis 3X hydrastis canadensis 3X kali bichromicum 3X phosphoricum acidum 3X
Hemorrhoids	Hylands Hemorrhoids	Hylands	Itching and burning pains	tablet	aesculus hippocastanum 3X calcarea fluorica 6X nux vomica 3X ratanhia 3X

Disease/Condition	Product	Manufacturer	Recommended Use	Dosage Form	Active Ingredients
Hyperactivity	Calms Forté	Hylands	Nervous tension	tablet	avena sativa 1X calcerea phosphorica 3X chamomilla 2X ferrum phospharica 3X humulus lupulus 1X kali phosphoricum 3X magnesia phosphoricum 3X natrum phosphoricum 3X passiflora incarnata 1X
	Calms Forté 4 Kids	Hylands	Mental and physical restlessness in children ages 2 and up	tablet	aconitum nap. 6X calc. phos 6X chamomilla 6X cina 6X lycopodium 6X nat. mur. 6X pulsatilla 6X sulphur 6X
Insect Bites	Dapis Gel	Boiron	Insect bites, itching	gel	apis mellifica 6X ledum palustre MT
Insomnia	Calms Forté	Hylands	Insomnia	caplet	avena sativa 1X calcarea phosphorica 3X chamomilla 2X humulus lupulus 1X kali phosphoricum 3X magnesia phosphoricum 3X natrum phosphoricum 3X passiflora 1X
	Calms Forté 4 Kids	Hylands	Mental and physical restlessness in children ages 2 and up	tablet	aconitum nap. 6X calc. phos 12X chamomilla 6X cina 6X lycopodium 6X nat. mur. 6X pulsatilla 6X sulphur 6X
	Hylands Insomnia	Hylands	Insomnia	tablet	hyoscyamus 3X ignatia amara 3X kali phosphoricum 3X
	Insomnia	Homeocan	Insomnia, anxiety	granules	avena sativa 4X hyoscyamus niger 9X passiflora inc. 4X valeriana officinalis 4X
Menopause	Menopause	Homeocan	Hot flashes, irritability, mood swings	granules	amyl nitrosum 9X aurum metallicum 9X bryonia alba 4X lachesis 10X sanguinaria canadensis 9X
Motion Sickness	Cocculine	Boiron	Motion sickness	tablet	cocculus 4CH colubrina 4CH petroleum 4CH tabacum 4CH
	Hylands Motion Sickness	Hylands	Nausea, dizziness	tablet	cocculus indicus 30X nux vomica 6X petroleum 12X tabacum 6X

Disease/Condition	Product	Manufacturer	Recommended Use	Dosage Form	Active Ingredients
Pain	Arthritic Pain	Homeocan	Arthritic pain	granules	apis mellifica 6X arnica montana 7X benzoicum acidum 3X causticum 6X colchicum autumnale 4X natrum carbonicum 4X
	Magnesium+	Homeocan	Nocturnal cramps, fatigue	tablet	ambra grisca 5X kalium phos. 5X magnesii chloras 1X magnesii phosphas 1X magnesii stereate 3X plumbum metallicum 8X
Sinus	Echinacea	Homeocan	Sinusitis, immunity, repeated infections	granules	echinacea purpurea, herba 6X and 12X echinacea purpurea, radix 6X and 12X zincum metallicum 10X
	Sinus	Homeocan	Sinus head pain, congestion and sinus pressure	granules	allium cepa 9X euphrasia officinalis 9X hepar sulfuris calcareum 9X hydrastis 3X sticta pulmonaria 9X thuja occidentalis 4X
Snoring	Snore Stop	Nutravite	Reduces snoring	spray	belladonna 6X ephedra vulgaris 6X histaminum hydrochloride 12X hydrastis canadensis 6X kali bichromium 6X nux vomica 4X teucrium marum 6X
Urinary Tract Health	EnurAid	Hylands	Involuntary urination in adults	tablet	apis mellifica 6X allium cepa 6X arnica montana 6X belladonna 6X cantharis 6X equisetum hyemale 3X rhus aromatica 6X

Product	Product	Manufacturer	Features
Intermittent Catheters for Men	Cysto-Care Red Rubber	Coloplast	Available as regular tip or coude
Intermittent Catheters for Men	Self-Cath Intermittent Catheters	Coloplast	Siliconized catheters with fire-polished eyelets Available with straight tip, coude-tapered tip, or coude olive tip Latex-free
Intermittent Catheters for Men	Self-Cath Plus	Coloplast	Siliconized catheters with fire-polished eyelets Hydrophilic coating activates with water for low friction catheterization Has uncoated grip zone Latex-free
Intermittent Catheters for Men	SpeediCath Complete for Men	Coloplast	Ready-to-use design with a non-touch handle and insertion guide Complete with an integrated collection bag Latex and PVC free
Intermittent Catheters for Men	SpeediCath Intermittent Catheter	Coloplast	Available in nelaton and coude Latex and PVC free
Intermittent Catheters for Women	Self-Cath Intermittent Catheters	Coloplast	Siliconized catheters with fire-polished eyelets Available with straight tip and straight tip with Luer end Latex-free
Intermittent Catheters for Women	SpeediCath Compact for Women	Coloplast	Designed for women Catheter length is 7 cm Non-touch insertion guide About the size of a highlighter
Intermittent Catheters for Women	SpeediCath Complete for Women	Coloplast	Ready-to-use design With a non-touch handle and insertion guide Complete with an integrated collection bag Latex and PVC free
Intermittent Catheters for Women	SpeediCath Intermittent Catheter	Coloplast	Available in nelaton Latex and PVC free
Intermittent Catheters for Children	Self-Cath Intermittent Catheters	Coloplast	Siliconized catheters with fire-polished eyelets Latex-free
Intermittent Catheters for Children	SpeediCath Intermittent Catheter	Coloplast	Available in nelaton Latex and PVC free
Unisex Catheters	Advance Hydro Soft	Hollister	Slippery hydrophilic coating Secure grip section Silicone construction Latex-free
Unisex Catheters	Advance Plus Closed System	Hollister	Available in straight tip or coude tip Latex-free
Unisex Catheters	Hollister Intermittent Catheter	Hollister	Available in straight tip, straight tip with luer end, straight tip with curved packaging, coude tip Ultra-smooth eyelets Latex-free
Male External Catheters	Conveen Security + External Catheter and Liner	Coloplast	2-piece catheter Adhesive can be placed to accommodate shorter shaft lengths Double-sided adhesive liner Available in latex and also in latex-free silicone
Male External Catheters	Active Cath Latex Catheter	Coloplast	Extended wear One-piece catheter
Male External Catheters	Clear Advantage	Coloplast	Self-adhering Made from silicone
Male External Catheters	Conveen Optima	Coloplast	Self-sealing Features push ring for secure connection to a leg bag and an anti-kink bulb to prevent backflow Latex-free

Product	Product	Manufacturer	Features
Male External Catheters	Conveen Security + Self-Sealing Catheter	Coloplast	1-piece catheter has integrated band of adhesive; has pull tabs to facilitate application Available in latex and also in latex-free silicone
Male External Catheters	Everyday Male External Catheter	Hollister	Self-adhesive Easy applicator collar
Male External Catheters	Extended Wear Latex External Catheter	Hollister	Self-adhesive Inner flap Easy applicator collar
Male External Catheters	Freedom Cath Latex Catheter	Coloplast	For standard every day use
Male External Catheters	Freedom Clear	Coloplast	Self-adhering Made from silicone
Male External Catheters	Freedom Clear LS (long seal)	Coloplast	Longer length adhesive seal
Male External Catheters	Freedom Clear SS (sport sheath)	Coloplast	Useful for men with penis retractions
Male External Catheters	InView	Hollister	Self-adhesive Available in 3 styles: special (shorter catheter length), standard and extra (70% more adhesive for added security) Latex-free
Pelvic Muscle Electric Stimulators	Cefar Peristim Pro	Empi (division of DJO Canada)	A dual channel incontinence stimulator Features nine preset incontinence program for use with a vaginal probe, anal probe and with surface electrodes Channels are simultaneous, which means that a selected program applies to both channels
Pelvic Muscle Electric Stimulators	Femetone Trophic Continence Stimulator	Biomation	Neuromuscular stimulator for treatment of incontinence Not programmable
Pelvic Muscle Electric Stimulators	FemiScan E-Stim	Mega Electronics	Electrical muscle stimulator for treatment of incontinence Suitable for men and women who have difficulty identifying their pelvic muscles Includes default programs for the treatment of stress incontinence, urge incontinence and pelvic floor pain
Pelvic Muscle Electric Stimulators	FemiScan Home Trainer	Mega Electronics	Interactive biofeedback device for women Designed for pelvic floor exercises Monitors muscle activity during every contraction and saves data from every session
Pelvic Muscle Electric Stimulators	ISIS ETS 290 Pelvic Floor Stimulator	Biomation	Neuromuscular stimulator for treatment of incontinence Has an automatic mode, with pre-set programs and a manual mode, to select the stimulation parameters
Pelvic Muscle Electric Stimulators	Minnova	Empi (division of DJO Canada)	Neuromuscular stimulator Manual mode only Comes with vaginal and rectal probe
Pelvic Muscle Electric Stimulators	Neuro-4 Trophic Muscle Stimulator	Biomation	Neuromuscular stimulator for treatment of incontinence Available with pre-programmed treatment cards for various uses
Fecal Incontinence	Drainable Fecal Collector with Flextend Barrier	Hollister	Flextend skin barrier provides strong ahderence and conforms to body contour Tapered skin barrier edge Barrier can be cut to fit Drain valve Can be left in place for up to 7 days as long as skin barrier is intact and adherent
Fecal Incontinence	Drainable Fecal Collector with Softflex skin barrier	Hollister	Softflex skin barrier provides gentle adherence that is essential when frequent removal of device is necessary Tapered skin barrier edge Barrier can be cut to fit Drain valve

Product	Product	Manufacturer	Features
Fecal Incontinence	Peristeen Anal Plug	Coloplast	Anal plug made from foam Conforms to the shape of the rectal cavity and protects against leakage May be left in rectum for up to 12 hours Comes with a lubricant
Various Devices	ActiCuf Compression Pouch	GT Urological	Disposable absorbent pouch designed to treat and manage light to moderate male incontinence Padded closure presses down on the urethra to control urinary flow Not to be used at night
Various Devices	Aquaflex Plevic Floor Exercise Cone System	Biomation	Designed to help target and strengthen pelvic floor muscles through passive contraction.
Various Devices	C3 Penile Clamp	SRS Medical	Designed to manage mild to moderate male incontinence Clamps around penis and puts pressure on the urethra
Various Devices	Conveen Drip Collector	Coloplast	Disposable absorbent pouch designed for moderate male incontinence Holds up to 3 oz of urine Adheres to underwear
Various Devices	Dribblestop Penile Clamp	Rennich Industries	Fully adjustable links to change size Safe to use at night for 24 hour control
Various Devices	Female Urinary Pouch	Hollister	Cut-to-fit, skin barrier Odour barrier film Alternative to indwelling catheter for bedbound females
Various Devices	FemSoft Female Urethral Insert	Rochester Medical	Disposable insert available by prescription only Made from silicone and mineral oil Designed to conform to her individual shape Creates a soft seal at the bladder neck Not recommended for use at night
Various Devices	Hodge Vaginal Pessary with Knob	Milex (Cooper Surgical)	Has wires that allow it to be shaped for different anatomies
Various Devices	Hodge Vaginal Pessary with Knob	Superior Medical	Has wires that allow it to be shaped for different anatomies
Various Devices	Incontinence Dish Vaginal Pessary	Milex (Cooper Surgical)	Available with and without support Made from silicone Latex-free
Various Devices	Incontinence Dish Vaginal Pessary	Superior Medical	Available with and without support Made from silicone Latex-free
Various Devices	Incontinence Ring Vaginal Pessary	Milex (Cooper Surgical)	Available with and without support Made from silicone Latex-free
Various Devices	Incontinence Ring Vaginal Pessary	Superior Medical	Available with and without support Made from silicone Latex-free
Various Devices	LadySystem	Duchesnay	Designed to help target and strengthen pelvic floor muscles through passive contraction.
Various Devices	Retracted Penis Pouch External Collection Device	Hollister	Cut-to-fit, skin barrier Odour barrier film Convenience drain
Various Devices	Uresta Vaginal Pessary Kit	EastMed	Stops leaking from the bladder by supporting the urethra, tapered end makes insertion easier Made from latex-free rubber

Product	Manufacturer	Absorbency	Comments
AMG Protective Underwear Unisex	AMG Medical	moderate to heavy	Tear-away sides for easy removal
Attends Bariatric Briefs	Attends Healthcare Products	maximum	Breathable side panels Extra wide easy-fit tape tabs Cloth-like inner liner Poly outer covering
Attends Breathable Briefs	Attends Healthcare Products	moderate to heavy	Breathable side panels Non-woven cloth-like inner and outer covering Comfort flex-tabs can refasten anywhere on the brief
Attends Breathable Briefs Extra Absorbent	Attends Healthcare Products	maximum	Breathable side panels Non-woven cloth-like inner and outer covering Comfort flex-tabs can refasten anywhere on the brief
Attends Briefs Waistband Style	Attends Healthcare Products	moderate	Stretchable waistband and 6 tape tabs for custom fit Cloth-like inner liner Poly outer covering
Attends Light Pads	Attends Healthcare Products	light	
Attends Male Guard	Attends Healthcare Products	light	Form-fitting shape Adhesive peel strip to keep it in place
Attends Shaped Pads	Attends Healthcare Products	heavy to maximum	Form-fitting shape Color-coded for every level of absorbency
Attends Pads	Attends Healthcare Products	light to moderate	Cloth-like inner and outer covering Adhesive patch for secure fit Available in Regular, Extra, Plus and Ultimate Absorbency
Attends Poly Briefs	Attends Healthcare Products	heavy	Breathable side panels Cloth-like inner liner Comfort flex-tabs can refasten anywhere on the brief
Attends Protective Underwear Overnight	Attends Healthcare Products	heavy	Pull-on design Breathable side panels Non-woven cloth-like inner and outer covering
Attends Protective Underwear Extra Absorbency	Attends Healthcare Products	moderate to heavy	Pull-on design Breathable side panels Non-woven cloth-like inner and outer covering
Attends Protective Underwear Regular Absorbency	Attends Healthcare Products	moderate	Pull-on design Breathable side panels Non-woven cloth-like inner and outer covering
Attends Undergarment Belted Style	Attends Healthcare Products	moderate to heavy	Pads with reusable belts Rapid-lock system
Depend Adjustable Underwear	Kimberly-Clark	moderate to heavy	Can be slipped on and off like regular underwear Has tabs that can be re-adjusted for a custom fit
Depend Belted Shields	Kimberly-Clark	moderate	Available as button strap or velcro strap Fits large hip sizes (up to 65 inches) Can be worn with underwear for additional protection and discretion
Depend Fitted Briefs Maximum Protection	Kimberly-Clark	maximum	For people with limited mobility Concentrates material in the centre for nighttime leakage protection Wetness indicator line disappears when brief requires removing
Depend Guards for Men	Kimberly-Clark	light to moderate	Designed for men Temporary or long-term loss of bladder control after surgery

Product	Manufacturer	Absorbency	Comments
Depend Overnight Fitted Brief	Kimberly-Clark	overnight	Concentrates material in the centre for nighttime leakage protection
Depend Protection with Tabs	Kimberly-Clark	maximum	Breathable side panels 6 easygrip tape tabs for custom fit Wetness indicator line disappears when brief requires removing
Depend Real Fit Briefs for Men	Kimberly-Clark	maximum	Finished waistband cloth-like inner and outer covering slim side profile
Depend Silhouette Briefs for Women	Kimberly-Clark	maximum	Finished waistband cloth-like inner and outer covering slim side profile
Depend Underwear for Men	Kimberly-Clark	moderate to heavy	
Depend Underwear for Women - Extra Absorbency	Kimberly-Clark	moderate	
Depend Underwear for Women - Super Plus Absorbency	Kimberly-Clark	moderate to heavy	
Poise Liners Extra Coverage	Kimberly-Clark	very light	
Poise Liners Regular	Kimberly-Clark	very light	
Poise Pads Maximum	Kimberly-Clark	moderate to heavy	
Poise Pads Maximum Extra coverage	Kimberly-Clark	moderate to heavy	Longer pad for extra coverage
Poise Pads Moderate	Kimberly-Clark	moderate	
Poise Pads Moderate Extra Coverage	Kimberly-Clark	moderate	Longer pad for extra coverage
Poise Pads Moderate with Wings	Kimberly-Clark	moderate	
Poise Pads Ultimate	Kimberly-Clark	maximum	
Poise Pads Ultimate Extra Coverage	Kimberly-Clark	maximum	
Poise Pads Ultra Thin Light	Kimberly-Clark	light	
Poise Pads Ultra Thin Light with Wings	Kimberly-Clark	light	
TENA Heavy Pads Long (formerly Ultra Plus)	SCA Hygiene Products	heavy	
TENA Men Protective Guards	SCA Hygiene Products	moderate	Adheres to underwear
TENA Men Underwear Super Plus	SCA Hygiene Products	moderate to heavy	
TENA Moderate Pads Long(formerly Extra Plus)	SCA Hygiene Products	moderate but frequent	
TENA Moderate Pads Long with Aloe Vera	SCA Hygiene Products	moderate but frequent	
TENA Moderate Pads Regular Length (formerly Extra)	SCA Hygiene Products	light to moderate	
TENA Pantiliners Long	SCA Hygiene Products	very light	
TENA Pantiliners Regular Length	SCA Hygiene Products	very light	
TENA Protective Underwear Ultimate Extra Absorbency	SCA Hygiene Products	maximum	
TENA Ultimate Pads Overnight	SCA Hygiene Products	overnight	
TENA Ultimate Pads Regular Length	SCA Hygiene Products	heavy	
TENA Ultra Thin Pads	SCA Hygiene Products	light	
TENA Ultra Thin Pads Long	SCA Hygiene Products	light	Longer pad for extra coverage
TENA Women Protective Underwear Super Plus	SCA Hygiene Products	moderate to heavy	

Product	Manufacturer	Features
Deluxe Pull-On Incontinence Pants	AMG Medical	Pull-on type Made from nylon tricot Machine washable and boilable
Deluxe Snap-On Incontinence Pants	AMG Medical	Has snap closures on both sides Made from nylon tricot Machine washable
Economy Pull-On Incontinence Pants	AMG Medical	Made from poly-vinyl materials to make them less noisy Can be used over regular or disposable underwear
Incontinence Pants with Snap Closures	Mansfield	Snap closures on both sides Designed to be worn under clothing with a liner Machine washable

Product	Manufacturer	Dosage Form	Active Ingredients
Ben's 30 Wilderness Spray	Tender	spray	DEET plus related toluamides 30%
Ben's 30 Wipes	Tender	towelette	DEET plus related toluamides 30%
Buzz Away Extreme Spray	Quantum Health	pump spray	castor oil cedarwood oil citronella oil coconut oil geranium oil glycerin lemongrass oil peppermint oil soybean oil
Buzz Away Original	Quantum Health	gel	cedarwood citronella oil eucalyptus lemongrass peppermint
Citronella Insect Repellent Lotion	Laboratoires Druide	lotion	citronella terpene 5% essential oil of citronella 10%
Citronella Insect Repellent Milk	Laboratoires Druide	milk	citronella terpene 5% essential oil of citronella 10%
Muskol Aerosol	Schering-Plough	aerosol spray	DEET 25%
Muskol Classic Liquid	Schering-Plough	lotion	DEET plus related toluamides 30%
Muskol Pump Spray	Schering-Plough	pump spray	DEET plus related toluamides 30%
Natrapel Lotion	Tender	lotion	citronella 10%
Natrapel Pump Spray	Tender	pump spray	citronella 10%
OFF! Active Aerosol	S.C. Johnson	aerosol spray	DEET plus related toluamides 15%
OFF! Active Lotion	S.C. Johnson	lotion	DEET plus related toluamides 7.5%
OFF! Active Pump Spray	S.C. Johnson	pump spray	DEET plus related toluamides 25%
OFF! Deep Woods Aerosol	S.C. Johnson	spray	DEET plus related toluamides 25%
OFF! Deep Woods Pump Spray	S.C. Johnson	pump spray	DEET plus related toluamides 25%
OFF! Deep Woods Sportsmen	S.C. Johnson	aerosol	DEET plus related toluamides 25%
OFF! Deep Woods Towelettes	S.C. Johnson	towelette	DEET plus related toluamides 25%
OFF! Skintastic	S.C. Johnson	pump spray	DEET plus related toluamides 7%
OFF! Skintastic for Kids	S.C. Johnson	pump spray	DEET plus related toluamides 5%
OFF! Skintastic Smooth & Dry	S.C. Johnson	spray	DEET plus related toluamides 15%
OFF! Skintastic Towelettes for Kids	S.C. Johnson	towelette	DEET plus related toluamides 7%
Skin So Soft Bug Guard plus Icaridin	Avon	spray	icaridin 10%
Watkins Insect Repellent Lotion	Watkins	lotion	DEET plus related toluamides 28.5%
Watkins Insect Repellent Spray	Watkins	spray	DEET plus related toluamides 23.75%

Product	Manufacturer	Dosage Form	Ingredients
EMLA Cream	AstraZeneca	cream	lidocaine 2.5% prilocaine 2.5%

Product	Manufacturer	Warranty	Power Source	Contents
BOSS 2000-3	Pos-T-Vac	Lifetime warranty on all major components	pump	Vacuum pump Cylinder Rings Mounting cone Personal lubricant Video instructions Carrying case
Encore VTU1	Encore Medical Products	Lifetime warranty on all hard plastic parts	pump	Vacuum pump Cylinder 4 numbered revive rings Mounting cone Lubricant
Encore VTUE	Encore Medical Products	Lifetime warranty on all hard plastic parts	battery	Vacuum pump Cylinder 4 numbered revive rings Mounting cone Lubricant
Osbon ErecAid Classic Vacuum Therapy System	Auto Control Medical	Lifetime warranty on cylinder and pump handle only against defective workmanship or materials	pump	Hand pump Cylinder 4 pressure-point tension rings Connecting tube Osbon personal lubricant Bilingual user's manual Bilingual video
Pos-T-Vac MVP 700	Pos-T-Vac	Lifetime warranty on all major components	pump	Vacuum pump Cylinder Rings Mounting cone Personal lubricant Video instructions Carrying case

Product	Manufacturer	Dosage Form	Anesthetic	Other Active Ingredients
Abreva	GlaxoSmithKline Consumer Healthcare	gel		docosanol 10%
Anbesol Gel	Paladin	gel	benzocaine 10%	
Anbesol Gel Extra Strength	Paladin	gel	benzocaine 20%	
Anbesol Liquid Maximum Strength	Paladin	liquid	benzocaine 20%	
Bionet Lozenge	Church & Dwight	lozenge	benzocaine 7.5 mg	cetalkonium chloride 5 mg
Blistex DCT Medicated Lip Balm	Blistex	ointment		camphor 0.38% menthol 0.6% octinoxate 7.3% oxybenzone 4.5% phenol 0.48%
Blistex Five Star Lip Protection	Blistex	ointment		homosalate 9.6% octinoxate 7.5% octisalate 5% oxybenzone 5% petrolatum 30.1%
Blistex Fruit Smoothies Lip Balm	Blistex	stick		dimethicone 2% octinoxate 7.5% oxybenzone 2.5%
Blistex Herbal Answer Lip Balm	Blistex	ointment		octinoxate 7.5% oxybenzone 2.5% petrolatum 43%
Blistex Lip Balm Regular/Berry/Mint	Blistex	ointment		dimethicone 2% oxybenzone 2.5% padimate O 6.6%
Blistex Lip Medex	Blistex	ointment		camphor 1% menthol 1% phenol 0.54%
Blistex Medicated Lip Conditioner SPF 15	Blistex	ointment		camphor 0.38% menthol 0.6% meradimate 2.5% octinoxate 6.6% phenol 0.45%
Blistex Medicated Lip Ointment	Blistex	ointment		allantoin 1% camphor 0.5% phenol 0.5%
Blistex Moisture Melt	Blistex	ointment		octinoxate 7.5% oxybenzone 2.5% petrolatum 31.7%
Blistex Silk & Shine Lip Balm	Blistex	stick		dimethicone 2% octinoxate 7.5% oxybenzone 2.5%
Blistex Raspberry Lemonade Blast	Blistex	ointment		dimethicone 1% octinoxate 7.5% oxybenzone 2.5%
Canker Care +	Quantum Health	gel		menthol 0.5%
Canker Cover Patch	Quantum Health	patch		menthol 2.5 mg
Canker-X	Sunstar GUM	gel		aloe vera polyvinyl pyrrolidone (PVP) sodium hyaluronate
Cold Sore Lotion	Rougier	liquid		benzoin 10% camphor 4% menthol 2%
Fletcher's Sore Mouth Medicine	Advantage CKN	liquid		potassium alum 1.28% potassium chlorate 2.5%

▶

Product	Manufacturer	Dosage Form	Anesthetic	Other Active Ingredients
Herpestat Lip Shield	Origin BioMed	ointment		self-heal extract (prunella vulgaris) 0.2% vitamin C 0.09% vitamin E 0.1% zinc 0.8 %
Kank-A	Blistex	liquid	benzocaine 20%	cetylpyridinium chloride 0.1%
Korner's Cold Sore Remedy (Dr. Krane)	Taiga Bioactives	ointment		geranium extract 5%
L-Lysine 500 mg Tablets	Various Manufacturers	capsule		lysine hydrochloride 500 mg
Lipactin	Novartis Consumer Health	gel		heparin sodium 160 IU/g zinc sulfate 5 mg/g
Lipclear Lysine Plus Ointment	Quantum Health	ointment		lysine zinc oxide 1.2 %
Lipsorex	Canderm	gel		benzethonium chloride 0.26% menthol 0.9% thymol 0.34%
Nature's Harmony L-Lysine 500 mg	SunOpta	capsule		lysine 500 mg
Orabase Paste	ConvaTec	paste		gelatin 13.3% pectin 13.3% sodium carboxymethyl cellulose 13.3%
Orajel Maximum Strength	Church & Dwight	gel	benzocaine 20%	
Orajel Maximum Strength Liquid	Church & Dwight	liquid	benzocaine 20%	
Orajel Maximum Strength PM	Church & Dwight	paste	benzocaine 20%	
Orajel Maximum Strength Swabs	Church & Dwight	swab	benzocaine 20%	
Orajel Mouth Sore Gel	Church & Dwight	gel	benzocaine 20%	zinc chloride 0.1%
Orajel Regular Strength	Church & Dwight	gel	benzocaine 10%	
Orajel Ultra Canker Sore Gel	Church & Dwight	gel	benzocaine 15%	menthol 2%
Polysporin Lip Therapy	Johnson & Johnson	ointment		camphor 1.5% menthol 0.75% phenol 0.5%
Super Lysine + Coldstick	Quantum Health	stick		benzophenone - 3 lysine octinoxate
Tanac Liquid	Insight	liquid	benzocaine 10%	benzalkonium chloride 0.12% tannic acid 6%
Viractin Gel	Medibrands	gel	tetracaine hydrochloride 2%	
Zilactin Cold Sore Gel	Blairex	gel		benzyl alcohol 10%
Zilactin-B	Blairex	gel	benzocaine 10%	

Product	Manufacturer	Dosage Form	Other Active Ingredients
Biotene Dry Mouth Mouthwash	GlaxoSmithKline	liquid	glucose oxidase 167 units/mL lactoferrin 1 mg/mL lactoperoxidase 167 units/mL lysozyme 2.7 mg/mL
Biotene Dry Mouth Toothpaste Original/ Gentle Mint	GlaxoSmithKline	gel	glucose oxidase 10,000 units lactoferrin 16 mg lactoperoxidase 15,000 units lysozyme 16 mg sodium monofluorophosphate (0.14% w/v fluoride ion)
Moi-Stir Spray	Pendopharm	spray	calcium chloride 0.15 mg/mL magnesium chloride 0.05 mg/mL potassium chloride 1.2 mg/mL sodium chloride 0.05 mg/mL sodium phosphate dibasic 0.28 mg/mL
Mouth Kote Oral Moisturizer	Alcon	liquid	yerba santa
OraMoist Dry Mouth Disc	Quantum Health	time-released gel disc	carbomer homopolymer glucose oxidase lactoferrin lysozyme polyvinyl pyrrolidone
Oral Balance Gel	GlaxoSmithKline	gel	glucose oxidase lactoferrin lactoperoxidase lysozyme
Oral Balance Liquid	GlaxoSmithKline	liquid	glucose oxidase lactoferrin lactoperoxidase lysozyme water
OralMedic Barrier Solution	Epien Medical	swabstick	HybenX (a mixture of hydroxybenzenesulfonic acid, hydroxymethylbenzenesulfonic acid, sulfuric acid and water)
Sialor	Pendopharm	tablet	anethole trithione 25 mg

Product	Manufacturer	Dosage Form	Fluoride	Other Active Ingredients
Antiseptic Mouthwash Alcohol Free	Atlas	mouthwash		cetylpyridinium chloride 0.05%
Antiseptic Mouthwash Regular/Coolmint/ Freshmint	H.J. Sutton	mouthwash		
Antiseptic Mouthwash Cool-Mint	Scott Chemical	mouthwash		eucalyptol 0.09% menthol 0.04% thymol 0.06%
Antiseptic Mouthwash Cool Mint/Mint	Trillium	mouthwash		eucalyptol 0.091% menthol 0.042% thymol 0.063%
Betadine Mouthwash & Gargle	Purdue Pharma	mouthwash		povidone-iodine 1%
Cepacol Mouthwash & Gargle	GlaxoSmithKline Consumer Healthcare	mouthwash		cetylpyridinium chloride 0.05%
Cepacol with Fluoride Mint/Peppermint	GlaxoSmithKline Consumer Healthcare	mouthwash	sodium fluoride 0.05%	cetylpyridinium chloride 0.05%
Crest Pro Health Complete	Procter & Gamble	mouthwash	sodium fluoride 0.021%	
Listerine Antiseptic Original/Cool Mint/Fresh Burst	Johnson & Johnson	mouthwash		eucalyptol 0.091% menthol 0.042% thymol 0.063%
Listerine Advanced Plus / Listerine Tartar Control / Listerine Total Care	Johnson & Johnson	mouthwash		eucalyptol 0.091% menthol 0.042% thymol 0.063% zinc chloride 0.09%
Listerine Fluoride / Listerine Platinum / Listerine Ultraclean Anti-Cavity	Johnson & Johnson	mouthwash	sodium fluoride 0.022%	eucalyptol 0.091% menthol 0.042% thymol 0.063%
Listerine Smart Rinse for Kids	Johnson & Johnson	mouthwash	sodium fluoride 0.0221%	
Listerine Total Care for Sensitive Teeth	Johnson & Johnson	mouthwash	sodium fluoride 0.022%	eucalyptol 0.091% menthol 0.042% potassium nitrate 2.4% thymol 0.063%
Listerine Whitening plus Restoring	Johnson & Johnson	mouthwash	sodium fluoride 0.022%	
Listerine Whitening Extreme	Johnson & Johnson	mouthwash	sodium fluoride 0.02%	
Oral-B Anti-Bacterial with Fluoride	Procter & Gamble	mouthwash	sodium fluoride 0.05%	cetylpyridinium chloride 0.05%
Oral-B Anti-Cavity Dental Rinse	Procter & Gamble	liquid	sodium fluoride 0.05%	
Oro NaF Daily Rinse	Germiphene	liquid	fluoride (as sodium fluoride) 0.023%	
Peroxyl Mouth Rinse	Colgate Oral Pharmaceuticals	mouthwash		hydrogen peroxide 1.5%
Plax Anti-Plaque Dental Rinse	Johnson & Johnson	liquid		sodium benzoate 2% sodium lauryl sulfate 0.25% sodium salicylate 0.2%
SteriSol	Johnson & Johnson	mouthwash		hexetidine 0.1%

Product	Manufacturer	Size	Support	Comments
Abdominal Belt	Formedica	small/medium large/x-large xx-large	moderate	Recommended for the relief of lumbo-sacral pain due to weakness of the abdominal muscles Can also hold dressings in place
Ankle Brace	Formedica	small, medium, large, x-large, xx-large		
Ankle Brace Laced	Formedica	x-small, small, medium, large, x-large	moderate - stabilizing	With removable side stabilizers for lateral protection
Ankle Elastic Criss-Crossed Support	Formedica	small, medium, large, x-large	mild	
Ankle Lastrap Brace	Coopercare	1 size	moderate	Adjustable fit with Thermovibe pads Designed to absorb vibrations and to provide extra warmth to the affected area
Ankle Support 8-shaped	Formedica	1 size		
Ankle Support Neoprene Ergo Sport	Formedica	small, medium, large, x-large		
Ankle Wrap	Coopercare	1 size	mild	Woven nylon reinforced
Arm Support	Formedica			Arm sling
Back Lastrap Brace	Coopercare	small, medium, large, x-large	moderate	With Thermovibe pads, designed to absorb vibrations and to provide extra warmth to the affected area
Cervical Collar Plasti-Forme	Formedica	baby, pediatric, x-small, small, medium, large	firm - stabilizing	
Cervical Collars	Formedica	various heights and neck circumferences	moderate	Recommended in cases where light support or heat is required Made of medium density polyurethane foam
Cervical Collars - Firm	Formedica	various heights and neck circumferences	firm - stabilizing	Provides firm support in case of muscular contusions or severe inflammation Made of high density polyurethane foam
Conforming Stretch, Non-Sterile Bandage	AMD-Ritmed	5/7.5/10/15 cm		
Conforming Stretch, Sterile Bandage	AMD-Ritmed	5/7.5/10/15 cm		
Elastic Bandage	AMD-Ritmed	5/7.5/10/15 cm x 4.6 m		
Elastic Bandage	Formedica	5/7.5/10/15 cm x 4.6 m		
Elastic Bandage-Self-Adhering	Formedica	5/7.5/10 cm		Available in beige and blue
Elbow Brace Ergo Sport	Formedica	small/medium large/x-large	moderate	Made from neoprene Velcro-type closures
Elbow Elastic Support	Formedica	small, medium, large		
Elbow Lastrap Brace	Coopercare	x-small, small, medium, large, x-large	moderate	With Thermovibe pads, designed to absorb vibrations and to provide extra warmth to the affected area
Flexible Ankle Support	Coopercare	small, medium, large	mild	
Flexible Elbow Support	Coopercare	small, medium, large	mild	
Flexible Hand Support	Coopercare	small, medium, large	mild	
Flexible Knee Support	Coopercare	small, medium, large	mild	
Futuro Ankle Support Wrap Around	3M Canada	small, medium, large	moderate	Adjustable straps

▶

Product	Manufacturer	Size	Support	Comments
Futuro Arm Sling Pouch	3M Canada	youth, adult		
Futuro Back Support	3M Canada	small/medium large/x-large	moderate	
Futuro Comfort Lift Ankle Support	3M Canada	small, medium, large	mild	Breathable material Contains natural rubber latex
Futuro Comfort Lift Elbow Support	3M Canada	small, medium, large	mild	Breathable material Contains natural rubber latex
Futuro Comfort Lift Knee Support	3M Canada	small, medium, large, x-large	mild	Breathable material Contains natural rubber latex
Futuro Deluxe Ankle Stabilizer	3M Canada	1 size	moderate - stabilizing	Provides rigid support and protection Side stabilizers help limit lateral motion Ankle straps lift and support arch
Futuro Deluxe Thumb Stabilizer	3M Canada	small/medium large/x-large	moderate - stabilizing	Has two metal stabilizers for stability of lower thumb joints Open design allows free movement of hand and fingers
Futuro Deluxe Wrist Stabilizer Right Hand/ Left Hand	3M Canada	small/medium large/x-large	firm - stabilizing	Palmar stabilizer allows for custom fit Dorsal stabilizers for additional support 3-strap design Breathable materials Latex-free Recommended for wrist immobilization
Futuro Elastic Bandage	3M Canada	5/7.5/10 cm		
Futuro Elbow Support with Pressure Pads	3M Canada	small, medium, large	moderate - stabilizing	Adjustable compression strap for custom fit Provides moderate support and stabilization to help prevent re-injury Contains natural rubber latex
Futuro Energizing Support Glove	3M Canada	small, medium, large	mild	
Futuro Energizing Wrist Support Right Hand/Left Hand	3M Canada	small/medium large/x-large	moderate - stabilizing	3 adjustable straps for custom fit Gel pad in palm for comfort Breathable
Futuro Infinity Active Knit Knee Stabilizer	3M Canada	small, medium, large	moderate - stabilizing	Strong side stabilizers Patella gel ring for cushioning Extra length for improved fit
Futuro Infinity Adjustable Elbow Support	3M Canada	1 size	moderate	Adjustable fit Easy-sleeve design for ease to put on and take off
Futuro Infinity Precision Fit Ankle Support	3M Canada	1 size	moderate	Flexible comfort straps for custom fit
Futuro Night Knee Sleep Support	3M Canada	1 size	mild	Adjustable fit For overnight use, provides support and cushioning Breathable, moisture-wicking materials Use for discomfort related to knee contact
Futuro Night Plantar Fasciitis Sleep Support	3M Canada	1 size	firm - stabilizing	Stabilizes foot in the proper therapeutic position all night long Use on either foot, with or without a sock
Futuro Night Wrist Sleep Support	3M Canada	1 size	mild	Adjustable straps For overnight use, provides support and cushioning Breathable, moisture-wicking materials Removable palmar stabilizer
Futuro Sport Ankle Support	3M Canada	small/medium large/x-large	moderate	

Product	Manufacturer	Size	Support	Comments
Futuro Sport Ankle Support Adjustable	3M Canada	1 size	moderate - stabilizing	Adjustable fit, recommended for ankle sprain with acute swelling Adjust strap as swelling decreases
Futuro Sport Knee Stabilizer Adjustable	3M Canada	1 size	moderate - stabilizing	Adjustable fit Dual stabilizers provide medial and lateral support Open kneecap design
Futuro Sport Knee Support Adjustable	3M Canada	1 size	moderate	Adjustable straps Open kneecap Side ventilation for breathability
Futuro Sport Moisture Control Knee Support	3M Canada	small, medium, large, extra large	moderate	Breathable moisture-wicking in back panel for comfort Open kneecap design
Futuro Sport Neoprene Elbow Support	3M Canada	1 size	moderate	Adjustable fit
Futuro Sport Tennis Elbow Support	3M Canada	1 size	firm - stabilizing	Adjustable fit Tendon pad allows for targeted compression
Futuro Sport Wrist Support Wrap Around	3M Canada	1 size	moderate	Adjustable foam pad for additional stability Contains natural latex rubber
Futuro Stabilizing Knee Support	3M Canada	small, medium, large	moderate - stabilizing	Dual side stabilizers provide support without limiting movement Open kneecap design
Futuro Stirrup Ankle Brace	3M Canada	1 size	firm - stabilizing	Plastic shell designed to help limit lateral motion post-cast or after acute injury Inflatable air cells help with circulation and swelling
Futuro Surgical Binder & Abdominal Support	3M Canada	small, medium, large, extra large	moderate	Support for post-surgery use
Futuro Wrist Support Adjustable	3M Canada	1 size	moderate	Adjustable fit with thumb loop Made from neoprene blend Available in beige and black
Futuro Wrist Wrap Brace	3M Canada	small, medium, large	moderate - stabilizing	Adjustable fasteners and thumb strap Removable, adjustable stabilizer Reversible to be used in either wrist
Golf and Tennis Elbow Bracelet	Formedica	small/medium large/x-large	moderate	
Knee and Leg Immobilizers	Formedica	small, medium, large, x-large, xx-large	firm - stabilizing	Has 4 removable aluminum rods for lateral and medial support Recommended in case of sprains, dislocations, simple fractures, and before or after surgery
Knee Brace Criss-Crossed Back	Formedica	small, medium, large, x-large, xx-large	moderate	Flexible spiral stays on each side
Knee Brace Neoprene	Formedica	small, medium, large, x-large, xx-large		
Knee Brace with Side Stabilizers	Formedica	small, medium, large, x-large, xx-large	moderate - stabilizing	
Knee Elastic Support	Formedica	small, medium, large, x-large, xx-large	mild	
Knee Lastrap Brace	Coopercare	small, medium, large, x-large	moderate	With Thermovibe pads, designed to absorb vibrations and to provide extra warmth to the affected area

Product	Manufacturer	Size	Support	Comments
Knee Support Neoprene-Patella	Formedica	small, medium, large, x-large		
Knee Support-Open Patella	Formedica	small, medium, large, x-large		
Knee Wrap	Coopercare	1 size	mild	Woven nylon reinforced
Leg Lastrap Brace	Coopercare	small, medium, large	moderate	With Thermovibe pads, designed to absorb vibrations and to provide extra warmth to the affected area
Lumbo-Sacral Support Sacro-Forme	Formedica	small/medium large/x-large xx-large	moderate	Designed to support the lower back postoperatively or post trauma for sprains, strains, muscle spasms, intra-abdominal pressure, lumbar disk syndrome or certain defined conditions which produce postural deformities or lower back pain Lateral stays for additional support
Lycragel Knee Support Gel	Formedica	small, medium, large, x-large, xx-large		
Maternity Support Belt	Formedica	small/medium large/x-large		
Neoprene Elbow Brace	Coopercare	1 size	mild	
Neoprene Knee Brace	Coopercare	small, medium, large, x-large	moderate	Available with open or padded knee
Neoprene Knee Stabilizer Brace	Coopercare	small, medium, large, x-large	moderate	Open knee Terry lined
Neoprene Open Knee Brace	3M Canada	1 size		Open knee prevents slippage
Neoprene Wrist Brace Left/Right	Coopercare	1 size	mild	Adjustable fit Terry lined
Rib Belt for Men/Women	Formedica	small/medium large/x-large	moderate - stabilizing	Supports the rib cage and helps relieve pain caused by respiratory movements after fractures or intercostal sprains May also be used post-operatively to hold dressings in place Soft stays keep it in place
Tennis Elbow Support Ergo Sport	Formedica	small/medium large/x-large	moderate	
Tensor Elastic Bandage	3M Canada	5/6.3/7.5/10/15 cm		Comes with E-Z clip Washable
Tensor Ankle Brace	3M Canada	small, medium, large	moderate	Contoured shape
Tensor Ankle Brace with Gel Cushions	3M Canada	small/medium large/x-large	firm	Has dual gel cushions around ankle joint for added comfort Mesh panels Lace-up design
Tensor Back Belt with Magnets	3M Canada	1 size	moderate	Adjustable fit Can be worn under clothing Permits full range of movement
Tensor Back Wrap with Gel Pack	3M Canada	1 size	moderate	Has re-usable hot & cold pack
Tensor Elasto-Preene Ankle support	3M Canada	small/medium large/x-large	moderate	Provides compression to reduce swelling to injured areas Retains therapeutic heat
Tensor Elasto-Preene Elbow Support	3M Canada	small/medium large/x-large	moderate	Provides compression to reduce swelling to injured areas Retains therapeutic heat

Product	Manufacturer	Size	Support	Comments
Tensor Elasto-Preene Knee Support	3M Canada	small/medium large/x-large	moderate	Provides compression to reduce swelling to injured areas Retains therapeutic heat
Tensor Elbow Brace	3M Canada	small, medium, large		
Tensor Knee Brace	3M Canada	small, medium, large, x-large		
Tensor Neoprene Ankle Brace	3M Canada	small, medium, large	moderate	Retains therapeutic heat Can be used during physical activity to prevent injury
Tensor Neoprene Ankle Wrap	3M Canada	1 size	moderate	Adjustable fit Retains therapeutic heat
Tensor Neoprene Elbow Brace	3M Canada	1 size	moderate	Adjustable for controlled compression Retains therapeutic heat
Tensor Neoprene Knee Brace	3M Canada	1 size		
Tensor Neoprene Open Patella Knee Brace	3M Canada	small, medium, large	moderate	Open knee prevents slippage Retains therapeutic heat
Tensor Neoprene OSFA Knee Brace	3M Canada	1 size	moderate	Adjustable fit Retains therapeutic heat Available as regular & open knee design
Tensor Neoprene Plus Knee Brace	3M Canada	small, medium, large	moderate	Flexible metal stabilizers for support Open knee prevents slippage
Tensor Neoprene Wrist Brace	3M Canada	1 size		Adjustable for controlled compression Retains therapeutic heat
Tensor Plus Knee Brace with Side Stabilizers	3M Canada	small, medium, large	moderate - stabilizing	Flexible metal side stabilizers provide medial/lateral support and stability
Tensor Plus Rigid Wrist Brace	3M Canada	small, medium, large		Preshaped plastic splint
Tensor Self-Adhesive Bandage	3M Canada	5/7.5/10 cm		
Tensor Tennis Elbow Brace	3M Canada	1 size	moderate	Adjustable Velcro strap
Thumb Stabilizer Ergo Select	Formedica	small/medium large/x-large	firm - stabilizing	Maximal support Ambidextrous Washable
Trufit Back Support	3M Canada	1 size	moderate - stabilizing	Dual adjustments provide support and stability Support stays provide added protection Breathable mesh fabric
Wrist Dorsal Immobilizers Ergo Select	Formedica	small/medium large/x-large	moderate	Allows free movement of fingers 4 Velcro closures
Wrist Immobilizer Left-Right Hand	Formedica	small, medium, large, x-large, xx-large	moderate - stabilizing	Removable aluminum support can be re-shaped to desired angle when necessary
Wrist Immobilizer Left-Right Hand with Self-Adhesive Closures	Formedica	small, medium, large, x-large	firm - stabilizing	Designed to be used following sprains, strains, cast removal or whenever restriction of wrist motion is required
Wrist Lastrap Brace for Left/ Right Hand	Coopercare	small, medium, large	moderate	With Thermovibe pads, designed to absorb vibrations and to provide extra warmth to the affected area
Wrist Support Ergo Sport	Formedica	small/medium large/x-large	mild	Made from neoprene Stabilizes and supports weak wrist muscles and ligaments after sprains and stress injuries
Wrist Wrap Lastrap	Coopercare	1 size	moderate	Ideal for people who do not want a rigid brace

Type	Product	Manufacturer	Energy (kcal)	Total Fat (g)	Sat Fat (g)	Protein (g)	Carbo-hydrate (g)	Fibre (g)	Sodium (mg)	Potassium (mg)	Iron (mg)	Comments
Meal Replacement	Boost Fruit Flavoured Beverage (per 237 mL)	Mead Johnson	180	0.4	0.2	8.8	36		70	10	2.25	Lactose-free Milk protein concentrate
	Boost High Protein (per 237 mL)	Mead Johnson	240	6	0.7	15	33		260	390	3.8	50% more protein than Boost liquid Lactose-free Milk protein concentrate Suitable for people recovering from surgery, injuries or fractures and people at risk for pressure ulcers
	Boost Liquid (per 237 mL)	Mead Johnson	240	4	0.5	10	41		253	409	3.8	Lactose-free Milk protein concentrate Canola oil High oleic sunflower oil Corn oil
	Boost Plus Calories (per 237 mL)	Mead Johnson	360	14	1.5	14	45		260	378	3.8	50% more calories than Boost Liquid Lactose-free Milk protein concentrate Sodium and calcium caseinates Canola oil High oleic sunflower oil Corn oil
	Boost Pudding (per 142 g)	Mead Johnson	240	9		6.8	33		125	250	2.7	Lactose-free Milk protein concentrate Sodium and calcium caseinates Canola oil High oleic sunflower oil Corn oil
	Carnation Instant Breakfast Vanilla/ Strawberry/ Chocolate/ Mocha (per 295 mL)	Nestlé	300	8.8		15.5	41		192	405	7	Gluten-free low residue Excellent source of iron, calcium, vitamin C and protein Available in powder and in ready-to-feed
	Ensure Hi-Protein Liquid (per 235 mL)	Abbott Nutrition	225	6	0.5	12	31		290	428	3.5	25% more protein than regular ensure Gluten-free Lactose-free Suitable for people recovering from surgery, injuries or fractures and people at risk for pressure ulcers

Type	Product	Manufacturer	Energy (kcal)	Total Fat (g)	Sat Fat (g)	Protein (g)	Carbo-hydrate (g)	Fibre (g)	Sodium (mg)	Potassium (mg)	Iron (mg)	Comments
Meal Replacement	Ensure Liquid (per 235 mL)	Abbott Nutrition	250	6.7	1	9.4	38.1		250	375	3.8	Gluten-free Lactose-free Milk protein concentrate For oral feeding only
	Ensure Prebiotic Formula	Abbott Nutrition	250	6.7	1	9.4	38.1		250	375	3.8	Same as Ensure Regular Has 3 g of NutraFlora scFOS (short chain fructooligosaccharides) to help maintain intestinal flora
	Ensure Plus Liquid	Abbott Nutrition	355	11	1	13.5	50.5		250	400	3.8	44% more protein and 105 more calories than regular Ensure Gluten-free Lactose-free For people who need to gain or maintain weight, and for those who have fluid restrictions or volume-limited feedings
	Ensure Pudding (per 113 g)	Abbott Nutrition	170	5	1	4	30		85	110	1.8	Gluten-free Lactose-free Milk protein concentrate For oral feeding only Contains 1 g of FOS to stimulate growth of beneficial bacteria in the colon
	Ensure with Fiber (per 235 mL)	Abbott Nutrition	250	7.8	3.3	9.4	38	3.4	250	375	3.8	Gluten-free Lactose-free Milk protein concentrate For oral feeding only 3.4 g of dietary fibre from soy fibre
	Fast Track Apple Cranberry	President's Choice	225	5.3	1.1	14	33	3.3	250	375		
	Fast Track Chocolate Fudge	President's Choice	229	6.6	4	14	35	2.1	250	375		
	Fast Track Honey-Nougat	President's Choice	229	5.5	3	14	34	1.9	250	375		
	Nutribar Original Meal Bar	Stella	260	8.6	4.4	13	33	1.7	250	375		Available in various flavours
	Nutribar Original Powder	Stella	259	7.0	3.6	14	35	2	290	600		When mixed with 250 mL (1 cup) 2% milk Available in various flavours, nutritional information can vary from flavour to flavour

Type	Product	Manufacturer	Energy (kcal)	Total Fat (g)	Sat Fat (g)	Protein (g)	Carbo-hydrate (g)	Fibre (g)	Sodium (mg)	Potassium (mg)	Iron (mg)	Comments
Meal Replacement	Slim-Fast Optima Meal Bar	Unilever	230	6	3.5	12	33	3	270	380	3.5	Designed as a weight-loss meal replacement, various flavours
	Slim-Fast Optima Powdered Shakes	Unilever	262	7.4	3.9	15	34	2.5	270	870	3	When mixed with 250 mL (1 cup) 2% milk. Available in various flavours, nutritional information can vary from flavour to flavour
	Ultra Shake Chocolate (per 235 mL)	President's Choice	353	12	1.2	18	44	0.4	258	491		
	Ultra Shake Strawberry	President's Choice	235	5.4	0.5	10	37	0.1	258	491		
	Ultra Shake Vanilla	President's Choice	353	12	1.2	12	44		258	491		
Energy Bar	Luna Bar	Clif Bar	170	3.5	0	9	29	3	115	170		Designed specifically for women Variety of flavours Nutritional information may vary from flavour to flavour
	Myoplex Energy Bar	Abbott Nutrition	190	4.5	3	15	26	4	260	320		Available in a variety of flavours Nutritional information may vary from flavour to flavour
	PowerBar Fruit Energize	PowerBar Foods	220	3.5	0.3	6	46	1	180	40		
	PowerBar Harvest	PowerBar Foods	220	4	0.8	8.3	40	4	80	390	3.5	High carbohydrate Moist and crunchy energy bar for recreational sport Made with real fruit/grains Fortified with 17 vitamins and minerals
	PowerBar ProteinPlus	PowerBar Foods	300	6	3.5	24	39	1	210	110	3.5	High protein Moderate carbohydrate energy bar Use after workout for body recovery
	PowerBar Recovery Bar	PowerBar Foods	260	10	4.5	12	30	0	180	105	3.5	Formulated to be used post-exercise to aid in recovery after endurance exercise Higher fat content
	PowerBar Sport	PowerBar Foods	200	1.6	0.6	9	43	3.5	200	400	3.5	High carbohydrate Sport nutrition for sustained energy Fortified with 17 vitamins and minerals

Type	Product	Manufacturer	Energy (kcal)	Total Fat (g)	Sat Fat (g)	Protein (g)	Carbo-hydrate (g)	Fibre (g)	Sodium (mg)	Potassium (mg)	Iron (mg)	Comments
Energy Bar	Zone Perfect Bar	Abbott	210	7	4	15	22	1	240	140	3	Available in a variety of flavours Nutritional information may vary from flavour to flavour
Enteral	Compleat (per 250 mL)	Nestlé	265	10.1		12	32	1.5	250	430	3.83	Ready-to-use blended mix of traditional foods such as chicken, peas, carrots, tomatoes and cranberry juice For tube feeding only
	Isosource 1.5 (per 250 mL)	Nestlé	375	16.2		16.9	42	2	322	536	4.82	High-calorie High-nitrogen With fibre For oral or tube feeding use
	Isosource HN (per 250 ml)	Nestlé	300	10.5		13.3	37.9	0	280	450	3	High nitrogen formula Designed for tube feeding only
	Isosource HN with Fibre	Nestlé	300	10.5		13.3	39.3	3	280	450	3	High nitrogen formula with 3 g of FOS as added fibre (is also a prebiotic) Designed for tube feeding only
	Isosource VHN (per 250 mL)	Nestlé	250	7.2		15.6	32	2.5	320	400	3.6	Very high protein formula With added fibre (FOS) For tube or oral feeding use
	Jevity (per 235 mL)	Abbott	250	8.4	8.5	10.3	33.1	3.3	173.9	291.4	3.2	High-oleic sunflower oil or high-oleic safflower oil Canola oil Fractionated coconut oil (MCT)
	Jevity Plus (per 235 mL)	Abbott	285	9.2		13	41	2.8	317	435	4.2	High-oleic safflower oil Canola oil Fractionated coconut oil (MCT)
	MCT Oil (per 15 mL)	Nestlé	115	14.1								Medium chain triglycerides oil
	Microlipid (per 89 mL)	Nestlé	400	45								50% safflower oil emulsion Rich source of polyunsaturated fat
	Nutren 1.5 (per 250 mL)	Nestlé	375	17	7.7	15	42		292	468	4.5	For long-term tube feeding/oral use for patients with a functioning GI tract Lactose-free Gluten-free Low residue Milder vanilla flavour available

Type	Product	Manufacturer	Energy (kcal)	Total Fat (g)	Sat Fat (g)	Protein (g)	Carbo-hydrate (g)	Fibre (g)	Sodium (mg)	Potassium (mg)	Iron (mg)	Comments
Enteral	Nutren 2.0 (per 250 mL)	Nestlé	500	26	17.2	20	49		325	480	6	For very high energy requirements/for shorter feeding times, Lactose-free, gluten-free, For long-term feeding/oral use
	Optimental (per 237 mL)	Abbott	237	6.7	2.4	12.2	32.9		265	405	3	For patients with metabolic stress, acute trauma or malabsorption conditions (e.g., Crohn's disease), For oral or tube feeding
	Osmolite 1 CAL (per 235 mL)	Abbott	250	8.4	1.96	10.4	33		181	310	3.22	High-oleic sunflower oil or high-oleic safflower oil Canola oil Fractionated coconut oil (MCT)
	Osmolite 1.2 CAL (per 235 mL)	Abbott	285	9.2	2.04	13	37		317	425	4.2	High-oleic safflower oil Canola oil Fractionated coconut oil (MCT)
	Peptamen (per 250 mL)	Nestlé	250	9.8	6.4	10	32		140	376	4.5	Lactose-free Gluten-free 100% whey peptide elemental diet For easy digestion and absorption by patients with impaired gastrointestinal function For oral/tube feeding Flavour packages available
	Peptamen 1.5 (per 250 mL)	Nestlé	375	14		17	47		265	485	6.75	100% whey peptides Lactose-free Gluten-free Energy dense for patients who require shortened feeding times Flavour package available
	Peptamen AF (per 250 mL)	Nestlé	300	13.75		17	47		255	465	6.75	Lactose free Gluten free For oral or tube feeding use Has less volume than Peptamen so can be used when fluid restriction is necessary

Type	Product	Manufacturer	Energy (kcal)	Total Fat (g)	Sat Fat (g)	Protein (g)	Carbo-hydrate (g)	Fibre (g)	Sodium (mg)	Potassium (mg)	Iron (mg)	Comments
Enteral	Peptamen with Prebio1 (per 250 mL)	Nestlé	250	9.8		10	31		140	375	4.5	Contains Prebio1, a blend of fructooligosaccharides (FOS) and inulin to restore tha balance of colonic microflora Lactose free Gluten free
	Perative (per 237 mL)	Abbott	308	8.8	4.05	15.8	42	1.6	250	410	3.7	Designed for metabolically stressed patients with pressure ulcers, fractures, wounds, burns, or surgery Contains 2 g of added arginine, peptide-based, semi-elemental protein for easier absorption
	Polycose Powder (per 100 g)	Abbott	380				94		120	10		Carbohydrate source For patients who are unwilling or unable to consume necessary energy for optimum recovery or maintenance of normal health Contains no protein, fat, or vitamins
	Promote (per 235 mL)	Abbott	235	6.1	1.48	14.8	30.2	0	210	419	4.2	High-protein liquid formula for people with increased protein needs relative to their estimated calorie requirements Can be used as an oral supplement For sole-source feeding, oral or tube feeding
	Scandishake (per 240 mL)	Aptalis	600	21	8	15	69		230	651		High caloric liquid preparation for weight gain, when mixed with 250 mL (1 cup) of whole milk
	Suplena (per 235 mL)	Abbott	470	23	2.03	7	60		183	7	4.5	High-calorie, low protein, low electrolyte formula Designed for people with chronic or acute renal failure who are not undergoing dialysis, oral or tube feeding

Type	Product	Manufacturer	Energy (kcal)	Total Fat (g)	Sat Fat (g)	Protein (g)	Carbo-hydrate (g)	Fibre (g)	Sodium (mg)	Potassium (mg)	Iron (mg)	Comments
	Tolerex (per 300 mL)	Nestlé	300	0.4		6.2	68		141	350	3	Nutritionally complete elemental diet for patients with impaired digestion and absorption, and specialized nutrient needs (e.g. allergies) For oral or tube feeding use
Disease Specific	Boost Diabetic (per 237 mL)	Mead Johnson	190	7	1	16	16		180	70	4.5	Designed for diabetics Contains a slow release energy system that optimizes glycemic control
	ExtendBar	AutoControl Medical	150	3	1	12	20	6	200	50		Designed for diabetics Sugar free Gluten-free Low glycemic index (41)
	Glucerna Bar Chocolate Graham	Abbott	144	4		6	24	4	60	65	1.82	Diabetic snack bar
	Glucerna Bar Lemon Crunch	Abbott	144	4		6	24	4	64	44	1.82	Diabetic snack bar
	Glucerna Oral (per 235 mL)	Abbott	211	8		11	28	1.9	209	366	3	Contains a slow release energy system that optimizes glycemic control Lactose-free
	Glucerna Tube Feeding (per 235 mL)	Abbott	235	13		9.9	23	3.4	196	329	3	For patients with diabetes and other forms of abnormal glucose tolerance Tube feeding or oral formula
	Pulmocare (per 235 mL)	Abbott	355	21.8		14.8	25		246	358	4.5	For patients with acute or chronic respiratory insufficiency, especially with CO_2 retention Oral and tube feeding
	Resource Diabetic (per 250 mL)	Nestlé	265	11.8		15.9	23.8	3	240	350	2.38	High-protein, fibre-containing formulation for diabetics For oral or tube feeding use
	Vital HN (per 100 mL)	Abbott	100	1.1		4.2	18.5		57	140	1.2	Nutritionally complete, partially hydrolyzed diet for patients with impaired gastrointestinal function

Type	Product	Manufacturer	Energy (kcal)	Total Fat (g)	Sat Fat (g)	Protein (g)	Carbohydrate (g)	Fibre (g)	Sodium (mg)	Potassium (mg)	Iron (mg)	Comments
Enteral	Compleat Pediatric (per 250 mL)	Nestlé	250	9.7		9.5	31	1.7	190	410	3.3	Ready-to-use blended mix of traditional foods such as chicken, peas, carrots, tomatoes and cranberry juice Designed for children 1-12 y of age For tube feeding only
	Nutren Junior (per 250 mL)	Nestlé	250	12.4	3.3	7.5	27.5		115	330	3.5	For children 1-13 y of age, for mild to moderate reflux, growth failure, or inadequate oral intake For tube feeding or oral use Can be used when transitioning from a semi-elemental diet Lactose-free Gluten-free Low-residue
	Nutren Junior with Fibre (per 250 mL)	Nestlé	250	12.4	3.3	7.5	27.5	1.5	115	330	3.5	For children 1-13 y of age 50:50 ratio whey:casein protein Improved digestion, gastric emptying Lactose-free Gluten-free Low-residue
	Pediasure (per 235 mL)	Abbott	235	12	3	7	31	1	90	310	3.3	Complete pediatric nutrition for children 1-10 y of age For tube feeding or oral use
	Pediasure with Fibre (per 235 mL)	Abbott	235	11.7	3.3	7.1	26	1.1	87	306	3.3	The benefits of fibre at no extra cost provide an ideal product for the tube-fed child
	Peptamen Junior (per 250 mL)	Nestlé	250	9.6	5.6	7.5	34		115	330	3.5	For children 1-13 y of age 100% whey peptide formulation Lactose-free Gluten-free For oral/tube feeding
	Peptamen Junior 1.5 (per 250 mL)	Nestlé	375	17		11.3	45		183	495	5.2	For children 1-13 y of age 100% whey peptide formulation Lactose-free Gluten-free For tube feeding only
	Resource Just for Kids 1.5 Cal with Fibre (per 237 mL)	Nestlé	355	17.8	9.8	10	39	2.1	164	309	3.3	For children 1-12 y of age For oral or tube feeding use

Type	Product	Manufacturer	Protein (g/dL)	Whey: Casein Ratio	Calories (per mL)	Iron mg/L	Dosage Form	Comments
Regular	Enfamil A+	Mead Johnson	demineralized whey powder, skim milk powder (1.42)	60:40	0.74	12.2	Ready-to-feed Liquid concentrate Powder	For infants 0-12 months Contains Omega-3 (DHA) and Omega-6 (ARA), similar to those found in breast milk Iron-fortified
	Enfamil Lower Iron	Mead Johnson	demineralized whey powder, skim milk powder (1.42)	60:40	0.68	7.4	Ready-to-feed Liquid concentrate Powder	For infants 0-12 months, routine formula Cow's milk based Iron-fortified but has less iron than other brands
	Enfamil with Iron	Mead Johnson	demineralized whey powder, skim milk powder (1.42)	60:40	0.67	12	Ready-to-feed Liquid concentrate Powder	For infants 0-12 months, routine formula Cow's milk based Iron-fortified
	Good Start	Nestlé	partially hydrolyzed reduced minerals whey protein concentrate (1.5)	100:0	0.67	10	Ready-to-feed Liquid concentrate Powder	For infants 0-12 months Cow's milk based Iron-fortified Contains 100% partially hydrolyzed whey protein
	Good Start with Omega-3 and Omega-6	Nestlé	partially hydrolyzed reduced minerals whey protein concentrate (1.5)	100:0	0.67	10	Ready-to-feed Liquid concentrate Powder	For infants 0-12 months Cow's milk based Iron-fortified Contains 100% partially hydrolyzed whey protein Contains Omega-3 (DHA) and Omega-6 (ARA), similar to those found in breast milk
	Good Start Probiotic	Nestlé	partially hydrolyzed reduced minerals whey protein concentrate (1.5)	100:0	0.67	10	Ready-to-feed Liquid concentrate Powder	For infants 0-12 months Supplemented with Bifidobacterium lactis (Bifidus BL), Omega-3 (DHA), and Omega-6 (ARA) Contains partially hydrolyzed protein Designed to be easier to digest and may reduce the risk of allergy in infants with a family history of allergy
	Similac	Abbott Nutrition	nonfat milk & whey protein concentrate (1.4)		0.68	4.7	Liquid concentrate Powder	For infants 0-6 months
	Similac Advance with Omega-3 & Omega-6	Abbott Nutrition	nonfat milk & whey protein concentrate (1.4)		0.68	12	Ready-to-feed Liquid concentrate Powder	For infants 0-12 months Contains Omega-3 (DHA) and Omega-6 (ARA), similar to those found in breast milk
	Similac Iron-Fortified	Abbott Nutrition	nonfat milk & whey protein concentrate (1.4)		0.68	12	Liquid concentrate Powder	For infants 0-6 months Iron-fortified formulation
Lactose-free	Enfamil A+ Lactose Free	Mead Johnson	milk protein (1.42)	18:82	0.68	12.2	Liquid concentrate Powder	For infants 0-12 months with common feeding problems due to lactose intolerance Cow's milk based Lactose free Sucrose-free Contains Omega-3 (DHA) and Omega-6 (ARA)
	Similac Sensitive Lactose-Free	Abbott Nutrition	total milk protein (1.5)		0.68	12	Ready-to-feed Liquid concentrate Powder	For infants 0-12 months For lactose intolerance or lactase deficiency

Compendium of Products for Minor Ailments

Type	Product	Manufacturer	Protein (g/dL)	Whey: Casein Ratio	Calories (per mL)	Iron mg/L	Dosage Form	Comments
Milk-free/Lactose-free	Alsoy with Omega-3 & Omega-6	Nestlé	soy protein isolate (1.7)		0.67	12	Liquid concentrate Powder	For infants 0-12 months Soy-based Iron-fortified formula Contains Omega-3 (DHA) and Omega-6 (ARA)
Milk-free/Lactose-free	Alsoy 2 with Omega-3 & Omega-6	Nestlé	soy protein isolate (1.9)		0.67	12	Powder	For infants 6-24 months Soy-based Iron-fortified formula Contains Omega-3 (DHA) and Omega-6 (ARA)
	Enfamil Soy A+	Mead Johnson	soy protein isolate (1.69)		0.68	12.2	Powder	Soy-based Iron-fortified formula for infants 0-12 months Contains Omega-3 (DHA) and Omega-6 (ARA)
	Isomil	Abbott Nutrition	soy protein isolate (1.7)		0.68	12	Ready-to-feed Liquid concentrate Powder	For infants 0-12 months with intolerance to cow's milk protein, intolerance to lactose and infants with galactosemia
	Isomil Advance with Omega-3 and Omega-6	Abbott Nutrition	soy protein isolate (1.7)		0.68	12	Ready-to-feed Liquid concentrate Powder	For infants 0-12 months Contains Omega-3 (DHA) and Omega-6 (ARA), similar to those found in breast milk
	Isomil Step 2	Abbott Nutrition	soy protein isolate (1.66)		0.68	12	Ready-to-feed Liquid concentrate Powder	For infants 6-24 months with intolerance to cow's milk protein, intolerance to lactose or galactosemia
Follow On	Enfagrow	Mead Johnson	nonfat milk & whey protein concentrate (3.5)	60:40	0.85	13.5	Ready-to-feed Liquid concentrate Powder	Nutritional supplement for children 12-36 months
	Enfapro A+	Mead Johnson	nonfat milk (1.76)		0.68	13.5	Powder	For infants 6-18 months Cow's milk based, Iron, protein, fat, sodium content nutritionally superior to cow's milk Contains Omega-3 (DHA) and Omega-6 (ARA) similar to those found in breast milk
	Enfapro Regular	Mead Johnson	nonfat milk (1.7)		0.68	12	Liquid concentrate Powder	For infants 6-18 months Cow's milk based Fat, sodium content nutritionally superior to cow's milk
	Follow-Up	Nestlé	skim milk powder (1.7)	18:82	0.67	12	Ready-to-feed Liquid concentrate Powder	Designed for babies 6-18 months of age eating baby foods Excellent source of calcium
	Good Start 2	Nestlé	partially hydrolyzed reduced minerals whey protein concentrate (1.5)	100:0	0.67	13	Liquid concentrate Powder	For infants 6-18 months Cow's milk based Iron fortified Calcium enriched

Type	Product	Manufacturer	Protein (g/dL)	Whey:Casein Ratio	Calories (per mL)	Iron mg/L	Dosage Form	Comments
Follow On	Good Start 2 with Omega-3 and Omega-6	Nestlé	partially hydrolyzed reduced minerals whey protein concentrate (1.5)	100:0	0.67	13	Liquid concentrate Powder	For infants 6-18 months Cow's milk based, iron fortified, calcium enriched, contains Omega-3 (DHA) and Omega-6 (ARA)
	Good Start 2 Probiotic	Nestlé	partially hydrolyzed reduced minerals whey protein concentrate (1.5)	100:0	0.67	10	Ready-to-feed Liquid concentrate Powder	For infants 6-18 months Supplemented with Bifidobacterium lactis (Bifidus BL), Omega-3 (DHA), and Omega-6 (ARA) Contains partially hydrolyzed protein Designed to be easier to digest and may reduce the risk of allergy in infants with a family history of allergy
	Similac Go & Grow Step 2	Abbott Nutrition	nonfat milk & whey protein concentrate (1.4)		0.68	12	Liquid concentrate Powder	For infants 6-24 months Contains extra calcium for development
	Similac Go & Grow Step 2 with Omega-3 and Omega-6	Abbott Nutrition	nonfat milk & whey protein concentrate (1.4)		0.68	12	Liquid concentrate Powder	Added Omega-3 (DHA) and Omega-6 (ARA), similar to those found in breast milk
Specialty	Alimentum	Abbott Nutrition	casein hydrolysate (60% free amino acids, 40% small peptides) (1.9)		0.68	12	Ready-to-feed	Pre-digested, lactose-free and corn-free formulation For infants allergic to cow's milk or soy protein, sensitive to intact proteins and/or with multiple food allergies, or for prevention of developing allergies in high-risk infants
	Enfamil Enfacare A+	Mead Johnson	nonfat milk & whey protein concentrate (2.1)		0.74	13.3	powder	For premature or low birth weight infants 0-12 months Cow's milk based Contains Omega-3 (DHA) and Omega-6 (ARA), similar to those found in breast milk
	Enfamil Gentlease A+	Mead Johnson	partially hydrolyzed nonfat milk, whey protein concentrate (1.56)	100:0	0.68	12.2	Powder	For infants 0-12 months Designed for infants with fussiness or gas Partially broken-down protein blend Contains Omega-3 (DHA) and Omega-6 (ARA)
	Nutramigen	Mead Johnson	hydrolyzed casein, amino acid premix (1.9)	0:100	0.68	12.2	Ready-to-feed Powder	For infants 0-12 months Hypoallergenic formula for infants with a sensitivity or allergy to intact proteins or colic caused by milk protein allergy 100% hydrolyzed casein Lactose free, sucrose free Unique 4-oil fat blend patterned after human milk
	Pregestimil	Mead Johnson	hydrolyzed casein amino acid premix (1.9)		0.69	12.2	Powder	For infants 0-12 months Contains Omega-3 (DHA) and Omega-6 (ARA) Specialized semi-elemental formula for infants with disorders of fat metabolism 100% hydrolyzed casein 55% MCT oil Lactose free, sucrose free

Type	Product	Manufacturer	Protein (g/dL)	Whey:Casein Ratio	Calories (per mL)	Iron mg/L	Dosage Form	Comments
Specialty	Similac Advance Neosure	Abbott Nutrition	nonfat milk & whey protein concentrate (2.1)	18:82	0.75	14	powder	Designed for premature babies To be used as a pre-term, post-discharge formula Contains Omega-3 (DHA) and Omega-6 (ARA), higher levels of protein, vitamins, and minerals than standard term formula
Thickened	Enfamil Thickened A+	Mead Johnson	nonfat milk & whey protein concentrate (1.69)	18:82	0.68	12.2	powder	For infants 0-12 months Thickened with added rice starch Cow's milk based Carbohydrate blend of lactose, rice starch, and maltodextrin Contains Omega-3 (DHA) and Omega-6 (ARA)

Product	Manufacturer	Dosage Form	Active Ingredients	Comments
Dairyaid	Tanta	tablet	4500 FCC lactase units	
Dairy Digest Extra Strength	Vita Health	tablet	4500 FCC lactase units	
Lactaid	McNeil Consumer Healthcare	tablet	3000 FCC lactase units	
Lactaid Drops for Milk	McNeil Consumer Healthcare	liquid	5000 FCC lactase units/mL	To be added to milk 24 hours before consumption
Lactaid Extra Strength	McNeil Consumer Healthcare	tablet	4500 FCC lactase units	
Lactaid Fast Act	McNeil Consumer Healthcare	caplet	9000 FCC lactase units	
Lactaid Fast Act Chewable	McNeil Consumer Healthcare	chewable tablet	9000 FCC lactase units	
Lacteeze Drops for Milk	Aurium	liquid	16 FCC lactase units/drop	To be added to milk 24 hours before consumption
Lacteeze Extra Strength	Aurium	tablet	4000 FCC lactase units	
Lacteeze for Children	Aurium	tablet	3000 FCC lactase units	
Lacteeze Ultra	Aurium	tablet	9000 FCC lactase units	
LactoMax	SteriMax	tablet	3000 FCC lactase units	
LactoMax Extra Strength	SteriMax	tablet	4500 FCC lactase units	
LactoMax Ultra Strength	SteriMax	tablet	9000 FCC lactase units	

Product	Manufacturer	Dosage Form	Active Ingredients	Comments
Daily Lean Tonalin	Valeant	capsule	conjugated linoleic acid (CLA) 800 mg	
Green Tea	Naka Herbs	capsule	standardized green tea extract 400 mg (available in 2 concentrations: 30% catechin content and 80% catechin content)	Dairy-free Does not contain any starch, wheat or yeast
Lean+	Genuine Health	capsule	alpha lipoic acid 25 mg coleus 50 mg (10% forskohlin) garcinia cambogia 348 mg (50% hydroxycitric acid) green tea extract 228 mg guggulipid extract 75 mg	
MetaSlim CLA	WN Pharmaceuticals	softgel	conjugated linoleic acid (CLA) 1000 mg	Derived from safflower seed oil Designed to be used for body fat weight loss
MetaSlim CLA with Green Tea Extract	WN Pharmaceuticals	softgel	green tea extract 180 mg conjugated linoleic acid (CLA) 567 mg	Designed to support increased fat burning and lean muscle development
MetaSlim Kit - Weight Reduction Formula	WN Pharmaceuticals	tablet	bitter orange extract (citrus aurantium) cayenne pepper ginger green tea extract yerba maté extract	Designed to stimulate themogenic fat-weight reduction
NutriTrim	Naka Herbs	softgel	conjugated linoleic acid (CLA) 500 mg fish oil 200 mg green tea extract 50 mg pine nut oil 10 mg grapefruit 20 mg iodine 100 mcg chromium 75 mcg	
PGX Daily	WN Pharmaceuticals	softgel	PGX (PolyGlycopleX) 750 mg medium chain tryglycerides 600 mg	Designed to help people reduce appetite
Phytoslim	Nutripur	ampoule	Day Ampoule: calcium gluconate 500 mg chicory 25 mg dandelion 25 mg essential oil of mandarin 10 mg fennel 50 mg green anise 50 mg green tea 150 mg lemon juice concentrate 100 mg meadowsweet 50 mg nopal (opuntia ficus-indica) 75 mg passiflora 25 mg passionfruit juice concentrate 200 mg pear juice concentrate 454 mg pineapple juice concentrate 908 mg yerba maté 50 mg Night Ampoule: acacia 50 mg basil 40 mg bitter orange (citurs aurantium) 240 mg chromium chloride 12.5 mg corn 40 mg kelp 160 mg parsley 80 mg pear juice concentrate 1.36 mg wax bean 240 mg	10 day kit package combines different active ingredients to achieve action over a 24 hour period Day ampoule is designed to prevent absorption of dietary fat, help drain and eliminate, and help control appetite Night ampoule is designed to act as a fat deposit reducer and help tone the figure
Shape+	Genuine Health	capsule	calcium 125 mg green tea extract 84.4 mg (40% EGCG) garcinia cambogia 187.5 mg (50% hydroxycitric acid)	Designed to suppress fat production and to increase fat burning and loss

▶

Product	Manufacturer	Dosage Form	Active Ingredients	Comments
Slim Styles	Natural Factors	softgel	PGX (PolyGlycopleX) 820 mg	Designed to help lower the glycemic index of meal; will promote satiety, curb food cravings.
Slimdown Green Tea with Apple Cider Vinegar Complex	Jamieson	caplet	green tea extract leaves 113 mg caffeine 37.5 mg EGCG 68 mg	
Weider Green Tea Capsules	Weider Nutrition Group	capsule	green tea extract 500 mg guarana extract 50 mg	
X-Trim	Bill Beauty & Health Products	capsule	green tea extract 650 mg (contains EGCG 15% & caffeine 7%)	Contains no preservatifves, flavours, sugars, starches, wheat, yeast or milk products

Product	Manufacturer	Dosage Form	Decongestant	Antihistamine	Other Active Ingredients
Albalon	Allergan	drops	naphazoline hydrochloride 0.1%		
Allergy Drops	Bausch & Lomb	drops	naphazoline hydrochloride 0.012%		
Clear Eyes	Prestige Brands	drops	naphazoline hydrochloride 0.012%		
Clear Eyes Allergy	Prestige Brands	drops	naphazoline hydrochloride 0.012%		glycerin 0.26% zinc sulfate 0.25%
Clear Eyes Redness Relief	Prestige Brands	drops	naphazoline hydrochloride 0.012%		glycerin 0.26% hypromellose 0.8%
Clear Eyes Triple Action	Prestige Brands	drops	tetrahydrozoline hydrochloride 0.05%		polyvinyl alcohol 0.5% povidone 0.6%
Cromolyn Eye Drops	Pharmascience	liquid			sodium cromoglycate 2%
Minims Phenylephrine Drops 2.5%	Bausch & Lomb	drops	phenylephrine hydrochloride 2.5%		
Mydfrin Drops	Alcon	drops	phenylephrine hydrochloride 2.5%		
Naphcon-A	Alcon	liquid	naphazoline hydrochloride 0.025%	pheniramine maleate 0.3%	
Naphcon Forte	Alcon	drops	naphazoline hydrochloride 0.1%		
Opcon-A	Bausch & Lomb	drops	naphazoline hydrochloride 0.02675%	pheniramine maleate 0.315%	
Opticrom	Allergan	liquid			sodium cromoglycate 2%
Optrex Drops	Schering-Plough	drops			allantoin 0.08% borax 0.22% boric acid 1.08% glycerol 1% witch hazel 12.5%
Refresh Eye Allergy Relief	Allergan	drops	naphazoline hydrochloride 0.051%	antazoline phosphate 0.51%	
Visine Advance Allergy	Johnson & Johnson	drops	naphazoline hydrochloride 0.025%	pheniramine maleate 0.3%	
Visine Advance Triple Action	Johnson & Johnson	liquid	tetrahydrozoline hydrochloride 0.05%		dextran 70 0.1% polyethylene glycol 400 1% povidone 1%
Visine Allergy Eye Drops	Johnson & Johnson	liquid	tetrahydrozoline hydrochloride 0.05%		zinc sulfate 0.25%
Visine Cool Eye Drops	Johnson & Johnson	drops	tetrahydrozoline hydrochloride 0.05%		polyethylene glycol 1%
Visine Original Eye Drops	Johnson & Johnson	liquid	tetrahydrozoline hydrochloride 0.05%		
Visine Workplace Eye Drops	Johnson & Johnson	liquid	oxymetazoline hydrochloride 0.025%		

Product	Manufacturer	Dosage Form	Anti-infective
Optimyxin Eye/Ear Drops	Sandoz	drops	gramicidin 0.025 mg/mL polymyxin B sulfate 10 000 IU/mL
Optimyxin Ointment	Sandoz	ointment	bacitracin 500 IU/g polymyxin B sulfate 10 000 IU/g
Polysporin Eye/Ear Drops	Johnson & Johnson	drops	gramicidin 0.025 mg/mL polymyxin B sulfate 10 000 IU/mL
Polysporin Ophthalmic Ointment	Johnson & Johnson	ointment	bacitracin 500 IU/g polymyxin B sulfate 10 000 IU/g

Product	Manufacturer	Dosage Form	Active Ingredients
Artificial Tears	Pendopharm	liquid	polyvinyl alcohol 1.4%
Artificial Tears Extra	Pendopharm	liquid	polyvinyl alcohol 1.4% povidone 0.6%
Bion Tears	Alcon	liquid	dextran 70 0.1% hypromellose 0.3%
Celluvisc	Allergan	drops	sodium carboxymethylcellulose 1%
Eyelube 0.5%	Sandoz	drops	hypromellose 0.5%
Eyelube 1%	Sandoz	drops	hypromellose 1%
Genteal	Novartis Ophthalmics	liquid	hypromellose 0.3%
Genteal	Novartis Ophthalmics	gel	hypromellose 0.3%
Hypotears	Novartis Ophthalmics	drops	polyvinyl alcohol 1%
Isopto Tears 0.5%	Alcon	drops	hypromellose 0.5%
Isopto Tears 1%	Alcon	drops	hypromellose 1%
Liquifilm Forte	Allergan	drops	polyvinyl alcohol 3%
Moisture Drops	Bausch & Lomb	drops	glycerin 0.2% hypromellose 0.5% polyvinyl pyrrolidone 0.1%
Murine Eye Care	Abbott	drops	polyvinyl alcohol 0.5% povidone 0.6%
Murine Supplemental Tears	Abbott	liquid	benzalkonium chloride 0.01% disodium edetate 0.05%
Refresh	Allergan	drops, unit dose	polyvinyl alcohol 1.4%
Refresh Liquigel	Allergan	solution	sodium carboxymethylcellulose 1%
Refresh Plus	Allergan	drops, unit dose	sodium carboxymethylcellulose 0.5%
Refresh Tears	Allergan	drops	sodium carboxymethylcellulose 0.5%
Systane	Alcon	drops	polyethylene glycol 400 0.4% propylene glycol
Tear Drops	Novartis Ophthalmics	drops	polyvinyl alcohol 1.4% povidone 0.6%
Tear-Gel	Novartis Ophthalmics	gel	carbomer 980 disodium edetate sorbitol
Tears Naturale	Alcon	liquid	dextran 70 0.1% hypromellose 0.3%
Tears Naturale Free	Alcon	drops, unit dose	dextran 70 0.1% hypromellose 0.3%
Tears Naturale II Lubricant Eye Drops	Alcon	drops	dextran 70 0.1% hypromellose 0.3%
Tears Plus	Allergan	liquid	polyvinyl alcohol 1.4%
Theratears	Advanced Vision Research	liquid	sodium carboxymethylcellulose 0.25%
Visine Advance True Tears	Johnson & Johnson	liquid	glycerin 0.2% hypromellose 0.3%
Visine Contact Lens Drops	Johnson & Johnson	liquid	glycerin 0.2% hypromellose 0.2%
Visine True Tears Eye Drops	Johnson & Johnson	liquid	polyethylene glycol 400 1%

Product	Manufacturer	Dosage Form	Active Ingredients
Eye Stream	Alcon	liquid	calcium chloride 0.048% magnesium chloride 0.03% potassium chloride 0.075% sodium chloride 0.64%
Eye Wash	Zee Medical	liquid	sodium chloride 0.47% sodium citrate 0.1% sodium phosphate dibasic 0.47% sodium phosphate monobasic 0.46%
Lid-Care Towelettes	Novartis Ophthalmics	pad	benzyl alcohol cocamidoproprylamine oxide disodium edetate disodium laureth sulfosuccinate polyethylene glycol-200 glyceryl tallowate polyethylene glycol-80 glyceryl cocoate
Optrex Wash	Reckitt Benckiser	liquid	witch hazel 13%

Product	Manufacturer	Dosage Form	Active Ingredients
Duolube	Bausch & Lomb	ointment	petrolatum 80% petrolatum liquid 20%
Hypotears Eye Ointment	Novartis Ophthalmics	ointment	mineral oil 15% white petrolatum 85%
Lacri-Lube S.O.P.	Allergan	ointment	petrolatum 55.5% mineral oil 42.5%
Lacrisert Ophthalmic Inserts	Aton	ophthalmic insert	hydroxypropyl cellulose (hyprolose) 5 mg
Optilube	Dioptic	ointment	lanolin 2% mineral oil 42.5% petrolatum 55%
Tears Naturale P.M.	Alcon	ointment	lanolin 3% mineral oil 3% petrolatum 94%

Product	Manufacturer	Dosage Form	Sodium (mmol/L)	Potassium (mmol/L)	Chloride (mmol/L)	Other Ingredients
Gastrolyte Regular/Fruit	sanofi-aventis	powder	60	20	60	dextrose 17.8 g/L
Hydralyte Electrolyte Freezer Pops	Hydration Pharmaceuticals	freezer pop	45	20	35	dextrose 16 g/L
Hydralyte Electrolyte Powder	Hydration Pharmaceuticals	powder	45	20	35	dextrose 16 g/L
Hydralyte Electrolyte Solution	Hydration Pharmaceuticals	liquid	45	20	35	dextrose 16 g/L
Pedialyte Liquid	Abbott	liquid	45	20	35	dextrose 25 g/L
Pediatric Electrolyte Freezer Pops	Pendopharm	freezer pop	45	20	35	dextrose 20 g/L fructose 5 g/L
Pediatric Electrolyte Solution	Pendopharm	liquid	45	20	35	dextrose 20 g/L fructose 5 g/L

Product	Manufacturer	Dosage Form
Allkare Adhesive Remover	ConvaTec	wipe
Allkare Protective Barrier	ConvaTec	wipe
Eakin Cohesive Seals	ConvaTec	seals
Hollihesive Paste	Hollister	tube
Karaya Paste	Hollister	tube
Karaya Powder	Hollister	puff bottle
Karaya Seal Ring	Hollister	ring
Medical Adhesive	Hollister	spray/can
Medical Adhesive Remover	Hollister	spray/can
Premium Paste	Hollister	tube
Premium Powder	Hollister	puff bottle
Skin Barrier Powder	Hollister	powder
SoftFlex Skin Barrier Rings	Hollister	20-50 mm
Stomahesive Paste	ConvaTec	tube
Stomahesive Powder	ConvaTec	plastic dispensing bottle
Universal Remover Wipes	Hollister	wipe

Product	Manufacturer	Size	Form	Comments
Accuseal Adapter	ConvaTec		adapter	
Active Life Convex Drainable Pouch, Pre-cut, Durahesive	ConvaTec	19, 22, 25, 28, 32, 35, 38, 45 mm	pouch	Transparent With Tape Collar With Comfort panels With Tail Clip
Active Life Closed-End Pouch, Cut-to-fit	ConvaTec	fits stoma sizes: 19 to 50 mm	pouch	Available opaque or transparent With Tape collar With Comfort panels
Active Life Convex Urostomy Pouch, Pre-Cut	ConvaTec	13, 16, 19, 22, 25, 28, 32, 35, 38 mm	pouch	Transparent Standard With Bendable Tap Durahesive
Active Life Drainable Pouch, Cut-to-fit, Stomahesive	ConvaTec	fits stoma sizes: 19 to 100 mm	flange	Available opaque or transparent With Tape collar With Tail clip With Comfort panels
Active Life Drainable Pouch, Pre-cut, Stomahesive	ConvaTec	19, 25, 32, 38, 45, 50 mm	pouch	Available opaque or transparent With Tape collar With Tail clip With Comfort panels
Active Life One-Piece Closed-End Pouch, Pre-cut, with filter	ConvaTec	25, 32, 38, 45, 50 mm	pouch	Opaque No Tape collar With Comfort panels With Filter
Active Life One-Piece Stoma Cap, Cut-to-fit	ConvaTec	fits stoma sizes up to 50 mm	cap	Opaque With Filter With Comfort panels
Active Life One-Piece Urostomy Pouch, Cut-to-fit, Stomahesive	ConvaTec	fits stoma sizes up to 45 mm	pouch	Transparent With Bendable Tap
Active Life One-Piece Urostomy Pouch, Pre-Cut, Durahesive	ConvaTec	19, 22, 25, 28, 32, 38 mm	pouch	Transparent Accuseal Tap with Valve With Comfort panels
Assura Closed Pouch	Coloplast	40, 50, 60 mm	pouch	Odour-control filter Soft moisture-absorbent backing Opaque ot transparent
Assura Closed Pouch, Cut-to-Fit	Coloplast	non-convex (flat) : fits sizes 20-55 mm convex light: fits sizes 15-43 mm	pouch	Flexible adhesive Soft moisture-absorbing backing & odour-control filter
Assura Closed Pouch, Pre-Cut	Coloplast	non-convex (flat): 25, 30, 35, 40 mm convex light: 21, 25, 28, 31 mm	pouch	Flexible adhesive Soft moisture-absorbing backing & odour-control filter
Assura Drainable Pouch	Coloplast	40, 50, 60 mm	pouch	Includes 5 pouch clamps and 10 twist-ties, without filter
Assura EasiClose Wide Outlet Drainable Pouches	Coloplast	40, 50, 60 mm	pouch	With integrated filter Optional slim line filter enhances discretion while controlling odour
Assura Extra-Extended Wear Drainable Pouch, Cut-to-Fit	Coloplast	non-convex (flat): fits sizes 10-70 mm convex: fits sizes 15-43 mm	pouch	Longer lasting wear time than traditional systems Transparent adhesive preserves integrity of surrounding skin Available flat or convex Without filter Includes 5 pouch clamps and 10 twist-tie closures

Product	Manufacturer	Size	Form	Comments
Assura Extra-Extended Wear Skin Barrier with Flange, Cut-to-Fit	Coloplast	40, 50, 60 mm	flange	Longer lasting wear time than traditional systems Has transparent adhesive that preserves the integrity of the skin With spiral technology, belt loops on all skin barriers Available flat, convex light (shallow convexity), and convex (deep convexity)
Assura Extra-Extended Wear Skin Barrier with Flange, Pre-Cut	Coloplast	40, 50, 60 mm	flange	Longer lasting wear time than traditional systems Has transparent adhesive that preserves the integrity of the skin With spiral technology Belt loops on all skin barriers Available flat, convex light (shallow convexity), and convex (deep convexity)
Assura Extra-Extended Wear Urostomy Pouch, Cut-to-Fit	Coloplast	non-convex (flat): fits sizes 10-55 mm convex light: fits sizes 15-43 mm	pouch	Multiple chambers to provide a more discreet and quiet pouch Soft moisture-absorbent backing and anti-reflux valve Secure outlet closure and simple locking connector for night drainage bag attachment Includes 5 adaptors
Assura Multi-Chamber Urostomy Pouch	Coloplast	40, 50, 60 mm	pouch	Soft moisture-absorbent backing With anti-reflux valve Secure outlet closure and simple connector for night drainage Includes 10 adaptors
Assura Skin Barrier with Flange, Cut-to-Fit	Coloplast	40, 50, 60 mm	flange	Flexible With spriral technology for long lasting wear Belt loops on all skin barriers Available flat, convex light (shallow convexity), and Convex (deep convexity)
Assura Skin Barrier with Flange, Pre-Cut	Coloplast	40, 50, 60 mm	flange	Flexible With spiral technology for long lasting wear Belt loops on all skin barriers Available flat, convex light (shallow convexity), and Convex (deep convexity)
Assura Standard Drainable Pouch, Cut-to-Fit	Coloplast	non-convex (flat): fits sizes 10-70 mm convex/convex light: fits sizes 15-43 mm	pouch	Flexible With spiral technology for long lasting wear Available flat, convex light (shallow convexity), and convex (deep convexity) Includes 5 pouch clamps and 10 twist-tie closures Without filter
Assura Standard Wear Drainable Pouch with EasiClose, Cut-to-Fit	Coloplast	non-convex (flat): fits sizes 10-70 mm convex/convex light: fits sizes 15-43 mm	pouch	Available flat, convex light (shallow convexity), and convex (deep convexity)
Assura Standard Wear Drainable Pouch with EasiClose, Pre-Cut	Coloplast	non-convex (flat): 25, 30, 35 mm convex/convex light: 21, 25, 28, 31 mm	pouch	Available flat, convex light (shallow convexity), and convex (deep convexity)
Assura Stoma Cap	Coloplast	20 to 55 mm	cap	With odour-control filter Designed as an alternative for discreet situations
Assura Stoma Cap	Coloplast	40, 50, 60 mm	cap	Designed as an alternative for discreet situations Mini security pouch with filter
Assura Uro Minicap	Coloplast	40, 50 mm	cap	Designed as an alternative for discreet situations Holds up to 100 mL of urine, lasting 30-60 minutes With odour barrier

Product	Manufacturer	Size	Form	Comments
Assura Urostomy Pouch, Pre-Cut	Coloplast	15, 18, 21, 25, 28, 31, 35 mm	pouch	Flexible adhesive Soft moisture-absorbing backing & odour-control filter Anti-reflux valve and simple closure with adaptor for night drainage bag Includes 5 adaptors
CenterPointLock Closed pouch	Hollister	38-70 mm	pouch	With Integraged Filter Odour-free rustle-free film With or without ComfortWear panels
CenterPointLock Closed, Pouch, Filter mini opaque, opaque, transparent	Hollister	38, 44, 57, 70 mm	mini pouch, pouch	Odour-barrier rustle-free film
CenterPointLock Convex Skin Barrier with floating flange	Hollister	13-51 mm	flange	Pre-sized in 12 sizes Floating flange
CenterPointLock Drainable Mini-Pouch, opaque	Hollister	38, 44, 57, 70 mm	mini-pouch	Pouch clamp closure Without ComfortWear panels
CenterPointLock Drainable Pouch with replaceable filter, transparent, opaque, regular or mini	Hollister	38-70 mm	pouch	Pouch clamp closure Odour-free rustle-free film 1 pack of 20 Hollister replacement filters and 2 plugs
CenterPointLock Drainable Pouch	Hollister	38-102 mm	pouch	Without integrated filter Pouch clamp closure Odour-barrier rustle-free film Available with or without ComfortWear panels
CenterPointLock Flat Skin Barriers	Hollister	38, 44, 57, 70 mm	flange	Flextend skin barrier Floating flange Cut-to-fit With tape border
CenterPointLock Stoma Cap	Hollister	38, 44, 57, 70 mm	stoma cap	With integrated filter Odour-free rustle-free film Without ComfortWear panels
CenterPointLock Stoma Irrigator Sleeve	Hollister	38, 44, 57, 70, 102 mm	drain	
CenterPointLock Urostomy Pouch	Hollister	38, 44, 57, 70 mm	pouch	Odour-barrier rustle-free film With or without ComfortWear panels
CenterPointLock, pre-sized, Skin Barrier with tape border	Hollister	38, 44, 57 mm for stoma opening 22 to 44 mm	flange	FlexWear skin barrier-flat With tape border
Closed Mini Pouch, pre-sized, with Tape Adhesive	Hollister	25, 32, 38, 44, 51 mm	pouch	With integrated filter Odour-barrier film Without ComfortWear panels
Contour I Stoma Cap, pre-sized	Hollister	50 mm	stoma cap	SoftFlex Skin Barrier-flat Without tape border With integrated filter Odour-barrier film Without ComfortWear film
Esteem Synergy Drainable Pouch	ConvaTec	35, 48, 61 mm	pouch	With Adhesive Coupling Technology Opaque or transparent With Comfort panels With Tail clip With filter
Esteem Synergy Straight Pouch	ConvaTec	35, 61, 89 mm	pouch	No filter With Adhesive Coupling Technology Transparent With Comfort panels With Tail clip

Product	Manufacturer	Size	Form	Comments
Esteem Synergy Adhesive Coupling Technology Closed-End Pouch, with filter	ConvaTec	35, 48, 61 mm	pouch	Opaque Available in mini-pouch size (16.3 cm) and standard (22.6 cm) With Filter With Comfort panels
Esteem Synergy Adhesive Coupling Technology Convex Moldable Durahesive Skin Barrier	ConvaTec	small: fits stoma sizes 13 to 22 mm medium: fits stoma sizes 22 to 33 mm large: fits stoma sizes 33 to 45 mm	flange	White With Flexible tape collar With Landing Zone flange
Esteem Synergy Adhesive Coupling Technology Stomahesive Skin Barrier, Cut-to-fit	ConvaTec	small: fits up to 35 mm stoma medium: fits up to 48 mm stoma large: fits up to 61 mm stoma	flange	White With Flexible tape collar With Landing Zone flange
Esteem Synergy Adhesive Coupling Technology Stomahesive Skin Barrier, Cut-to-fit	ConvaTec	small: fits up to 35 mm stoma medium: fits up to 48 mm stoma large: fits up to 61 mm stoma extra large: fits up to 89 mm stoma	flange	No Tape collar With Landing Zone flange
Esteem Synergy Adhesive Coupling Technology Stomahesive Skin Barrier, Pre-cut	ConvaTec	small: 13, 16, 19, 25, 28, 32, 35, 38 mm medium: 38, 41, 45 mm	flange	With Flexible Tape collar With Landing Zone flange
Esteem Synergy Drainable, Left-side Pouch, with InvisiClose Clipless Closure	ConvaTec	35, 48, 61 mm	pouch	Opaque With filter With Adhesive Coupling Technology With Comfort panels
Esteem Synergy Drainable, Right-side pouch, with InvisiClose Clipless Closure	ConvaTec	35, 48, 61 mm	pouch	Available opaque or transparent With filter With InvisiClose Clipless Closure With Comfort panels
Esteem synergy Urostomy Pouch, Accuseal Tap with valve, with 1-sided comfort panel	ConvaTec	35, 48, 61 mm	pouch	Available opaque or transparent
First Choice, cut-to-fit, 19 cm Closed Pouch	Hollister	up to 64 mm	pouch	
First Choice, cut-to-fit, 30 cm Drainable Pouch	Hollister	up to 64 mm	pouch	With tape border Without integrated filter Pouch clamp clousre Odour-barrier rustle-free film Without ComfortWear panels Available with FlexWear or SoftFlex skin barrier
First Choice, pre-sized, 19 cm Closed Pouch	Hollister	25, 32, 38, 44, 51, 64 mm	pouch	
First Choice, pre-sized, 30 cm Drainable Pouch with FlexWear Skin Barrier-Convex	Hollister	19,22, 25, 29, 32, 35, 38, 41 mm	pouch	With tape border Without integrated filter Pouch clamp closure Odour-barrier rustle-free film Without ComfortWear Panels
First Choice, pre-sized, 30 cm Drainable Pouch with SoftFlex Skin Barrier-flat	Hollister	25,32, 38, 44, 51 mm	pouch	With tape border Without integrated filter Pouch clamp closure Odour-barrier rustle-free film Without ComfortWear panels
First Choice Urostomy Pouch, cut-to-fit, with Flat Barriers	Hollister	up to 64 mm	pouch	

Product	Manufacturer	Size	Form	Comments
First Choice Urostomy Pouch, pre-sized, with Convex Barriers	Hollister	16, 19, 22, 25, 29, 32, 35, 38 mm	pouch	
Gentle Touch Colostomy Postoperative Discharge Kit	ConvaTec	100 mm		Each kit includes: 5 Stomahesive wafers with Sur-Fit flanges; 5 Sur-Fit Drainable postoperative pouches with Gentle Touch flange, Transparent; 1 tail closure
Gentle Touch Colostomy/Ileostomy Postoperative Discharge Kit	ConvaTec	45, 70 mm		Each kit includes: 5 Sur-Fit Flexible wafers-White Collar; 5 Sur-Fit Drainable postoperative pouches with Gentle Touch flange, Standard, Transparent; 1 tail closure
Gentle Touch Colostomy/Ileostomy Postoperative System, sterile	ConvaTec	45, 70 mm		Each set includes: 1 Stomahesive wafer with Sur-Fit flange; 1 Sur-Fit Drainable postoperative pouch, 1 tail closure
Gentle Touch Loop Ostomy Postoperative System, sterile	ConvaTec	70 mm		Each set includes: 1 Stomahesive wafer with Sur-Fit flange; 1 Sur-Fit Drainable postoperative pouch, 1 tail closure, 1 rod 90 mm
Gentle Touch Loop Ostomy Postoperative System, sterile	ConvaTec	100 mm		Each set includes: 1 Stomahesive wafer with Sur-Fit flange; 1 Sur-Fit Drainable postoperative pouch, 1 tail closure, 1 rod 65 mm
Gentle Touch Urostomy Postoperative Discharge Kit	ConvaTec	45, 70 mm		Each kit includes: 5 Durahesive wafers; 5 Sur-Fit Urostomy postoperative pouches with GentleTouch flange, Standard Transparent; 1 night drainable adapter
Gentle Touch Urostomy Postoperative System, sterile	ConvaTec	45, 70 mm		Each set includes: 1 Stomahesive wafer with Sur-Fit flange; 1 Sur-Fit Urostomy postoperative pouch; 1 night drainage adapter
Hollihesive Skin Barrier Blanket	Hollister	10 x 10 cm 20 x 20 cm		Non-sterile
Karaya 5 Closed Pouch, Pre-sized, with or without Integrated Filter	Hollister	22, 29, 35, 38, 51, 64 mm	pouch	With tape border Odour-barrier film, without ComfortWear panels
Karaya 5 Drainable Pouch, Pre-sized, with Odour-Barrier Film	Hollister	15, 22, 29, 35, 38 mm	pouch	With tape border Without integrated filter Pouch clamp closure Without ComfortWear panels Availalble in 3 pouch lengths: 23 cm (mini), 30 cm, & 40 cm
Karaya 5 Drainable Pouch, pre-sized, with replaceable filter	Hollister	15, 22, 29, 35, 38, 51 mm	pouch	With tape border Pouch clamp closure Odour-barrier rustle-free film Without ComfortWear panels Includes 20 replacement filters and 2 plugs
Karaya 5 Drainable Pouch, pre-sized, without integrated filter, with odour-barrier rustle-free film	Hollister	22, 29, 35, 38, 51, 64 mm	pouch	With tape border Pouch clamp closure Odour-barrier rustle-free film Without ComfortWear panels
Karaya 5 Urostomy Pouch	Hollister	16, 22, 29, 35, 38 mm	pouch	Karaya 5 skin barrier With tape border Odour-barrier film Without ComfortWear panels
New Image Closed Pouch, with odour-barrier rustle-free film	Hollister	44, 57, 70 mm	pouch	ComfortWear Panel(s) With integrated filter Transparent or opaque Available in 18 (mini), 19 and 23 cm pouch length

Product	Manufacturer	Size	Form	Comments
New Image Convex Skin Barrier	Hollister	44, 57, 70 mm	skin barrier/ flange	FlexWear, convex, floating flange Cut-to-fit With or without tape border
New Image Convex Skin Barrier	Hollister	22, 25 mm Flange size: 44 mm 29, 32 mm Flange size: 57 mm	skin barrier/ flange	FlexWear, convex, floating flange Pre-sized With or without tape border
New Image Convex Skin Barrier	Hollister	44, 57, 70 mm	skin barrier/ flange	FlexWear, convex, floating flange Cut-to-fit With or without tape border
New Image Convex Skin Barrier	Hollister	22, 25 mm flange size: 44 mm 29, 32 mm flange size: 57 mm	skin barrier/ flange	FlexWear, convex, floating flange Pre-sized With or without tape border
New Image Drainable Mini-pouch, odor-barrier rustle-free film	Hollister	44, 57, 70 mm	pouch	
New Image Drainable Pouch, odour-barrier rustle-free film	Hollister	44, 57, 70 mm	pouch	
New Image Drainable Pouch, with Pouch Clamp closure	Hollister	44, 57, 70 mm	pouch	ComfortWear Panel(s) Pouch clamp closure Transparent or beige With or without integrated filter
New Image High Output Drainable Pouch	Hollister	44, 57, 70, 102 mm	pouch	ComfortWear Panel Soft Tap Without integrated filter Odour-barrier film
New Image Irrigator Drain	Hollister	44, 57, 70 mm	drain	1 pouch clamp Odour-barrier film
New Image Skin Barrier with floating flange	Hollister	44, 57, 70, 102 mm	skin barrier/ flange	FlexWear skin barrier With or without tape border Cut-to-fit
New Image Skin Barrier with floating flange	Hollister	44, 57, 70, 102 mm	skin barrier/ flange	Flextend skin barrier With or without tape border Cut-to-fit
New Image Skin Barrier with floating flange	Hollister	44 mm: fits 16, 19, 22, 25, 29, 32 mm 57 mm: fits 35, 38 mm	skin barrier/ flange	FlexWear skin barrier With or without tape border Pre-sized
New Image Skin Barrier with floating flange	Hollister	45 mm: fits 16, 19, 22, 25, 29, 32 mm 57 mm: fits 35, 38 mm	skin barrier/ flange	Flextend skin barrier With or without tape border Pre-sized
New Image Skin Barrier with stationary 44 mm flange	Hollister	16-38 mm	skin barrier/ flange	FlexWear skin barrier Stationary flange Without tape border Pre-sized
New Image Skin Barrier with stationary 44 mm flange	Hollister	16-38 mm	skin barrier/ flange	FlexWear skin barrier Stationary flange Without tape border Pre-sized
New Image Skin Barrier with stationary flange	Hollister	44, 57, 70 mm	skin barrier/ flange	FlexWear skin barrier Stationary flange Cut-to-fit Without tape border
New Image Skin Barrier with stationary flange	Hollister	44, 57, 70 mm	skin barrier/ flange	Flextend skin barrier Stationary flange Cut-to-fit Without tape border

Product	Manufacturer	Size	Form	Comments
New Image Urostomy Pouch, transparent or opaque odour-barrier film	Hollister	44, 57, 70 mm	pouch	Comfort Wear Panel(s)
Ostomy Appliance Belt	ConvaTec	up to 100 cm	belt	Specially designed for light, cool and long-wearing patient comfort
Premier Closed Pouch, Cut-to-Fit, with SoftFlex Skin Barrier	Hollister	up to 55 mm	pouch	Without tape border With integrated filter Odour-barrier rustle-free film With ComfortWear panels
Premier Closed Pouch, Pre-sized, with SoftFlex Skin Barrier	Hollister	25, 30, 35 mm	pouch	Without tape border With integrated filter Odour-barrier rustle-free film With ComfortWear panels
Premier Drainable Pouch, cut-to-fit, with Convex Flextend Skin Barrier	Hollister	25, 38, 51 mm	pouch	With tape border Without integrated filter With odour-barrier, rustle-free film With ComfortWear panels Available with Pouch Clamp Closure or Lock n'Roll Integrated Closure
Premier Drainable Pouch, cut-to-fit, with Lock n' Roll Integrated Closure	Hollister	up to 64 mm	pouch	With tape border Without integrated filter With Flextend Skin Barrier -flat With ComfortWear panels Available with odour-barrier film, or odour-barrier rustle-free film
Premier Drainable Pouch, cut-to-fit, with Lock n' Roll Integrated Closure, with SoftFlex Skin Barrier	Hollister	up to 55 mm	pouch	Without tape border With integrated filter Odour-barrier rustle-free film With ComfortWear panels Available transparent or beige
Premier Drainable Pouch, cut-to-fit, with Pouch Clamp Closure	Hollister	up to 64 mm	pouch	
Premier Drainable Pouch, pre-sized, with Convex Flextend Skin Barrier	Hollister	19, 22, 25, 29, 32, 35, 38, 41, 44, 51 mm	pouch	With tape border Without integrated filter With odour-barrier, rustle-free film With ComfortWear panels Available with Pouch Clamp Closure or Lock n'Roll Integrated Closure
Premier Drainable Pouch, pre-sized, with Lock n' Roll Integrated Closure, with Flextend Skin Barrier	Hollister	25, 32, 38, 44 mm	pouch	With tape border Without integrated filter Odour-barrier rustle-free film With ComfortWear panels
Premier Drainable Pouch, pre-sized, with Lock n' Roll Integrated Closure, with SoftFlex Skin Barrier	Hollister	25, 30, 35, 40 mm	pouch	Without tape border With integrated filter Odour-barrier rustle-free film With ComfortWear panels Available transparent or beige In 18cm (mini) or 30 cm pouch length
Premier Drainable Pouch, pre-sized, with Pouch Clamp Closure	Hollister	23 cm length: 19, 25, 32, 38, 44, 51 mm 30 cm length: 19, 25, 32, 38, 44, 51, 64 mm	pouch	With tape border Without integrated filter With Flextend Skin Barrier With ComfortWear panels With odour-barrier rustle-free film Available in 23 (mini), and 30 cm pouch length
Premier Urostomy Pouch, Cut-to-Fit	Hollister	up to 64 mm	pouch	

Product	Manufacturer	Size	Form	Comments
Premier Urostomy Pouch, Cut-to-Fit, with Convex Skin Barrier	Hollister	25, 38, 51 mm	pouch	With tape border Odour-barrier rustle-free film With ComfortWear panels
Premier Urostomy Pouch, Pre-sized	Hollister	19, 25, 32, 38, 44, 51 mm	pouch	
Premier Urostomy Pouch, Pre-sized, with Convex Skin Barrier	Hollister	13, 16, 19, 19, 22, 25, 29, 32, 35, 38, 44 mm	pouch	With tape border Odour-barrier rustle-free film With ComfortWear panels
SenSura Click Closed Pouch	Coloplast	40, 50, 60, 70 mm	pouch	With odour filter
SenSura Click EasiClose Wide-Outlet Drainable Pouch	Coloplast	40, 50, 60, 70 mm	pouch	Available opaque or transparent With filter or without filter
SenSura Click Skin Barriers with Flange, Cut-to-Fit or Pre-Cut	Coloplast	40, 50, 60, 70 mm	flange	Sensura click with audible click-lock security ring Double layer technology for long-lasting wear Available flat or convex light (shallow convexity)
SenSura Click Urostomy Pouch	Coloplast	40, 50, 60 mm	pouch	Opaque or transparent
SenSura Click Xpro Skin Barriers with Flange, Cut-to-Fit or Pre-Cut	Coloplast	40, 50, 60, 70 mm	flange	Sensura Click locking ring Double layer technology for long-lasting wear and two extra ingredients to protect against aggressive output Belt loop Available flat or convex light (shallow convexity)
SenSura Closed Pouch, Cut-to-Fit	Coloplast	flat: fits sizes 10 to 76 mm convex light: fits sizes 15 to 43 mm	pouch	With New Wave filter Available flat or convex light (shallow convexity) Opaque or transparent
SenSura Closed Pouch, Pre-Cut	Coloplast	21, 25, 28, 31 mm	pouch	With New Wave filter Available flat or convex light (shallow convexity) Opaque or transparent
SenSura Drainable Pouch, Cut-To-Fit	Coloplast	flat: fits sizes 10 to 76 mm convex light: fits sizes 15 to 43 mm	pouch	With New Wave filter With EasiClose Wide outlet Available flat or convex light (shallow convexity) Opaque or transparent
SenSura Drainable Pouch, Pre-Cut	Coloplast	21, 25, 28, 31 mm	pouch	With New Wave filter With EasiClose Wide outlet Available flat or convex light (shallow convexity) Opaque or transparent
SenSura Flex Closed Pouch	Coloplast	35, 50, 70, 90 mm	pouch	Opaque With New Wave odour filter
SenSura Flex EasiClose Wide-Outlet Drainable Pouch	Coloplast	35, 50, 70, 90 mm	pouch	With New Wave filter Opaque or transparent
SenSura Flex Skin Barrier with Flange, with Adhesive Coupling, Cut-to-Fit or Pre-Cut	Coloplast	35, 50, 70, 90 mm	flange	Low profile Double layer adhesive
SenSura Flex Urostomy Pouch	Coloplast	35, 50 mm	pouch	Opaque or transparent
SenSura Flex Xpro Barrier with Flange, Cut-to-Fit	Coloplast	35, 50, 70 mm	pouch	Low profile Double layer adhesive Available flat or convex light (shallow convexity)
Sensura Xpro Urostomy Pouch, Cut-to-Fit	Coloplast	flat: fits sizes 10 to 76 mm convex light: fits sizes 15 to 43 mm	pouch	With odour-proof film Anti-reflux valve Simple adaptor for night drainage bag Opaque or transparent

Product	Manufacturer	Size	Form	Comments
Stoma Cap, Pre-sized	Hollister	51, 76 mm	cap	Tape adhesive With integrated filter Odour-barrier film Without ComfortWear panels
SUR-FIT AutoLock Closed-End Pouch	ConvaTec	35, 45, 57, 70 mm	pouch	With filter Opaque With Comfort panels
SUR-FIT Autolock Durahesive Skin Barrier, Cut-to-fit, with flexible tape collar	ConvaTec	35, 45, 57, 70, 100 mm	flange	Available with Flexible tape collar or without tape collar White
SUR-FIT Autolock Two-Piece Disposable Convex Insert	ConvaTec	Inner Diameter Opening 19 mm	insert	For use with 35 mm SUR-FIT AutoLock Durahesive Flexible and SUR-FIT AutoLock Stomahesive Flexible Skin Barriers
SUR-FIT Autolock Two-Piece Disposable Convex Insert	ConvaTec	Inner Diameter Opening 32 mm	insert	For use with 45 mm SUR-FIT AutoLock Durahesive Flexible and SUR-FIT AutoLock Stomahesive Flexible Skin Barriers
SUR-FIT AutoLock Two-Piece Drainable Pouch	ConvaTec	35, 45, 57, 70, 100 mm	pouch	Available opaque or transparent With traditional Tail clip With Comfort panels No filter
SUR-FIT AutoLock Urostomy Pouch, standard	ConvaTec	35, 45, 57, 70 mm	flange	Available opaque or transparent With Accuseal Tap with valve With Comfort panel
SUR-FIT Natura Closed Mini-Pouch, with 1-sided comfort panel, no filter	ConvaTec	32, 38, 45, 57 mm	pouch	
SUR-FIT Natura Durahesive Skin Barrier with Convex-It Technology, Pre-Cut	ConvaTec	46 mm flange: fits stomas 13, 16, 19, 22, 25, 28, 32, 35 mm 57 mm flange: fits stomas 38, 41, 45, 50 mm	flange	With Flexible Tape collar 45 mm Flange
SUR-FIT Natura Durahesive Skin Barrier, Cut-to-Fit	ConvaTec	32, 38, 45, 57, 70, 100 mm	flange	Durahesive skin barriers are designed for people whose stoma output is mostly liquid; Durahesive skin barriers swell up or «Turtleneck» to further protect the stoma and peristomal skin Tan or white Available with Flexible Tape collar or without Tape collar
SUR-FIT Natura Low Pressure Adapter	ConvaTec	45, 57, 70, 100 mm	flange	Converts any Sur-Fit Natura ostomy system into a low-pressure solution post-surgery; product is an insert between pouch and skin barrier to create clearance for a nurse to insert fingers and snap the pouch coupling ring into place without applying force to abdomen
SUR-FIT Natura Moldable Skin Barrier Convex, Durahesive, with flexible tape collar	ConvaTec	45 mm flange: fits stoma sizes : 13-22 mm and 22-33 mm 57 mm flange: fits stoma sizes 33-45 mm	flange	
SUR-FIT Natura Moldable Skin Barrier, Durahesive, with hydrocolloid flexible collar	ConvaTec	45 mm flange: fits stoma sizes : 13-22 mm and 22-33 mm 57 mm flange: fits stoma sizes 33-45 mm 70 mm flange: fits stoma sizes 45-56 mm	flange	
SUR-FIT Natura Moldable Skin Barrier, Stomahesive, with hydrocolloid flexible collar	ConvaTec	45 mm flange: fits stoma sizes : 13-22 mm and 22-33 mm 57 mm flange: fits stoma sizes 33-45 mm 70 mm flange: fits stoma sizes 45-56 mm	flange	

Product	Manufacturer	Size	Form	Comments
SUR-FIT Natura Stomahesive Skin Barrier, Cut-to-Fit, with flexible tape collar, white	ConvaTec	32, 38, 45, 57, 70, 100 mm	flange	Stomahesive skin barriers are designed for people whose stoma output is semi-formed or formed Tan or white Available with Flexible Tape collar or without Tape collar
SUR-FIT Natura Two-Piece Closed-End Pouch, with 2-sided comfort panel	ConvaTec	38, 45, 57, 70 mm	pouch	Available with or without filter
SUR-FIT Natura Two-Piece Disposable Convex Inserts	ConvaTec	Inner diameter opening: 19, 22, 25, 29, 32, 35, 38, 41 mm	insert	For use with either 38 mm, 45 mm, or 57 mm skin barriers
SUR-FIT Natura Two-Piece Drainable Pouch	ConvaTec	32, 38, 45, 57, 70 mm	pouch	With Tail Clip Opaque With Comfort panels
SUR-FIT Natura Two-Piece Drainable Pouch with InvisiClose Clipless Closure	ConvaTec	38, 45, 57, 70 mm	pouch	With InvisiClose Clipless Closure Available opaque or transparent With Comfort panels
SUR-FIT Natura Two-Piece Drainable Pouch High Output	ConvaTec	45, 57, 70 mm	pouch	For high output With anti-reflux valve With replaceable filter With Outlet with Spout & Cap With Comfort panels
SUR-FIT Natura Two-Piece Drainable Pouch	ConvaTec	32, 38, 45, 57, 70 mm	pouch	With Tail Clip With filter Available opaque or transparent With comfort panels
SUR-FIT Natura Two-Piece Drainable Pouch, Extra Large (35.5 cm)	ConvaTec	100 mm	pouch	With Tail Clip Opaque With Comfort panels
SUR-FIT Natura Two-Piece Stomahesive Skin Barrier, Pre-Cut	ConvaTec	45 mm flange: fits stomas 13, 16, 19, 22, 25, 28, 32, 35 mm 57 mm flange: fits stomas 38, 41, 45 mm	flange	With Flexible Tape collar 45 mm Flange
SUR-FIT Natura Urostomy Pouch, with 1-sided comfort panel	ConvaTec	32, 38, 45, 57, 70 mm	pouch	Available opaque or transparent Available with Accuseal Tap with Valve or Bendable Tap

Product	Manufacturer	Size	Form	Comments
Assura Pediatric Pouch One-Piece, drainable or closed	Coloplast	10-35 mm	pouch	Flexible and skin friendly skin barrier With filter for odour control
Assura Pediatric Pouch Two-Piece	Coloplast		pouch	Soft backing comfort and odour-proof film Locking system reduces pressure to abdomen
Assura Pediatric Skin Barrier with Flange	Coloplast	10-35 mm	flange	
Assura Pediatric Urostomy Pouch	Coloplast	10-35 mm	pouch	Odour-proof film with anti-reflux valve and soft backing for comfort
Easiflex Pediatric Drainable Pouch with EasiClose	Coloplast	20-30 mm coupling size	pouch	With adhesive coupling Integrated closure with filter
Easiflex Pediatric Skin Barrier with Flange, Cut-to-fit	Coloplast	20 mm coupling: 0-15 mm 30 mm coupling: 0-25 mm	flange	Flat barrier With adhesive coupling EasiClose outlet
Little Ones Drainable Pouch, Extra-small, with 1-sided comfort panel	ConvaTec	fits stoma opening 0 to 23 mm	pouch	Transparent
Little Ones Drainable Pouch, Cut-to-fit, with 1-sided comfort panel, tail clip	ConvaTec	fits sizes 8 to 50 mm	pouch	Transparent
Little Ones Drainable Pouch, Cut-to-fit, Standard 5" pouch with fold up tab	ConvaTec	fits sizes 8 to 25 mm	pouch	Transparent
Pouchkins Drain Tube	Hollister		tubing	
Pouchkins Newborn Ostomy	Hollister	up to 22 x35 mm	pouch	
Pouchkins Newborn Pouch, Cut-to-fit	Hollister	35 mm x 22 mm	pouch	SoftFlex Skin Barrier - flat Without tape border Without integrated filter Without ComfortWear panels Can be used with or without Drain Valve
Pouchkins One-Piece Drainable Pouch with Odour-Barrier Rustle-Free Film	Hollister	16 cm length: up to 38 mm 21 cm length: up to 51 mm	pouch	SoftFlex Skin Barrier - flat Without starter hole Without tape border Without integrated filter Soft wire closure Without ComfortWear panels
Pouchkins Pediatric Ostomy Belt	Hollister	26-43 cm	belt	Adjustable from 26 to 43 cm
Pouchkins Pediatric Two-Piece Urostomy Pouch, 44 mm flange size	Hollister	up to 21 cm pouch length	pouch	Odour-barrier rustle-free film Without ComfortWear panels
Pouchkins Pediatric Urostomy Pouch	Hollister	up to 38 mm	pouch	SoftFlex Skin Barrier - flat Without tape border Odour-barrier rustle-free film Without ComfortWear panels
Pouchkins Premie/Newborn Pouch, cut-to-fit	Hollister	up to 15mm	pouch	SoftFlex Skin Barrier - flat Without tape border Without integrated filter Without ComfortWear panels Can be used as a premie closed or drainable pouch
Pouchkins Two-Piece Pediatric Drainable Pouch with 44 mm flange size	Hollister	up to 21 cm pouch length	pouch	Without integrated filter Soft Wire Closure Odour-barrier rustle-free film Without ComfortWear Panels
Pouchkins Two-Piece Pediatric system with CenterPointLock Floating Flange	Hollister	44 mm flange size: up to 32 mm	flange	SoftFlex Skin Barrier - flat Without tape border

Product	Manufacturer	Form	Comments
Adapt Lubricating Deodorant	Hollister	wipe, bottle	
Allkare Adhesive Remover	ConvaTec	wipe	Iso-alcohol-free solution
Allkare Protective Barrier	ConvaTec	wipe	Non-water soluble
Barriere	WellSpring Pharma	tube, jar	dimethylpolysiloxane 20%
Coloplast Ostomy Paste	Coloplast	tube, strips	Low alcohol content Used to fill uneven skin areas to create flat pouching surface and to protect peristomal area
Coloplast Prep Protective Liquid Skin Barrier	Coloplast	wipes, bottle	Forms barrier against skin irritants No need to remove between applications
Coloplast Skin Barrier	Coloplast	patches	Can be used around stomas, draining wounds, and other areas subject to irritation
M9 Odour Eliminator Drops	Hollister	bottle	Available scented or unscented
Moisture Barrier Skin Ointment	Hollister	tube	Protects skin from irritating damage Petroleum based
Restore Barrier Creme	Hollister	tube	Skin protectant, breathable
Restore Clean N Moist	Hollister	spray bottle	Adjustable nozzle, 3-in-1 cleans, moisturizes and protects
Skin Cleanser	Hollister	spray/bottle	Cleans peristomal and perineal skin
Skin Conditioning Creme	Hollister	bottle	Vitamins A, D and E
Skin Gel	Hollister	wipe	Protects skin from adhesive trauma
Universal Remover Wipes	Hollister	wipe	For adhesives and barriers

Product	Manufacturer	Dosage Form	Active Ingredients
Auralgan	Pfizer Consumer Healthcare	liquid	antipyrine 5.4% benzocaine 1.4%
Auro-Dri Ear Water Drying Aid	Insight	liquid	isopropyl alcohol 95%
Cerumol	Paladin	liquid	chlorbutol 5% oil of terebinth 10% paradichlorobenzene 2%
Flents Ear Drops	Apothecary Products	liquid	carbamide peroxide 6.5%
Lidomyxin	Sandoz	liquid	lidocaine hydrochloride 50 mg/mL polymyxin B sulfate 10 000 IU/mL
Murine Ear Drops	Prestige	liquid	carbamide peroxide 6.5%
Murine Ear Wax Removal System	Prestige	liquid	carbamide peroxide 6.5%
Optimyxin Eye/Ear Drops	Sandoz	liquid	gramicidin 0.025 mg/mL polymyxin B sulfate 10 000 IU/mL
Personnel Liquid Ear Drops	Apothecary Products	liquid	carbamide peroxide 6.5%
Polysporin Eye/Ear Drops	Pfizer Consumer Healthcare	liquid	gramicidin 0.025 mg/mL polymyxin B sulfate 10 000 IU/mL

Product	Manufacturer	Warranty	PEF Scale (L/min)	Target Zones	Dimensions	Weight	Contents	Comments
AirZone	Clement Clarke	1 year	60-720	Adaptable to 3 or 4 zone system[ab] Locking markers	13.75 x 3.125 cm	42.5 g	Operating instructions Patient diary (English, French & Spanish)	Meets ATS, NAEPP & NHLBI standards Materials are latex-free
Asthma Digital Monitor	Microlife	2 years	50-900	3 zone system[a] Measures FEV_1	14.4 x 7.7 x 4.8 cm	150 g (including batteries	Manual Carrying case Wall holder Software and connection cable included	Can be used by children and adults 240 Reading memory Uses 2 x AAA batteries FEV_1 Range: 0.01-9.99 L total volume
AsthmaMentor	Philips Respironics	1 year	60-810	3 zone system[a] Built in AutoZone system	15.3 x 6.6 x 2 cm	99 g	Instructions Daily diary Asthma action plan sticker	Auto-zone system will automatically calculate colour-coded peak flow zones Meets NAEPP standards Dishwasher safe
Breath-Alert	Medical Developments International	2 years	50-800	3 zone system[a] Zone markers	18 x 3.5 x 3.5 cm	45 g	Manual Daily recording card	Dishwasher safe Can be used by children or adults Meets NAEPP standards
Breath-Alert Low Range	Medical Developments International	2 years	50-370	3 zone system[a] Zone markers	19 x 3.5 x 3.5 cm	45 g	Manual Daily recording card	Dishwasher safe Can be used by children or adults Meets NAEPP standards
Mini-Wright Standard	Clement Clarke	1 year	60-880	3 zone system[a] Zone markers	15 x 4.4 cm	82.2 g	Operating instructions Patient diary (English & French)	Meets ATS, NAEPP & NHLBI standards Materials are latex-free One-way valve
Mini-Wright AFS Low Range	Clement Clarke	1 year	30-400	3 zone system[a] Zone markers	14.4 x 3.4 cm	62.4 g	Operating instructions Patient diary (English & French)	Meets ATS, NAEPP & NHLBI standards Materials are latex-free One-way valve
PeakAir	Omron	3 years	50-750	Zone markers	15 x 10 cm	60 g	Instruction manual Reusable mouthpiece Children's stickers	Meets ATS standards

▶

Product	Manufacturer	Warranty	PEF Scale (L/min)	Target Zones	Dimensions	Weight	Contents	Comments
Piko-1 Electronic Monitor	Nspire Health	6 months	15-999	3 zone system[a] Measures FEV_1	7.5 x 3.5 x 2.0	35 g	Manual Software and USB interface cradle included	Meets ATS standards Warning & indicator for cough or abnormal blow Uses 2 x 357 silver oxide button batteries FEV_1 Range: 0.15-9.99 L total volume
Pocket Peak	Nspire Health	1 year	50-720	Adaptable to 3 or 4 zone system[ab] Locking markers	8.4 x 9.4 x 3 cm (with mouthpiece)	42.5 g	Operating instructions Patient diary (English, French & Spanish)	Meets ATS, NAEPP & NHLBI standards Materials are latex-free
TruZone	Trudell Medical	1 year	60-800	4 zone system[b] Tapes	17.4 x 3.2 x 3.2 cm	35 g	ColorZone tapes Daily record	One size fits all, can be used by children and adults Logarithmic scale Tamper-proof internal indicator User friendly design Portable Meets NAEPP standards

[a] **3 zone system:**
GREEN: 80-100% of personal best signals "all clear"
YELLOW: 50-80% of personal best signals "caution"
RED: below 50% of personal best signals "medical alerts"

[b] **4 zone system:**
GREEN: 80-100% of personal best signals "all clear"
HIGH YELLOW: 65-80% of personal best signals "caution"
LOW YELLOW: 50-65% of personal best signals "higher level of caution"
RED: below 50% of personal best signals "medical alerts"

Abbreviations:
PEF = Peak Expiratory Flow
FEV_1 = Forced Expiratory Volume in 1 second
ATS = American Thoracic Society
NAEPP = National Asthma Education and Prevention Program
NHLBI = National Heart, Lung, Blood Institute

     Compendium of Products for Minor Ailments

Product	Manufacturer	Warranty	Type	Power Source	Weight	Contents	Comments
AeroEclipse II Breath Actuated Nebulizer	Trudell Medical	none	Breath Actuated Nebulizer used with compressor	AC		Nebulizer Top Nebulizer Cup Mouthpiece Tubing	Features AeroControl System Regulator (SR) which provides true breath actuation for patient on-demand therapy The device may be used with a compressor capable of delivering a flow of 2.75 to 8 liters per minute (lpm) under an operating pressure of 15 to 50 pounds per square inch (psi). For 7 day use
AG Classic	Medel	3 year	compressor	AC	1.5 kg	Compressor unit Medel Jet nebulizer Tubing Angled mouthpiece Filter (5 pcs)	Built-in handle High pressure/flow system Operates all types of nebulizers
AG Edge	Medel	3 year	compressor	AC Battery pack Car adapter	0.3 kg	Microcompressor unit Medel Jet Pro nebulizer Tubing Mouthpiece Filter (5pcs) Universal adapter	Small compressor/nebulizer Handheld or tabletop operation
AG Plus	Medel	3 year	compressor	AC Battery pack Car adapter	0.4 kg	Microcompressor unit Medel Jet Pro nebulizer Tubing Mouthpiece Filter (5pcs) Universal adapter	Small, compact design Operates all typer of nebulizers
Comp-Air	Omron	5 year	compressor	AC	1.7 kg	Instruction manual Nebulizer kit Carrying case	Adult or child use CSA approved
Comp-Air Elite	Omron	5 year	compressor	AC Battery pack Car adapter	310 g	Instruction manual Nebulizer kit Carrying case	Adult or child use Optional battery pack Optional DC automobile adapter CSA approved
Inspiration 626	Philips Respironics	5 year	compressor	AC	2 kg	Instruction manual (English/ French/ Spanish) Nebulizer Child mask Mouthpiece Tee adapter Extension tube Storage compartment	Adult or child use Adult mask available Replacement parts available
Inspiration Elite	Philips Respironics	5 year	compressor	AC	1.5 kg	Compressor Sidestream Nebulizer mouthpiece Tubing Filter	Delivers treatment within 7 minutes Adult or child use Adult or child mask available Replacement parts available
MedPro AirPort Portable	AMG Medical	5 year	compressor	AC Car adapter	345 g	Carry/Storage bag Mouthpiece AC Adapter Car adapter Ni-Cd rechargeable battery pack Masks (adult & pediatric) Filter & spare parts	Adult or child use Fits comfortably in one hand

▶

Product	Manufacturer	Warranty	Type	Power Source	Weight	Contents	Comments
MedPro Compressor	AMG Medical	5 year	compressor	AC	2 kg	Instruction manual Nebulizer Air tube Mouthpiece 5 filters Adult mask	Built-in nebulizer kit and power cord storage Adult or child use
MicroAir Vibrating Mesh Nebulizer	Omron	2 year	ultrasonic	AC AA battery	227 g	Instruction video AC adapter Mouthpiece Adult mask Medicine cup Spare mesh cap Rinse bottle Soft case	Small nebulizer Pediatric mask is available
PARI Proneb Ultra II Adult	PARI Respiratory Equipment	5 year	compressor	AC DC (car battery)	1.3 kg	Instruction DVD PARI LC Sprint reusable nebulizer Tubing Deluxe carry case	Delivers treatment in 5 minutes (with LC sprint nebulizer) Other LC reusable nebulizers available Extra LC nebulizer included as backup
PARI Proneb Ultra II Pediatric	PARI Respiratory Equipment	5 year	compressor	AC DC (car battery)	1.3 kg	Instruction DVD PARI LC Sprint reusable nebulizer Bubbles the Fish II pediatric mask Tubing Deluxe carry case	Pediatric model Delivers treatment in 5 minutes (with LC sprint nebulizer) Other LC reusable nebulizers available Extra LC nebulizer included as backup
PARI Trek S Compact	PARI Respiratory Equipment	3 year (6 months on battery)	compressor	AC (110V & 240V) DC (car battery) Rechargeable internal battery	0.5 kg	Compressor Instruction DVD Deluxe carry case LC Sprint (reusable nebulizer) Multi Voltage charger-adapter DC car adapter	Delivers treatment in 5-6 minutes Battery delivers up to 8 treatments (of 2.5 mL normal saline solution) Available separately: Adult rigid mask, Bubbles the Fish pediatric mask, and baby conversion kit
Salter AIRE Plus	Salter Labs	5 year	compressor	AC	1.9 kg	Instruction manual Mouthpiece Tubing Nebulizer	Adult or child use Nebulizer available: disposable, PARI LC reusable, or PARI LC Sprint reusable Optional travel bag Treatment time 6-7 minutes

Product	Manufacturer	Dosage Form	Benzoyl Peroxide	Salicylic Acid	Sulfur	Other Active Ingredients
Acnomel Cream	Numark	cream			8%	resorcinol 2%
Acnomel Vanishing Cream	Numark	cream			8%	resorcinol 2%
Adasept Acne Gel	Odan	gel		2%		sodium thiosulfate 8% triclosan 0.5%
Adasept B.P.5 Acne Gel	Odan	gel	5%			
Adasept Skin Cleanser	Odan	liquid				triclosan 0.5%
Aveeno Acne Treatment	Johnson & Johnson	bar		0.5%		
Benzagel 5 Gel	Columbia	gel	5%			
Benzagel 5 Wash	Columbia	liquid	5%			
Clearasil Acne Cream - Skin Tone	Reckitt Benckiser	cream			8%	resorcinol 2%
Clearasil Acne Cream - Vanishing	Reckitt Benckiser	cream			3%	resorcinol 2%
Clearasil BP Plus Lotion	Reckitt Benckiser	lotion	5%			
Clearasil Cleanser	Procter & Gamble	liquid		2%		
Clearasil Clearstick	Procter & Gamble	liquid		2%		
Clearasil Deep Cleansing Wash	Reckitt Benckiser	suspension				triclosan 0.3%
Clearasil Stay Clear Deep Cleaning Pads	Reckitt Benckiser	pad		2%		
Clean & Clear BP Cleanser Continuous Control	Johnson & Johnson	lotion	5%			
Clean & Clear Continuous Control Acne Wash	Johnson & Johnson	liqid		2%		
Clean & Clear Deep Cleaning	Johnson & Johnson	liquid		2%		
Clean & Clear Deep Cleaning Sensitive	Johnson & Johnson	liquid		0.5%		
Clean & Clear Dual Action Moisturizer	Johnson & Johnson	cream		0.5%		
Clean & Clear Foaming Facial Cleanser	Johnson & Johnson	liquid				triclosan 0.25%
Clean & Clear Invisible Blemish Treatment	Johnson & Johnson	gel		2%		
Clean & Clear Persa Gel	Johnson & Johnson	lotion	5%			
Neo Strata Blemish Spot Gel	Canderm	gel	2%			
Neutrogena Acne Wash Cream Cleanser	Johnson & Johnson	cream		2%		
Neutrogena Acne Wash Oil-Free	Johnson & Johnson	liquid		2%		
Neutrogena Clear Pore Scrub	Johnson & Johnson	gel		2%		
Neutrogena Skin Cleaning Face Wash	Johnson & Johnson	lotion		1.5%		
Noxzema Triple Clean Antibacterial Cleanser	Alberto-Culver	lotion				triclosan 0.3%
Noxzema Triple Clean Pads	Alberto-Culver	pad		2%		
Oxy Cover Up Formula	Mentholatum	cream	5%			
Oxy Daily Cleaning Pads - Deep Cleaning	Mentholatum	pad		2%		
Oxy Daily Cleaning Pads - Sensitive	Mentholatum	pad		0.5%		
Oxy DeepClean Pore Daily Cleanser	Mentholatum	liquid		2%		
Oxy Vanishing Formula Acne	Mentholatum	lotion	5%			
Oxy Vanishing Formula Acne - Sensitive Skin	Mentholatum	lotion	2.5%			
PanOxyl 5 Bar	Stiefel	soap	5%			
PanOxyl 5 Wash	Stiefel	lotion	5%			
Snap Facial Soap	Stella	paste				pumice
Solugel 4	Stiefel	gel	4%			
Sulfur Soap	Valeo	soap			10%	
Tersaseptic	Stiefel	liquid				triclosan 0.5%
Trisan	Dermtek	gel				triclosan 0.25%

Product	Manufacturer	Type	Comments
Alldress	Molnlycke	square	Multi-layered absorptive waterproof cover
Band-Aid Brand Adhesive Bandages Advanced Cuts and Scrapes	Johnson & Johnson	strips	Multi-day protection
Band-Aid Brand Adhesive Bandages Advanced Healing	Johnson & Johnson	strips	Multi-day protection
Band-Aid Brand Adhesive Bandages Antibiotic	Johnson & Johnson	strips	Antibiotic on the pad
Band-Aid Brand Adhesive Bandages Antibiotic Waterproof	Johnson & Johnson	strips	Antibiotic on the pad
Band-Aid Brand Adhesive Bandages Clear	Johnson & Johnson	strips	Less noticeable than regular bandages
Band-Aid Brand Adhesive Bandages Clear Water Block Plus	Johnson & Johnson	strips	Clear Waterproof Four-sided adhesive
Band-Aid Brand Adhesive Bandages Comfort-Flex Clear	Johnson & Johnson	strips	Clear Waterproof
Band-Aid Brand Adhesive Bandages Comfort-Flex Plastic	Johnson & Johnson	strips	Waterproof
Band-Aid Brand Adhesive Bandages Flexible Fabric	Johnson & Johnson	strips	Stretchable
Band-Aid Brand Adhesive Bandages Flexible Fabric Extra Large	Johnson & Johnson	extra large pad	Stretchable
Band-Aid Brand Adhesive Bandages Flexible Fabric Knuckle & Fingertip	Johnson & Johnson	knuckle & fingertip	Stretchable
Band-Aid Brand Adhesive Bandages Gentle Care	Johnson & Johnson	strips	
Band-Aid Brand Adhesive Bandages Perfect Fit	Johnson & Johnson	strips	Waterproof Stretchable
Band-Aid Brand Adhesive Bandages Plastic	Johnson & Johnson	strips	
Band-Aid Brand Adhesive Bandages Tough-Strips	Johnson & Johnson	strips	Heavy duty fabric
Band-Aid Brand Adhesive Bandages Water Block Plus Clear	Johnson & Johnson	strips	Waterproof Four-sided adhesive
Band-Aid Brand Adhesive Bandages Water Block Plus Finger-Care	Johnson & Johnson	knuckle & fingertip	Waterproof Four-sided adhesive
Band-Aid Brand Adhesive Bandages Water Block Plus Finger-Wrap	Johnson & Johnson	tapered shape for fingers	Tapered design to stay on fingers Waterproof Four-sided adhesive
Band-Aid Brand Adhesive Bandages Water Block Plus Large	Johnson & Johnson	strips	Waterproof Four-sided adhesive
Band-Aid Brand Adhesive Bandages Wet-Flex	Johnson & Johnson	strips	Padded foam material gives extra protection Water resistant
Band-Aid Single Step Liquid Bandage	Johnson & Johnson	liquid	
Nexcare Bandages Active	3M	strips	Waterproof Latex-free Stretchable
Nexcare Comfort Fabric Bandages	3M	strips	Latex-free
Nexcare Heavy Duty Flexible Fabric Bandages	3M	strips	Late-free Four-sided adhesive
Nexcare Heavy Duty Waterproof Bandages	3M	strips	Latex-free Waterproof Clear
Nexcare No Sting Liquid Bandage Spray	3M	liquid	
Nexcare No Sting Liquid Bandage Drops	3M	liquid	
Nexcare Premium Bandage Pack	3M	strips	Assorted

Product	Manufacturer	Type	Comments
Nexcare Waterproof Clear Protection Bandages	3M		Waterproof Diamond shaped
Surepress Absorbent Padding	ConvaTec		Underpadding Viscose/super-absorbent fibres This padding protects the skin and provides additional absorption and even distribution of pressure under the SUREPRESS High Compression Bandage To be used with the SUREPRESS High Compression bandage
SurePress Bandage	ConvaTec		High compression bandage (30-40 mm Hg) Cotton-viscose, nylon, Lycra An extensible bandage designed for use over a wound dressing for patients with impaired venous return
Tubifast Retention Bandage	ConvaTec		Tubular retention bandage Viscose, elastane Used to hold dressings securely in place on any part of the body
Tubigrip Shaped Support Bandage	ConvaTec		Support bandage Elasticized cotton Anatomically-shaped Used in the management of venous disorders to aid venous and lymphatic return
Tubigrip Support Bandage	ConvaTec		Support bandage Cotton, elastodiene, polyamide Provides tissue support in the treatment of strains and sprains, soft tissue injuries and joint effusions
Tubinette Tubular Bandage	ConvaTec		Tubular retention bandage Viscose Stockinet use to hold dressings securely in place and to protect clothing from ointments and creams
Tubipad Limb Bandage	ConvaTec		Padded support bandage Cotton, elastodiene, polyamide For the prevention and treatment of pressure and friction ulcers

Product	Manufacturer	Dosage Form	Active Ingredients
Afterburn	Tender	jelly	lidocaine hydrochloride 0.5%
Betacaine	Canderm	gel	lidocaine 5%
EMLA Cream	AstraZeneca	cream	lidocaine 2.5% prilocaine 2.5%
EMLA Patch	AstraZeneca	pad	lidocaine 2.5% prilocaine 2.5%
Lidodan Ointment	Odan Labs	ointment	lidocaine 5%
Lidodan Viscous	Odan Labs	liquid	lidocaine hydrochloride 2%
Maxilene Cream 4%	RGR Pharma	cream	lidocaine 4%
Maxilene Cream 5%	RGR Pharma	cream	lidocaine 5%
Nupercainal Ointment	Novartis Consumer Health	ointment	dibucaine 1%
Solarcaine Lidocaine Lotion	Schering-Plough	lotion	lidocaine hydrochloride 0.5%
Solarcaine Lidocaine Medicated Gel	Schering-Plough	gel	lidocaine 0.5%
Solarcaine Lidocaine Spray	Schering-Plough	aerosol	lidocaine 0.5%
Xylocaine Jelly	AstraZeneca	gel	lidocaine hydrochloride 2%
Xylocaine Ointment	AstraZeneca	ointment	lidocaine 5%
Xylocaine Topical	AstraZeneca	ointment	lidocaine 4%
Xylocaine Viscous	AstraZeneca	liquid	lidocaine hydrochloride 2%

Compendium of Products for Minor Ailments

Product	Manufacturer	Dosage Form	Active Ingredients
Canesten Topical	Bayer Consumer	cream	clotrimazole 1%
Clotrimazole Cream	Various Manufacturers	cream	clotrimazole 1%
Fungicure Gel	Alva-Amco Pharmacal	gel	tolnaftate 1%
Fungicure Liquid	Alva-Amco Pharmacal	liquid	undecylenic acid 10%
Fungicure Professional	Alva-Amco Pharmacal	liquid	undecylenic acid 12.5%
Micatin Derm Cream	McNeil Consumer Healthcare	cream	miconazole nitrate 2%
Monistat Derm Cream	Johnson & Johnson	cream	miconazole nitrate 2%
Nyaderm Cream	Taro	cream	nystatin 100 000 IU/g
Nystatin Cream	Various Manufacturers	cream	nystatin 100 000 IU/g
Nystatin Ointment	Various Manufacturers	ointment	nystatin 100 000 IU/g
ratio-Nystatin cream	Teva	cream	nystatin 100 000 IU/g
ratio-Nystatin ointment	Teva	ointment	nystatin 100 000 IU/g
Tinactin Cream	Schering-Plough	cream	tolnaftate 1%

Product	Manufacturer	Dosage Form	Zinc Pyrithione	Tar Product	Other Active Ingredients
2-in-1 Conditioning Dandruff Shampoo	Scott	shampoo	1%		
Dandruff Shampoo	Scott	shampoo	1%		
Dan-Gard Shampoo	Valeo	shampoo	2%		
Denorex Extra Strength with Conditioner	Ultimark	shampoo		coal tar solution 10%	chloroxylenol 0.5% menthol 1.5%
Denorex Regular with Conditioner	Ultimark	shampoo		coal tar solution 7.5%	chloroxylenol 0.5% menthol 1.5%
Dermarest Medicated Shampoo	Church & Dwight	shampoo			salicylic acid 3%
Gillette Anti Dandruff Shampoo	Procter & Gamble	shampoo	1%		
Head & Shoulders Clinical Strength	Procter & Gamble	shampoo			selenium sulfide 1%
Head & Shoulders Dandruff Conditioner	Procter & Gamble	shampoo	0.5%		
Head & Shoulders Dandruff Shampoo	Procter & Gamble	shampoo	1%		
Herbal Essences No Flakin Way Anti Dandruff Shampoo	Procter & Gamble	shampoo	1%		
Medi-Dan Shampoo	Mahdeen	shampoo		coal tar 4.25%	benzalkonium chloride 0.2% salicylic acid 2%
Neutrogena T/Gel Extra	Johnson & Johnson	shampoo		coal tar 1%	
Neutrogena T/Gel Therapeutic Shampoo	Johnson & Johnson	shampoo		coal tar 0.5%	
Nizoral Shampoo	McNeil Consumer Healthcare	shampoo			ketoconazole 2%
Pantene Anti-Dandruff Shampoo	Procter & Gamble	shampoo	1%		
Pert-Plus Dandruff Away	Procter & Gamble	shampoo	1%		
Polytar AF Shampoo	Stiefel	shampoo		coal tar 0.5%	menthol 0.5% pyrithione disulfide 1% salicylic acid 2%
Sebcur	Dermtek	shampoo			salicylic acid 4%
Sebcur/T	Dermtek	shampoo		coal tar solution 10%	salicylic acid 4%
Selsun Blue	Chattem	shampoo			selenium sulfide 1%
Selsun Blue 2-in-1	Chattem	shampoo			selenium sulfide 1%
Selsun Blue Deep Cleansing	Chattem	shampoo			salicylic acid 3%
Selsun Suspension	Chattem	liquid			selenium sulfide 2.5%
Sterex Shampoo	International Dermatologicals	shampoo		coal tar 2%	salicylic acid 2% sulfur 2%
Tardan Shampoo	Odan	shampoo		coal tar 5%	salicylic acid 2% triclosan 0.3%
Tersaseptic	Stiefel	liquid			triclosan 0.5%
Z-Plus Shampoo	Dormer	shampoo	2%		menthol 0.3%

Product	Manufacturer	Dosage Form	Keratolytic	Anti-inflammatory	Other Active Ingredients
Aveeno Anti-Itch Cream	Johnson & Johnson	cream			calamine 3% pramoxine hydrochloride 1%
Aveeno Anti-Itch Lotion	Johnson & Johnson	lotion			calamine 3% pramoxine hydrochloride 1%
Aveeno Bath Relief Treatment	Johnson & Johnson	powder			oats 100%
Aveeno Moisturizing Bath	Johnson & Johnson	powder			oats 43%
Aveeno Shower & Bath Oil	Johnson & Johnson	liquid			oats 5%
Barriere	WellSpring	cream			dimethylpolysiloxane 20%
Benadryl Itch Relief Cream	Pfizer Consumer Healthcare	cream			diphenhydramine hydrochloride 2%
Calamine Lotion	Various Manufacturers	liquid			calamine 8% zinc oxide 8%
Calamine Lotion with Antihistamine	Various Manufacturers	suspension			calamine 8% diphenhydramine 1%
Cetaphil Gentle Cleansing Bar	Galderma	bar			nonmedicated cleanser for sensitive skin
Cetaphil Gentle Skin Cleanser	Galderma	lotion			nonmedicated cleanser
Cetaphil Moisturizing Lotion & Cream	Galderma	cream/lotion			nonmedicated emollient
Cetaphil Restoraderm Lotion	Galderma	lotion			ceramides nonmedicated emollient
Cetaphil Oily Skin Cleanser	Galderma	lotion			nonmedicated cleanser
Claritin Skin Itch Relief	Schering-Plough	cream		hydrocortisone 0.5%	
Complex 15 Face Cream	Schering-Plough	cream			dimethicone 0.5% lecithin 0.1%
Complex 15 Lotion	Schering-Plough	lotion			dimethicone 1% lecithin 0.3%
Cortate Cream	Schering-Plough	cream		hydrocortisone 0.5%	
Cortate Ointment	Schering-Plough	ointment		hydrocortisone 0.5%	
Cortef	Johnson & Johnson	cream		hydrocortisone acetate 0.5%	
Cortoderm	Taro	ointment		hydrocortisone 0.5%	
Curel Continuous Comfort Lotion	KAO	lotion			glycerin 12% petrolatum 4%
Dermaflex Hand Cream	Neolab	cream	urea 10%		
Dermaflex 20 Urea Cream	Neolab	cream	urea 20%		
Dermal Therapy Extra Strength Body Lotion	Dermal Therapy Research		urea 10%		
Dermal Therapy Finger Care	Dermal Therapy Research	cream	urea 20%		
Dermal Therapy Hand Elbow and Knee Cream	Dermal Therapy Research	cream	urea 15%		
Dermal Therapy Heel Care	Dermal Therapy Research	cream	urea 25%		
Dermalac Cream	Taro	cream/lotion	lactic acid 12%		
Dormer 211 Cream	Dormer	cream			hyaluronic acid complex lecithin
Dormer 211 Face Cream	Dormer	cream			hyaluronic acid complex lecithin

▶

Product	Manufacturer	Dosage Form	Keratolytic	Anti-inflammatory	Other Active Ingredients
Dormer 211 Lotion	Dormer	lotion			hyaluronic acid complex lecithin
Epi-Lyt Medicated Lotion	Valeo	lotion	lactic acid 5%		glycerin 25%
EpiCeram Skin Barrier Emulsion	Pediapharm	emulsion			ceramides cholesterol free fatty acids
Episec	Odan	lotion			petrolatum liquid 12% propylene glycol 4% triethanolamine stearate 4%
Eucerin Lotion	Beiersdorf	lotion	urea 10%		
Eurax	Columbia	cream			crotamiton 10%
Glaxal Base	WellSpring	cream/lotion			nonmedicated hypoallergenic base
Gold Bond Medicated Cream	Chattem				menthol 1% pramoxine hydrochloride 1%
Hyderm	Taro	cream		hydrocortisone acetate 0.5%	
Hydrocortisone Cream	Various Manufacturers	cream		hydrocortisone 0.5%	
Hydrocortisone Ointment	Various Manufacturers	ointment		hydrocortisone 0.5%	
Hydrophil Ointment	Omega	ointment	urea 5%		petrolatum liquid 64.5%
Hydrosone	ratiopharm	cream		hydrocortisone 0.5%	
Ihle's paste	Various Manufacturers	paste			zinc oxide 25%
Keri Bath & Shower Oil	Novartis Consumer Health	oil			moisturizing oil cleanser
Keri Lotion - Original	Novartis Consumer Health	lotion			lanolin 0.6% mineral oil 15.9%
Keri Lotion - Fast Absorbing	Novartis Consumer Health	lotion			dimethicone 3% petrolatum 6%
Lac-Hydrin	Novartis Consumer Health	lotion	lactic acid 12%		
Lassar's Paste	Atlas	paste	salicylic acid 2%		zinc oxide 24%
Lubriderm Advanced Moisture Therapy	Johnson & Johnson	cream			glycerin mineral oil vitamin A vitamin E
Lubriderm Lotion Scented/ Unscented	Johnson & Johnson	lotion			lanolin mineral oil
Lubriderm Sensitive Skin Lotion	Johnson & Johnson	lotion			fragrance-free, non-comedogenic lotion
Moisturel Cream	Novartis Consumer Health	cream			dimethicone 1% petrolatum 30%
Moisturel Lotion	Novartis Consumer Health	lotion			dimethicone 3% petrolatum 6%
Nutraderm Lotion	Galderma	lotion			light mineral oil
Oilatum Liquid	Stiefel	liquid			petrolatum liquid 63.4%
Palmers Cocoa Butter Cream	E.T. Browne	cream			cocoa butter
Palmers Cocoa Butter Lotion	E.T. Browne	lotion			cocoa butter
Prevex Cream	Stiefel	cream			petrolatum 67%
Reversa Oily Skin Solution	Dermtek	liquid	glycolic acid 8%		

Product	Manufacturer	Dosage Form	Keratolytic	Anti-inflammatory	Other Active Ingredients
Reversa Skin Smoothing Face & Neck Cream	Dermtek	cream	glycolic acid 8%		
Spectro Derm	GlaxoSmithKline Consumer Healthcare	liquid			hypoallergenic cleanser
Spectro Eczema Care Medicated Cream	GlaxoSmithKline Consumer Healthcare	cream		clobetasone butyrate 0.05%	
Taro Base	Taro	cream			nonmedicated base
Trisan	Dermtek	gel			triclosan 0.25%
Uree 20	Riva	cream	urea 20%		
Uremol 10% Cream	Stiefel	cream	urea 10%		
Uremol 10% Lotion	Stiefel	lotion	urea 10%		
Uremol 20% Cream	Stiefel	cream	urea 20%		
Urisec-10	Odan	cream	urea 10%		
Urisec-40	Odan	cream	urea 40%		
Urisec Cream	Odan	cream	urea 22%		
Urisec Lotion	Odan	lotion	urea 12%		
Vitamin E Cream with Vitamins A & D	Adams	cream			vitamin A 250 IU/mL vitamin D 50 IU/mL vitamin E 75 IU/mL
Zinc & Castor Oil Cream	Various Manufacturers	cream			castor oil 50% zinc oxide 7.5%
Zinc Cream	Various Manufacturers	cream			zinc oxide 15%
Zinc Ointment 15%	Various Manufacturers	ointment			zinc oxide 15%
Zinc Ointment 20%	Various Manufacturers	ointment			zinc oxide 20%

Product	Manufacturer	Comments
Acticoat	Smith & Nephew	Anti-microbial barrier dressing Composed of nanocrystalline silver Latex-free
Actisorb Silver	Johnson & Johnson	Primary wound dressing that combines anti-microbial action and odour control Composed of activated charcoal with silver
Adaptic	Johnson & Johnson	Composed of knitted cellulose acetate and petrolatum emulsion Non-adherent film dressing
Algisite	Smith & Nephew	Composed of calcium-alginate Forms a soft, integral gel when it comes into contact with wound exudate For moderate to high exudate
Alldress Wound Dressing	Johnson & Johnson	Composed of a polyurethane film and a polyester nonwoven coated with a polyacrylate adhesive The absorbent pad is covered with a low-adherent polyolefin net
Allevyn Cavity	Smith & Nephew	Composed of polyurethane foam Sterile Latex-free For high to very high exudate
Allevyn+ Cavity	Smith & Nephew	Composed of polyurethane foam Sterile Latex-free
Allevyn Compression	Smith & Nephew	Composed of polyurethane matrix and a polyurethane top film Gentle adhesive Sterile Latex-free For moderate to high exudate
Allevyn Hydrocellular Adhesive Foam Dressing	Smith & Nephew	Composed of 3-layer structure: wound contact layer, absorbent central hydrocellular layer, and waterproof outer film layer Wound contact layer is coated with an adhesive that adheres well to intact skin, but not to wounds For moderate to high exudate
Allevyn Hydrocellular Non-Adhesive Foam Dressing	Smith & Nephew	Composed of 3-layer structure: Non-adherent wound contact layer, absorbent central hydrocellular layer, and waterproof outer film layer For moderate to high exudate
Allevyn Sacrum	Smith & Nephew	Composed of 3-layer structure Wound contact layer is coated with an adhesive that adheres well to intact skin, but not to wound For moderate to high exudate Shaped to fit sacral area
Allevyn Thin	Smith & Nephew	Composed of polyurethane foam Gentle adhesive Sterile Latex-free
Aquacel	ConvaTec	Composed of sodium carboxymethylcellulose 100% For the management of heavily exudating wounds
Aquacel AG	ConvaTec	Composed of sodium carboxymethylcellulose 100% Dressing contains ionic silver, which is released in a controlled manner as wound exudate is absorbed For the management of heavily exudating wounds
Bactigras	Smith & Nephew	Composed of chlorhexidine acetate 0.5% Nonadherent tulle gras gauze
Biatain Adhesive and Non-Adhesive Polymer Dressing	Coloplast	Composed of 3D polymer Leaves no residue in the wound
Bioclusive Transparent Dressing	Johnson & Johnson	Hypo-allergenic adhesive Semi-occlusive polyurethane film

Product	Manufacturer	Comments
Carboflex	ConvaTec	Composed of calcium-sodium alginate, sodium carboxymethylcellulose and activated charcoal For wound odour control and exudate management
Carbonet	Smith & Nephew	Composed of an activated charcoal cloth Nonadherent Odour absorbent
Combiderm ACD	ConvaTec	Composed of extra absorbent polymers Non-adhesive and absorbent Used as a cover dressing over heavily exudating wounds with fragile peri-wound skin
Comfeel Plus	Coloplast	Composed of a semipermeable polyurethane film coated with sodium carboxy-methylcellulose, hydroxyethylcellulose and calcium alginate
Comfeel Purilon Hydrogel	Coloplast	Composed of water and some calcium-alginate Sterile Maintains optimal moist wound environment
Comfeel Seasorb Soft Alginate Dressing	Coloplast	Composed of calcium-alginate
Contreet	Coloplast	Composed of polyurethane foam bonded to a semipermeable film with silver complex Sustained silver released for up to 7 days
Cutinova Hydro	Smith & Nephew	Conformable Waterproof Provides a bacterial barrier, but is oxygen and water vapour permeable
Derma-gel	Medline	Semi-occlusive hydrogel dressing Non-adherent
Dermatix Ultra Gel	Valeant	Composed of ester C, cyclopentasolixane, polysilicone-11, dimethicone, phenyl trimethicone, and polymethylsilsesquioxane Scar care Lightweight Self-drying gel
DuoDERM CGF	ConvaTec	Composed of sodium carboxymethylcellulose, gelatin and pectin Moisture-retentive hydrocolloid dressing For use on wounds with low to moderate amounts of exudate
DuoDERM CGF Border	ConvaTec	Composed of sodium carboxymethylcellulose, gelatin and pectin Moisture-retentive hydrocolloid dressing For use on wounds located in hard-to-dress (sacrum/heel) areas with low to moderate amounts of exudate
DuoDERM Extra-Thin	ConvaTec	Composed of sodium carboxymethylcellulose, gelatin and pectin Moisture-retentive hydrocolloid dressing For use on reddened skin as a protector against friction and shear forces Can also be used on areas of superficial skin breakdown
DuoDERM Hydroactive Gel	ConvaTec	Facilitates autolytic debridement For management of partial and full-thickness wounds and as a filler for cavity wounds
DuoDERM Signal	ConvaTec	Composed of sodium carboxymethylcellulose, gelatin and pectin Moisture-retentive hydrocolloid dressing For use on wounds located in hard-to-dress (sacrum/heel) areas with low to moderate amounts of exudate
Ete Low-adherent Dressing	Molnlycke	Low-adherent, 'rayon-sil' cover dressing for moderate to high exudates Designed for absorption and protection Ideal when a moist wound environment is contraindicated
Exu-Dry	Smith & Nephew	Latex-free Non-adherent Multi-layer Designed to conform to the contours of the upper limbs

Product	Manufacturer	Comments
Fibracol Plus	Johnson & Johnson Medical	Composed of a combination of 90% collagen and 10% alginate Nonadherent
Hypergel	Molnlycke	Composed of 20% sodium chloride hydrogel Requires secondary cover dressing
IntraSite Gel	Smith & Nephew	Composed of water and fibres Provides a moist wound healing environment
Iodosorb	Smith & Nephew	Composed of cadexomer iodine Sterile
Kaltostat	ConvaTec	Composed of calcium-sodium alginate fibre For management of moderate to heavily exudating wounds Controls minor bleeding
Medipore+Pad	3M	Sterile Soft cloth wound dressing Medipore tape with absorbent non-stick gauze pad
Mefix	Molnlycke	Moisture vapour permeable Polyurethane film transparent film
Melgisorb	Molnlycke	Composed of calcium-alginate fibre Requires secondary cover dressing
Mepiform	Molnlycke	Composed of silicone Self-adherent Scar care
Mepilex	Molnlycke	Absorbent foam dressing with Safetac
Mepilex Border	Molnlycke	Self-adherent Absorbent foam dressing
Mepitel	Molnlycke	Transparent silicone coated Non-adherent Micro-adherent wound contact dressing
Mepore	Molnlycke	Self-adhesive island dressing Rectangular
Mepore Pro	Moynlycke	Waterproof self-adhesive Sterile island absorbent film dressing Rectangular shape
Mesalt	Molnlycke	Composed of sodium chloride Designed as an antibacterial/cleansing dressing, releases sodium chloride as it absorbs exudate Requires secondary cover dressing
Mesorb Absorbent and Wound Dressing	Molnlycke	High absorption capacity and retention capacity
Normlgel	Molnlycke	Contains sodium chloride 0.9% ingel form Designed to release sodium chloride into wound to maintain moist environment
Nu-Derm Alginate	Johnson & Johnson	Composed of guluronic acid alginate and carboxy methyl cellulose fiber
Nu-Derm Hydrocolloid	Johnson & Johnson	Hydrocolloid Dressing designed to maintain a optimum moist environment
Nu-Gel Hydrogel/Collagen	Johnson & Johnson	Sterile hydrogel formulation of preserved polyvinyl pyrrolidone in water
Opsite Flexifix	Smith & Nephew	Transparent moisture vapour permeable film dressing For moist wound healing
OpSite Wound/Flexigrid	Smith & Nephew	Polyurethane coated with acrylic adhesive Sterile Transparent moisture vapour permeable film dressing For moist wound healing
Promogran Protease Modulated Matrix	Johnson & Johnson	Composed of collagen, cellulose, and 1% silver Sterile

Product	Manufacturer	Comments
Restore Calcium Alginate Wound Care Dressing	Hollister	Composed of calcium sodium alginate Sterile To manage moderate to heavily exuding, partial- to full-thickness wounds
Restore Calcium Alginate Wound Care Dressing with Silver	Hollister	Composed of calcium sodium alginate Contains ionic silver that is slowly released
Restore Dressing for Psoriasis	Hollister	Sterile hydrocolloid Occlusive dressing with flexible film backing for the management of psoriasis
Restore Extra Thin Dressing	Hollister	Synthetic and hydrocolloid materials with tackifiers Sterile To manage superficial wounds with minimal or no exudate To protect skin or wounds that are at risk from friction injury
Restore Hydrogel Dressing	Hollister	Clear, viscous gel
Restore Plus Dressing	Hollister	Synthetic and hydrocolloid materials with tackifiers Sterile Absorbs excess wound exudates Facilitates autolytic debridement
Tegaderm/Tegaderm HP Transparent Dressings	3M	Composed of polyurethane coated with acrylic adhesive Transparent, semipermeable film dressing Polyurethane film
Tegaderm+ Pad	3M	Transparent dressing with absorbent pad Polyurethane film with absorbent non-stick gauze pad
Tegafoam Adhesive Dressing	3M	Composed of of a comformable, absorbent polyurethane foam pad, with a breathable film backing, and with soft cloth tape High absorption capacity and retention capacity
Tegafoam Non Adhesive Dressing	3M	A woven, nylon fabric with sealed edges Non-adherent, non-irritating To be used under gauze or other absorbent dressing
Tegagel Wound Filler	3M	Amorphous gel
Tegagen HI & HG	3M	Composed of calcium-sodium alginate fibre Needs secondary dressing to hold in place Available in high gelling or high integrity (HG & HI)
Tegasorb Ulcer Dressing/Tegasorb Thin Ulcer Dressing	3M	Composed of pectin, gelatin and carboxymethylcellulose The oval and sacral shape include a transparent film backing and border
Tielle/Tielle Plus Hydropolymer	Johnson & Johnson	Composed of a polyurethane foam and coated with an acrylic adhesive. Island dressing
Triad Hydrophillic Dressing	Coloplast	Hydrophyllic paste Composed of zinc oxide Paste that adheres to moist weeping wounds
Versiva with AG Hydrofibre	ConvaTec	Composed of carboxymethylcellulose Transforms to gel on contact with fluid
Wound'Dres Collagen Hydrogel	Coloplast	Composed of collagen, and allantoin Acts as a wound debriding catalyst of necrotic tissue and debris

Product	Manufacturer	Dosage Form	Antiseptic	Anti-infective	Antipruritic	Anesthetic	Other Active Ingredients
Adasept Skin Cleanser	Odan	liquid	triclosan 0.5%				
After-Bite	Tender	liquid					ammonia 3.5%
Afterburn	Tender	jelly				lidocaine hydrochloride 0.5%	
Allerject 0.15 mg	sanofi-aventis	liquid					epinephrine 0.15 mg/dose
Allerject 0.3 mg	sanofi-aventis	liquid					epinephrine 0.3 mg/dose
Aloe Vera	Various Manufacturers	gel					aloe vera 90%-98%
Antibiotic Cream	Various Manufacturers	cream		gramicidin 0.25 mg/g polymyxin B sulfate 10 000 IU/g			
Antibiotic Ointment	Various Manufacturers	ointment		bacitracin 500 IU/g polymyxin B sulfate 10 000 IU/g			
Aveeno Anti-Itch Cream	Johnson & Johnson	cream			calamine 3%	pramoxine hydrochloride 1%	
Aveeno Anti-Itch Lotion	Johnson & Johnson	lotion			calamine 3%	pramoxine hydrochloride 1%	
Bacitin	Pharmascience	ointment		bacitracin 500 IU/g			
Bactine	Bayer Consumer	nonaerosol	benzalkonium chloride 0.13%			lidocaine hydrochloride 2.5%	
Baxedin	Omega	liquid	chlorhexidine gluconate 0.05%				
Benadryl Cream	Pfizer Consumer Healthcare	cream			diphenhydramine hydrochloride 2%		
Benadryl Itch Stick	Pfizer Consumer Healthcare	stick			diphenhydramine hydrochloride 2%		zinc acetate 0.1%
Benadryl Itch Spray	Pfizer Consumer Healthcare	liquid			diphenhydramine hydrochloride 2%		zinc acetate 0.1%
Betadine Ointment	Purdue Pharma	ointment	povidone-iodine 10%				
Betadine Solution	Purdue Pharma	liquid	povidone-iodine 10%				
Betadine Surgical Scrub	Purdue Pharma	liquid	povidone-iodine 7.5%				
Bioderm	Odan	ointment		bacitracin 500 IU/g polymyxin B sulfate 10 000 IU/g			
Calamine Lotion	Various Manufacturers	liquid			calamine 8%		zinc oxide 8%
Calamine Lotion with Antihistamine	Various Manufacturers	suspension			calamine 8% diphenhydramine hydrochloride 1%		
Claritin Cream	Schering-Plough	cream					hydrocortisone 0.5%
Cortate Cream	Schering-Plough	cream					hydrocortisone 0.5%

Product	Manufacturer	Dosage Form	Antiseptic	Anti-infective	Antipruritic	Anesthetic	Other Active Ingredients
Cortate Ointment	Schering-Plough	ointment					hydrocortisone 0.5%
Cortef	McNeil Consumer Healthcare	cream					hydrocortisone acetate 0.5%
Dakin's Solution 0.5% Modified	Century	liquid	sodium hypochlorite solution 0.5%				
Dettol Liquid	Reckitt Benckiser	liquid	chloroxylenol 4.8%				
Dexidin 0.5%-70% Solution	Atlas	liquid	chlorhexidine gluconate 0.5% isopropyl alcohol 70%				
Dexidin 2% Detergent	Atlas	liquid	chlorhexidine gluconate 2%				
Dexidin 2% Solution	Atlas	liquid	chlorhexidine gluconate 2%				
Dexidin 4% Solution	Atlas	liquid	chlorhexidine gluconate 4%				
Dexidin 20% Solution	Atlas	liquid	chlorhexidine gluconate 20%				
Dovidine 7.5%	Atlas	liquid	povidone-iodine 7.5%				
Dovidine 10%	Atlas	liquid	povidone-iodine 7.5%				
EpiPen	King Pharma	liquid					epinephrine 0.3 mg/dose
EpiPen Jr	King Pharma	liquid					epinephrine 0.15 mg/dose
Eurax	Columbia	cream			crotamiton 10%		
Family Medic First Aid Treatment	Tender	liquid/lotion	benzalkonium chloride 0.13%			lidocaine hydrochloride 0.745%	
Hyderm	Taro	cream					hydrocortisone acetate 0.5%
Hydrocortisone Cream	Various Manufacturers	cream					hydrocortisone 0.5%
Hydrocortisone Ointment	Various Manufacturers	ointment					hydrocortisone 0.5%
Hydrogen Peroxide 10 Volume	Various Manufacturers	liquid	hydrogen peroxide 3%				
Hydrogen Peroxide 20 Volume	Various Manufacturers	liquid	hydrogen peroxide 6%				
Hydrosone	Teva	cream					hydrocortisone 0.5%
Iodine Tincture 2.5%	Various Manufacturers	tincture	iodine 2.5% potassium iodide 2.5%				
Iodine Tincture 5%	Various Manufacturers	liquid	iodine 5% potassium iodide 3.3%				
Isopropyl Alcohol 99%	Various Manufacturers	liquid	isopropyl alcohol 99%				

Product	Manufacturer	Dosage Form	Antiseptic	Anti-infective	Antipruritic	Anesthetic	Other Active Ingredients
Isopropyl Rubbing Alcohol	Various Manufacturers	liquid	isopropyl alcohol 70%				
Lanacane Medicated Cream	Combe	cream	resorcinol 2%			benzocaine 6%	
Lanacane Spray	Combe		benzethonium chloride 0.2%			benzocaine 20%	
Lassar's Paste	Atlas	paste					salicylic acid 2% zinc oxide 24%
Mercurochrome	Atlas	liquid	chlorhexidine gluconate 0.05%				
Nupercainal Cream	Novartis Consumer Health	cream				dibucaine 0.5%	domiphen bromide 0.05%
Nupercainal Ointment	Novartis Consumer Health	ointment				dibucaine 1%	
Nyaderm Cream	Taro	cream		nystatin 100 000 IU/g			
Nyaderm Ointment	Taro	ointment		nystatin 100 000 IU/g			
Nystatin Cream	Various Manufacturers	cream		nystatin 100 000 IU/g			
Nystatin Ointment	Various Manufacturers	ointment		nystatin 100 000 IU/g			
Osmopak Plus	Rougier	ointment				benzocaine 0.5%	magnesium sulfate 60%
Ozonol	Bayer Consumer	ointment		phenol 0.18%			zinc oxide 3.72%
Ozonol Antibiotic Plus	Bayer Consumer	ointment		bacitracin 500 IU/g polymyxin B sulfate 10 000 IU/g		lidocaine hydrochloride 40 mg/g	
Penaten Cream	Johnson & Johnson	cream					zinc oxide 18%
pHisoHex Skin Cleanser	sanofi-aventis	emulsion	hexachlorophene 3%				
Polyderm Ointment	Taro	ointment		bacitracin zinc 500 IU/g polymyxin B sulfate 10 000 IU/g			
Polysporin Complete Ointment	Johnson & Johnson	ointment		bacitracin 500 IU/g gramicidin 0.25mg/g polymyxin B sulfate 10 000 IU/g lidocaine 50mg/g			
Polysporin Cream	Johnson & Johnson	cream		gramicidin 0.25 mg/g polymyxin B sulfate 10 000 IU/g			
Polysporin For Kids Cream	Johnson & Johnson	ointment		gramicidin 0.25mg/g polymyxin B sulfate 10 000 IU/g		lidocaine hydrochloride 50 mg/g	

Product	Manufacturer	Dosage Form	Antiseptic	Anti-infective	Antipruritic	Anesthetic	Other Active Ingredients
Polysporin Ointment	Johnson & Johnson	ointment		bacitracin 500 IU/g polymyxin B sulfate 10 000 IU/g			
Polysporin Plus Pain Relief Cream	Johnson & Johnson	cream		gramicidin 0.25 mg/g polymyxin B sulfate 10 000 IU/g		lidocaine hydrochloride 50 mg/g	
Polysporin Triple Antibiotic Ointment	Johnson & Johnson	ointment		bacitracin 500 IU/g gramicidin 0.25 mg/g polymyxin B sulfate 10 000 IU/g			
Polytopic Cream	Sandoz	cream		gramicidin 0.25 mg/g polymyxin B sulfate 10 000 IU/g			
Polytopic Ointment	Sandoz	ointment		bacitracin 500 IU/g polymyxin B sulfate 10 000 IU/g			
Pramegel	Medicis	gel			menthol 0.5%	pramoxine hydrochloride 1%	
Proviodine Detergent	Teva	liquid	povidone-iodine 7.5%				
Proviodine Solution	Teva	liquid	povidone-iodine 10%				
ratio-Nystatin Cream	Teva	cream		nystatin 100 000 IU/g			
ratio-Nystatin Ointment	Teva	ointment		nystatin 100 000 IU/g			
Rubbing Alcohol	Various Manufacturers	liquid	isopropyl alcohol 70%				
Solarcaine First Aid Lidocaine Spray	Schering-Plough	aerosol				lidocaine 0.5%	
Solarcaine First Aid Spray	Schering-Plough	aerosol	triclosan 0.02%			benzocaine 3%	
Solarcaine Medicated Lidocaine Gel	Schering-Plough	gel				lidocaine hydrochloride 0.5%	
Solarcaine Medicated First Aid Lotion	Schering-Plough	lotion				lidocaine hydrochloride 0.5%	
Spectro Jel	GlaxoSmithKline Consumer Healthcare	liquid					polysiloxane cellulose complex
Stanhexidine 2%	Omega	liquid	chlorhexidine gluconate 2%				isopropyl alcohol 4%
Stanhexidine 4%	Omega	liquid	chlorhexidine gluconate 4%				isopropyl alcohol 4%
Tersaseptic	Stiefel	liquid	triclosan 0.5%				
Twinject 0.15 mg Auto-Injector	Paladin	liquid					epinephrine 0.15 mg/dose
Twinject 0.3 mg Auto-Injector	Paladin	liquid					epinephrine 0.3 mg/dose

Product	Manufacturer	Dosage Form	Antiseptic	Anti-infective	Antipruritic	Anesthetic	Other Active Ingredients
Vitamin E Ointment	Various Manufacturers	ointment					vitamin E 30 IU/g
Vitamin E Skin Oil	Various Manufacturers	liquid					vitamin E 28 000 IU/30 mL
Vitamin E with Vitamins A & D	Various Manufacturers	cream					vitamin A 250 IU/g vitamin D 100 IU/g vitamin E 75 IU/g
Watkins Petro-Carb First Aid Salve	Watkins	ointment			phenol 1.5%		
Zinaderm	ratiopharm	cream					zinc oxide 15%
Zinaderm	ratiopharm	ointment					zinc oxide 15%
Zinc & Castor Oil Cream	Various Manufacturers	cream					castor oil 50% zinc oxide 7.5%
Zinc Cream	Various Manufacturers	cream					zinc oxide 15%
Zincoderm Ointment	Taro	ointment					zinc oxide 40%
Zinc Ointment 15%	Various Manufacturers	ointment					zinc oxide 15%
Zinc Ointment 20%	Various Manufacturers	ointment					zinc oxide 20%

Product	Manufacturer	Dosage Form	Active Ingredient
Apo-Gain	Apotex	solution	minoxidil 2%
Rogaine Solution	Johnson & Johnson	solution	minoxidil 2%

Product	Manufacturer	Dosage Form	Lindane	Pyrethrins	Permethrin	Other Active Ingredients
Hexit Lotion	Odan	lotion	1%			
Hexit Shampoo	Odan	shampoo	1%			
Kwellada-P Creme Rinse	Prestige Brands	liquid			1%	
Nix Creme Rinse	Insight	cream			1%	
Nyda	Pediapharm	liquid				dimeticone 50%
Pronto Lice Control System	ANB	liquid		pyrethrins 0.33%		piperonyl butoxide 4%
Resultz	Nycomed	liquid				isopropyl myristate 50% w/w cyclomethicone 50%
R & C II Spray	Prestige Brands	aerosol		pyrethins 0.3%		piperonyl butoxide 1.5%
R & C Shampoo/Conditioner	Prestige Brands	shampoo		pyrethrins 0.33%		piperonyl butoxide 3%

Product	Manufacturer	Dosage Form	Salicylic Acid	Coal Tar	Other Active Ingredients
Anthraforte 2%	Medican Pharma	ointment			anthralin 2%
Anthrascalp Lotion	Medican Pharma	lotion			anthralin 0.4%
Denorex Extra Strength/Extra Strength with Conditioner	Ultimark	shampoo		10.4%	chloroxylenol 0.5% menthol 1.5%
Denorex Regular with Conditioner	Ultimark	shampoo		7.5%	chloroxylenol 0.5% menthol 1.5%
Dermarest Medicated Shampoo	Chuch & Dwight	shampoo	3%		
Polytar AF Shampoo	Stiefel	shampoo	2%	0.5%	pyrithione disulfide 1% menthol 0.5%
Psoriasin S/A Therapeutic Shampoo	Alva-Amco Pharmacal	shampoo	3%		
Sebcur	Dermtek	shampoo	4%		
Sebcur/T	Dermtek	shampoo	4%	10%	
Tardan Shampoo	Odan	shampoo	2%	5%	triclosan 0.3%
Targel	Odan	gel		10%	
Targel SA	Odan	liquid	3%	10%	

Product	Manufacturer	Dosage Form	lindane	permethrin	Other Active Ingredients
Eurax	Columbia	cream			crotamiton 10%
Hexit Lotion	Odan	lotion	1%		
Kwellada-P Lotion	Prestige Brands	lotion		5%	
Nix Dermal Cream	GlaxoSmithKline Consumer Healthcare	cream		5%	

Product	Manufacturer	Dosage Form	Active Ingredients	Other Ingredients
Esoterica Facial	Medicis	cream	hydroquinone 2%	oxybenzone 2.5% padimate O 3.3%
Esoterica Regular	Medicis	cream	hydroquinone 2%	
Esoterica Sunscreen Fade Cream	Medicis	cream	hydroquinone 2%	oxybenzone 2.5% padimate O 3.3%
Glyquin XM	Valeant	cream	hydroquinone 4%	avobenzone 3% octocrylene 8% oxybenzone 4%
Lustra	Taro	cream	hydroquinone 4%	
Lustra AF	Taro		hydroquinone 4%	avobenzone 3% octinoxate 7.5%
Neostrata HQ Gel	Canderm Pharma	gel	hydroquinone 2%	glycolic acid 10%
Neostrata HQ Plus Gel	Canderm Pharma	gel	hydroquinone 4%	glycolic acid 5% gluconolactone 5%
Ultraquin Cream with Sunscreen	Canderm Pharma	cream	hydroquinone 4%	homosalate 5% octinoxate 7.5% octocrylene 2% oxybenzone 4%
Ultraquin Gel	Canderm Pharma	gel	hydroquinone 4%	oxybenzone 2.5% padimate O 3.3%
Ultraquin Plain Cream	Canderm Pharma	emulsion	hydroquinone 4%	

Product	Manufacturer	SPF Value	Dosage Form	UVA Absorber[a]	UVB Absorber[a]
Alba Sun Aloe Vera Sunscreen SPF 15	Alba Botanica	15	cream	oxybenzone 4.5%	octinoxate 7.5%
Alba Sun Facial Mineral Sunscreen SPF 10	Alba Botanica	10	cream	titanium dioxide 5.9%	titanium dioxide 5.9%
Alba Sun Facial Sunscreen SPF 20	Alba Botanica	20	cream	avobenzone 1.5% oxybenzone 5%	octinoxate 7.5% octisalate 4%
Alba Sun Fragrance Free Sunscreen SPF 15	Alba Botanica	15	cream	oxybenzone 4.5%	octinoxate 7.5%
Alba Sun Green Tea SPF 30+ Sunscreen	Alba Botanica	30	cream	avobenzone 3% oxybenzone 6%	homosalate 5% octinoxate 7.5% octisalate 5%
Alba Sun Kids Mineral Sunscreen SPF 18	Alba Botanica	18	cream	titanium dioxide 7%	titanium dioxide 7%
Alba Sun Kids Sunscreen SPF 30+	Alba Botanica	30	cream	avobenzone 3% oxybenzone 6%	homosalate 5% octinoxate 7.5% octisalate 5%
Anthelios SP	La Roche-Posay	30	cream	avobenzone 2% Mexoryl SX 2% titanium dioxide 4%	enzacamene 5% titanium dioxide 4%
Anthelios Spray SPF 30	La Roche-Posay	30	spray	avobenzone 3% Mexoryl SX 0.5% titanium dioxide 5.6%	octocrylene 10% octisalate 5% titanium dioxide 5.6%
Anthelios XL SPF 45	La Roche-Posay	45	cream	avobenzone 3.5% Mexoryl SX 2% Mexoryl XL 3% titanium dioxide 3.3%	octocrylene 10% Mexoryl XL 3% titanium dioxide 3.3%
Anthelios XL SPF 60	La Roche-Posay	60	cream	avobenzone 3.5% Mexoryl SX 3% Mexoryl XL 3% titanium dioxide 4.15%	octocrylene 10% Mexoryl XL 3% titanium dioxide 4.15%
Anthelios XL SPF 60 Face Stick	La Roche-Posay	60	stick	avobenzone 3% Mexoryl XL 2% titanium dioxide 6.25%	octocrylene 10% Mexoryl XL 2% titanium dioxide 6.25%
Aveeno Baby Sunblock Lotion	Johnson & Johnson	55	lotion	avobenzone 3% oxybenzone 6%	homosalate 10% octocrylene 2.8% octisalate 5%
Aveeno Sunblock Lotion	Johnson & Johnson	45	lotion	avobenzone 3% oxybenzone 6%	homosalate 10% octocrylene 2.4% octisalate 5%
Aveeno Sunblock Lotion for the Face SPF 60	Johnson & Johnson	60	lotion	avobenzone 3% oxybenzone 6%	homosalate 15% octocrylene 2.8% octisalate 5%
Aveeno Sunblock Spray with SPF 45	Johnson & Johnson	45	spray	avobenzone 3% oxybenzone 6%	homosalate 15% octocrylene 4% octisalate 5%
Avéne Extreme Sunblock -Water Resistant SPF 50	Pierre Fabre	50	cream	titanium dioxide 10.78% zinc oxide 2.4%	titanium dioxide 10.78% zinc oxide 2.4%
Avon Sun Kids Disappearing Color Sunscreen	Avon	40	cream	avobenzone 3% oxybenzone 4%	homosalate 8% octinoxate 7.5% octisalate 5%
Avon Sun Lip Balm SPF 15	Avon	15		oxybenzone 2%	octinoxate 7.5%
Avon Sun Sunscreen Lotion SPF 40	Avon	40	cream	avobenzone 3% oxybenzone 4%	homosalate 8% octinoxate 7.5% octisalate 5%
Babies Sunscreen Lotion SPF 30	Norwood	30	lotion	avobenzone 2% oxybenzone 2%	homosalate 10.5% octocrylene 2% octisalate 5%

Product	Manufacturer	SPF Value	Dosage Form	UVA Absorber[a]	UVB Absorber[a]
Babies Sunscreen Lotion SPF 45	Norwood	45	lotion	oxybenzone 6%	homosalate 8% octinoxate 7.5% octisalate 5%
Babies Sunscreen Spray SPF 45	Norwood	45	spray	oxybenzone 6%	homosalate 8% octinoxate 7.5% octisalate 5%
Banana Boat Active Kids Sunblock	Banana Boat	50	cream	oxybenzone 6%	octocrylene 10% octinoxate 7.5% octisalate 5%
Banana Boat Baby Tear-Free Continuous Spray	Banana Boat	60	spray	avobenzone 3%	homosalate 15% octinoxate 7.5% octisalate 5% octocrylene 2.4%
Banana Boat Dark Tanning Dry Oil Continuous Spray SPF 4	Banana Boat	4	spray		octinoxate 2% padimate O 1.4%
Banana Boat Dark Tanning Oil	Banana Boat	4	liquid		octinoxate 2% padimate O 1.4%
Banana Boat Dark Tanning Oil	Banana Boat	8	liquid	oxybenzone 1%	octinoxate 3.5% padimate O 4.5%
Banana Boat Kids Tear-Free Lotion SPF 60	Banana Boat	60	cream	titanium dioxide 2.4%	homosalate 15% octinoxate 7.5% octisalate 5% titanium dioxide 2.4%
Banana Boat Kids Tear-Free Spray SPF 60	Banana Boat	60	spray	avobenzone 3%	homosalate 15% octocrylene 2.4% octinoxate 7.5% octisalate 5%
Banana Boat Sport Performance Spray Sunscreen SPF 15	Banana Boat	15	spray	avobenzone 3% oxybenzone 2%	homosalate 8.78% octinoxate 5% octisalate 5% octocrylene 2.5%
Banana Boat Sport Performance Spray Sunscreen SPF 30	Banana Boat	30	spray	avobenzone 3% oxybenzone 5%	homosalate 8.78% octinoxate 5% octisalate 5% octocrylene 2.5%
Banana Boat Sport Performance Spray Sunscreen SPF 60	Banana Boat	60	spray	avobenzone 3% oxybenzone 5%	octocrylene 10%
Banana Boat Sport Performance Sunscreen SPF 30	Banana Boat	30	lotion	avobenzone 1% oxybenzone 4%	homosalate 10% octocrylene 0.8% octisalate 5%
Banana Boat Sport Performance Sunscreen SPF 50	Banana Boat	50	lotion	avobenzone 1.5% oxybenzone 6%	homosalate 15% octocrylene 1.25% octisalate 5%
Banana Boat Sport Performance Sunscreen SPF 60	Banana Boat	60	lotion	avobenzone 3% oxybenzone 5%	octocrylene 10%
Banana Boat Sport Sunblock	Banana Boat	15	lotion	oxybenzone 3.4%	octinoxate 5.25% octisalate 3%
Banana Boat Ultra Defense Spray SPF 30	Banana Boat	30	spray	avobenzone 3% oxybenzone 5%	homosalate 8.78% octinoxate 5% octisalate 5% octocrylene 2.5%
Banana Boat Ultra Defense Spray SPF 60	Banana Boat	60	spray	avobenzone 3% oxybenzone 5%	octocrylene 10%
Banana Boat Ultra Defense Sunscreen Lotion SPF 15	Banana Boat	15	lotion	avobenzone 1% oxybenzone 2%	homosalate 6% octocrylene 0.8%

Product	Manufacturer	SPF Value	Dosage Form	UVA Absorber[a]	UVB Absorber[a]
Banana Boat Ultra Defense Sunscreen Lotion SPF 30	Banana Boat	30	lotion	avobenzone 1% oxybenzone 4%	homosalate 10% octocrylene 0.8% octisalate 5%
Banana Boat Ultra Defense Sunscreen Lotion SPF 50	Banana Boat	50	lotion	avobenzone 1.5% oxybenzone 6%	homosalate 15% octocrylene 1.25% octisalate 5%
Biotherm - Face Multi Protection SPF 15	Biotherm	15	cream	avobenzone 3% Mexoryl SX 0.25% Mexoryl XL 0.75% titanium dioxide 0.8%	octocrylene 9% octisalate 5% Mexoryl XL 0.75% titanium dioxide 0.8%
Biotherm - Face Multi Protection SPF 30	Biotherm	30	cream	avobenzone 3% Mexoryl SX 1% Mexoryl XL 1% titanium dioxide 4.15%	octocrylene 10% octisalate 5% Mexoryl XL 1% titanium dioxide 4.15%
Biotherm - Face Multi Protection SPF 50	Biotherm	50	cream	avobenzone 2% Mexoryl SX 2% Mexoryl XL 3% titanium dioxide 5%	octocrylene 10% Mexoryl XL 3% titanium dioxide 5%
Biotherm - Ultra-Fluid Body Milk Sun Protection SPF 15	Biotherm	15	lotion	avobenzone 1.5% Mexoryl SX 0.5% Mexoryl XL 1% titanium dioxide 1.65%	octocrylene 7.5% Mexoryl XL 1% titanium dioxide 1.65%
Biotherm - Ultra-Fluid Body Milk Sun Protection SPF 30	Biotherm	30	lotion	avobenzone 3.5% Mexoryl SX 0.25% Mexoryl XL 0.75% titanium dioxide 4.15%	octocrylene 9% Mexoryl XL 0.75% titanium dioxide 4.15%
Blistex DCT Medicated Lip Balm	Blistex	20	ointment	oxybenzone 4.5%	octinoxate 7.3%
Blistex Five Star Lip Protection	Blistex	30	ointment	oxybenzone 5%	homosalate 9.6% octinoxate 7.5% octisalate 5%
Blistex Fruit Smoothies Lip Balm	Blistex	15	stick	oxybenzone 2.5%	octinoxate 7.5%
Blistex Herbal Answer Lip Balm	Blistex	15	ointment	oxybenzone 2.5%	octinoxate 7.5%
Blistex Lip Balm Regular/Berry/Mint	Blistex	15	ointment	oxybenzone 2.5%	padimate O 6.6%
Blistex Medicated Lip Conditioner SPF 15	Blistex	15	ointment	meradimate 2.5%	padimate O 6.6%
Blistex Moisture Melt	Blistex	15	ointment	oxybenzone 2.5%	octinoxate 7.5%
Blistex Silk & Shine Lip Balm	Blistex	15	stick	oxybenzone 2.5%	octinoxate 7.5%
Blistex Raspberry Lemonade Blast	Blistex	15	ointment	oxybenzone 2.5%	octinoxate 7.5%
Burt's Bees Sunscreen Lotion with Hemp Seed Oil SPF 15	Burt's Bees	15	lotion	titanium dioxide 6.83%	titanium dioxide 6.83%
Burt's Bees Sunscreen Lotion with Hemp Seed Oil SPF 30	Burt's Bees	30	lotion	titanium dioxide 8.58%	titanium dioxide 8.58%
Cetaphil Daily Facial Moisturizer SPF 15	Galderma	15	liquid	avobenzone 3%	octocrylene 10%
Cetaphil Daily Facial Moisturizer SPF 50	Galderma	50	liquid	oxybenzone 6% titanium dioxide 5.7%	octinoxate 7.5% octisalate 5% octocrylene 7% titanium dioxide 5.7%
Chapstick Sunblock Lip Balm	Wyeth Consumer Healthcare	30	stick	oxybenzone 5%	octinoxate 7.5% octisalate 5% octocrylene 7%
Clarins Sun Care Cream High Protection for Children	Clarins	30	cream	titanium dioxide 15.2% zinc oxide 3%	titanium dioxide 15.2% zinc oxide 3%
Clarins Sun Care Cream for Rapid Tanning SPF 10	Clarins	10	cream	avobenzone 2.5%	octinoxate 7.5% octisalate 5% octocrylene 2%

Product	Manufacturer	SPF Value	Dosage Form	UVA Absorber[a]	UVB Absorber[a]
Clarins Sun Control Stick High Protection SPF 30	Clarins	30	stick	oxybenzone 5% titanium dioxide 4.9%	octinoxate 7.5% titanium dioxide 4.9%
Clear Continuous Spray Sunscreen SPF 30	Fruit of the Earth	30	spray	oxybenzone 5%	homosalate 9% octinoxate 7.5% octisalate 5%
Clear Continuous Spray Sunscreen for Kids SPF 50	Fruit of the Earth	50	spray	avobenzone 3% oxybenzone 6%	homosalate 15% octisalate 5%
Clinique - Face & Body Cream	Clinique	15	cream	avobenzone 3%	homosalate 10% octisalate 5% octocrylene 2.7%
Clinique - Sun Body Cream SPF 30	Clinique	30	cream	avobenzone 3% oxybenzone 3%	homosalate 10% octinoxate 7.5% octisalate 5%
Clinique - Sun Body Cream SPF 50	Clinique	50	cream	avobenzone 3% oxybenzone 5%	homosalate 10% octinoxate 7.5% octisalate 5%
Clinique - Sun Body Spray	Clinique	25	spray	avobenzone 3%	octocrylene 2.7% octisalate 5%
Clinique - Sun Face Cream SPF 30	Clinique	30	cream	avobenzone 3% oxybenzone 3%	homosalate 10% octinoxate 7.5% octisalate 5%
Clinique - Sun Face Cream SPF 50	Clinique	50	cream	avobenzone 3% oxybenzone 5%	homosalate 10% octinoxate 7.5% octisalate 5%
Continuous Spray Sunscreen SPF 15	Fruit of the Earth	15	spray	oxybenzone 3%	homosalate 5% octinoxate 7.5% octisalate 5%
Coppertone Continuous Spray Clear SPF 15	Schering-Plough	15	spray	oxybenzone 3%	homosalate 5% octinoxate 7.5% octisalate 5%
Coppertone Continuous Spray Clear SPF 30	Schering-Plough	30	spray	avobenzone 2% oxybenzone 4%	homosalate 15% octisalate 5%
Coppertone Continuous Spray Clear SPF 60	Schering-Plough	60	spray	avobenzone 3% oxybenzone 6%	homosalate 15% octocrylene 10% octisalate 5%
Coppertone Dry Oil Continuous Spray SPF 10	Schering-Plough	10	spray	oxybenzone 3%	homosalate 5% octinoxate 7.5% octisalate 5%
Coppertone Kids Continuous Spray Clear SPF 60	Schering-Plough	60	spray	avobenzone 3% oxybenzone 6%	homosalate 15% octocrylene 10% octisalate 5%
Coppertone Kids Sunscreen Lotion SPF 60	Schering-Plough	60	lotion	avobenzone 3% oxybenzone 6%	homosalate 15% octocrylene 10% octisalate 5%
Coppertone Oil Free Continuous Spray SPF 50	Schering-Plough	50	spray	avobenzone 3% oxybenzone 6%	homosalate 15% octocrylene 5% octisalate 5%
Coppertone Oil Free Sunscreen Lotion SPF 50	Schering-Plough	50	lotion	avobenzone 3% oxybenzone 6%	homosalate 13% octocrylene 5% octisalate 5%
Coppertone Sport Continuous Spray SPF 15	Schering-Plough	15	spray	oxybenzone 3%	homosalate 5% octinoxate 7.5% octisalate 5%

Product	Manufacturer	SPF Value	Dosage Form	UVA Absorber[a]	UVB Absorber[a]
Coppertone Sport Continuous Spray SPF 30	Schering-Plough	30	spray	oxybenzone 4.25%	homosalate 5% octinoxate 7.5% octisalate 5%
Coppertone Sport Continuous Spray SPF 60	Schering-Plough	60	spray	avobenzone 3% oxybenzone 6%	homosalate 15% octocrylene 10% octisalate 5%
Coppertone Sport Sunscreen Lotion SPF 15	Schering-Plough	15	lotion	avobenzone 2%	homosalate 8% octocrylene 5% octisalate 5%
Coppertone Sport Sunscreen Lotion SPF 30	Schering-Plough	30	lotion	avobenzone 2% oxybenzone 5%	homosalate 10% octocrylene 4% octisalate 5%
Coppertone Sunscreen Lotion SPF 8	Schering-Plough	8	lotion	oxybenzone 2%	octinoxate 7%
Coppertone Sunscreen Lotion SPF 15	Schering-Plough	15	lotion	avobenzone 2%	homosalate 10% octocrylene 5% octisalate 5%
Coppertone Sunscreen Lotion SPF 30	Schering-Plough	30	lotion	avobenzone 2% oxybenzone 2%	homosalate 10.5% octocrylene 2% octisalate 5%
Coppertone Sunscreen Lotion SPF 60	Schering-Plough	60	lotion	avobenzone 3% oxybenzone 6%	homosalate 15% octocrylene 10% octisalate 5%
Coppertone WaterBabies Continuous Spray SPF 60	Schering-Plough	50	spray	avobenzone 2.1% oxybenzone 2.8%	homosalate 9.1% octocrylene 10% octisalate 5%
Coppertone WaterBabies Sunscreen Lotion SPF 60	Schering-Plough	60	lotion	avobenzone 3% oxybenzone 6%	homosalate 15% octocrylene 10% octisalate 5%
Coppertone Water Babies Sunscreen Mousse SPF 60	Schering-Plough	60	mousse	avobenzone 2.7% oxybenzone 5.4%	homosalate 13.5% octocrylene 9% octisalate 4.5%
Dormer 211 Daily Protective Cream SPF 15	Dormer	15	cream	avobenzone 2% oxybenzone 3%	octinoxate 7.5%
Dormer 211 Daily Protective Cream SPF 30	Dormer	30	cream	avobenzone 2.5% oxybenzone 3% titanium dioxide 0.8%	octinoxate 7.5% octisalate 5% titanium dioxide 0.8%
Fruit of the Earth Block- Up Baby Sunblock with Aloe	Fruit of the Earth	30	lotion	oxybenzone 5%	octinoxate 7.5% octisalate 5%
Fruit of the Earth Block- Up Continuous Spray SPF 30	Fruit of the Earth	30	spray	oxybenzone 5%	homosalate 9% octinoxate 7.5% octisalate 5%
Fruit of the Earth Block- Up Kids SPF 45	Fruit of the Earth	45	lotion	oxybenzone 5%	homosalate 9% octinoxate 7.5% octisalate 5%
Fruit of the Earth Block- Up Kids SPF 50	Fruit of the Earth	50	lotion	avobenzone 2% oxybenzone 5%	homosalate 9% octinoxate 7.5% octisalate 5% octocrylene 1.5%
Fruit of the Earth Block-Up Sport	Fruit of the Earth	15	lotion	oxybenzone 4%	octinoxate 7.5%
Fruit of the Earth Continuous Spray SPF 30	Fruit of the Earth	30	spray	avobenzone 2% oxybenzone 4%	homosalate 15% octisalate 5%
Fruit of the Earth Continuous Spray SPF 50	Fruit of the Earth	50	spray	avobenzone 3% oxybenzone 6%	homosalate 15% octisalate 5%

Product	Manufacturer	SPF Value	Dosage Form	UVA Absorber[a]	UVB Absorber[a]
Fruit of the Earth Lotion SPF 50	Fruit of the Earth	50	lotion	avobenzone 2% oxybenzone 5%	homosalate 9% octinoxate 7.5% octisalate 5% octocrylene 1.5%
Fruit of the Earth Sport Continuous Spray SPF 15	Fruit of the Earth	15	spray	avobenzone 2% oxybenzone 3%	homosalate 10% octisalate 5%
Fruit of the Earth Sport Lotion SPF 15	Fruit of the Earth	15	lotion	avobenzone 2% oxybenzone 4%	octinoxate 7.5%
Glow Face Sunscreen Lotion SPF 45	Prime Enterprises	45	lotion	avobenzone 2%	octisalate 5% octocrylene 2.5%
Hawaiian Tropic Baby Faces Lotion	Tanning Research Labs	50	lotion	avobenzone 1% oxybenzone 3.5%	octocrylene 8%
Hawaiian Tropic Baby Sunscreen SPF 60	Tanning Research Labs	60	lotion	avobenzone 1% oxybenzone 3.5%	octocrylene 8%
Hawaiian Tropic Continuous Flow Cream SPF 10	Tanning Research Labs	10	cream	avobenzone 1% oxybenzone 1.5%	octocrylene 2%
Hawaiian Tropic Dark Tanning Lotion	Tanning Research Labs	4	lotion		octinoxate 5% octisalate 2%
Hawaiian Tropic Dark Tanning Oil	Tanning Research Labs	4	liquid		octinoxate 5%
Hawaiian Tropic Dry Oil Sunscreen Spray	Tanning Research Labs	10	spray	avobenzone 1% oxybenzone 3%	octocrylene 5%
Hawaiian Tropic Island Sport Sunscreen Lotion SPF 30	Tanning Research Labs	30	lotion	oxybenzone 5%	homosalate 8.5% octinoxate 7.5% octisalate 5%
Hawaiian Tropic Kids Sunscreen SPF 60	Tanning Research Labs	60	lotion	avobenzone 1% oxybenzone 3.5%	octocrylene 8%
Hawaiian Tropic Plus	Tanning Research Labs	15	lotion	titanium dioxide 0.65%	octinoxate 4% octisalate 4% titanium dioxide 0.65%
Hawaiian Tropic Sensitive Skin Face Sunscreen SPF 30	Tanning Research Labs	30	lotion	avobenzone 1% oxybenzone 3%	octocrylene 5%
Hawaiian Tropic Sheer Touch Sunscreen SPF 15	Tanning Research Labs	15	lotion	avobenzone 0.9% oxybenzone 3%	octocrylene 3%
Hawaiian Tropic Sheer Touch Sunscreen SPF 30	Tanning Research Labs	30	lotion	avobenzone 1% oxybenzone 3%	octocrylene 4.5%
Hawaiian Tropic Sheer Touch Sunscreen SPF 45	Tanning Research Labs	45	lotion	avobenzone 1% oxybenzone 3.5%	octocrylene 8%
Hawaiian Tropic Sunscreen SPF 4	Tanning Research Labs	4	lotion	oxybenzone 0.5%	octocrylene 1%
Hawaiian Tropic Sunscreen SPF 8	Tanning Research Labs	8	lotion	oxybenzone 1.5%	octocrylene 2%
Heiko Chemical Free Sunscreen SPF 30	Heiko	30	cream	zinc oxide 14%	zinc oxide 14%
Heiko Chemical Free Sunscreen SPF 40	Heiko	40	cream	zinc oxide 18%	zinc oxide 18%
Heiko Chemical Free Sunscreen SPF 40 Kids	Heiko	40	cream	zinc oxide 25%	zinc oxide 25%
High Protection Kids Sunscreen SPF 30	Norwood	29	lotion	avobenzone 3% oxybenzone 1% titanium dioxide 2.2%	octocrylene 12% titanium dioxide 2.2%
High Protection Sunscreen SPF 30	Norwood	30	lotion	avobenzone 3% oxybenzone 1% titanium dioxide 2.2%	octocrylene 12% titanium dioxide 2.2%

Product	Manufacturer	SPF Value	Dosage Form	UVA Absorber[a]	UVB Absorber[a]
Kids Sunscreen Spray SPF 45	Norwood	45	spray	oxybenzone 6%	homosalate 8% octinoxate 7.5% octisalate 5%
KINeSYS Cream Sunscreen SPF 30	KINeSYS Pharmaceutical	30	cream	oxybenzone 6% titanium dioxide 4%	octinoxate 7.5% titanium dioxide 4%
KINeSYS Cream Sunscreen Max SPF 45	KINeSYS Pharmaceutical	45	cream	avobenzone 1% oxybenzone 6%	octinoxate 8.5% octisalate 6%
KINeSYS Funscreen Spray SPF 50	KINeSYS Pharmaceutical	50	spray	avobenzone 3% oxybenzone 6%	homosalate 15% octisalate 5%
KINeSYS Kids Spray Sunscreen SPF 30 Fragrance-Free	KINeSYS Pharmaceutical	30	spray	avobenzone 2%	octinoxate 7.5% octocrylene 7% octisalate 4%
KINeSYS Spray Sunscreen SPF 15	KINeSYS Pharmaceutical	15	spray	avobenzone 2% octinoxate 7.5%	octisalate 5%
KINeSYS Spray Sunscreen SPF 30	KINeSYS Pharmaceutical	30	spray	avobenzone 2%	octinoxate 7.5% octocrylene 7% octisalate 4%
KINeSYS Sun Protection Stick	KINeSYS Pharmaceutical	30	stick	oxybenzone 4.5% titanium dioxide 1%	octinoxate 7.5% octisalate 5% titanium dioxide 1%
Lubriderm Lotion Daily UV Defense	Pfizer Consumer Healthcare	15	lotion	oxybenzone 3%	octinoxate 7.5% octisalate 4%
Mary Kay Lip Protector Sunscreen SPF 15	Mary Kay	15	stick	oxybenzone 3% zinc oxide 3.4%	octinoxate 7.5% zinc oxide 3.4%
Mary Kay Sunscreen SPF 30	Mary Kay	30	lotion	avobenzone 2% oxybenzone 4%	homosalate 10% octinoxate 7.5% octisalate 5%
Mary Kay Timewise Sunscreen SPF 15	Mary Kay	15	lotion	oxybenzone 2% zinc oxide 4%	octinoxate 7.5% zinc oxide 4%
Mary Kay Timewise Sunscreen SPF 25	Mary Kay	25	lotion	oxybenzone 3% zinc oxide 3.88%	octinoxate 7.5% octisalate 5% zinc oxide 3.88%
Mary Kay Tinted Lip Balm SPF 15	Mary Kay	15	stick	oxybenzone 5% zinc oxide 8%	octinoxate 5% octocrylene 3% zinc oxide 8%
Neutrogena Fresh Cooling Body Mist Sunscreen SPF 30	Johnson & Johnson	30	spray	avobenzone 3% oxybenzone 5%	homosalate 8% octisalate 5% octocrylene 2.35%
Neutrogena Fresh Cooling Body Mist Sunscreen SPF 45	Johnson & Johnson	45	spray	avobenzone 3% oxybenzone 6%	homosalate 15% octisalate 5% octocrylene 2.35%
Neutrogena Fresh Cooling Body Mist Sunscreen SPF 60	Johnson & Johnson	60	spray	avobenzone 3% oxybenzone 6%	homosalate 15% octisalate 5% octocrylene 10%
Neutrogena Lip Moisturizer	Johnson & Johnson	15	stick	oxybenzone 4%	octinoxate 7.5%
Neutrogena Ultimate Sport Sunscreen Spray SPF 45	Johnson & Johnson	45	spray	avobenzone 3% oxybenzone 6%	homosalate 15% octisalate 5% octocrylene 4%
Neutrogena Ultimate Sport Sunscreen Spray SPF 60	Johnson & Johnson	60	spray	avobenzone 3% oxybenzone 6%	homosalate 15% octisalate 5% octocrylene 10%

Product	Manufacturer	SPF Value	Dosage Form	UVA Absorber[a]	UVB Absorber[a]
Neutrogena Ultra Sheer Body Mist Sunscreen SPF 30	Johnson & Johnson	30	spray	avobenzone 3% oxybenzone 5%	homosalate 8% octisalate 4% octocrylene 2.35%
Neutrogena Ultra Sheer Body Mist Sunscreen SPF 45	Johnson & Johnson	45	spray	avobenzone 3% oxybenzone 6%	homosalate 15% octisalate 5% octocrylene 2.35%
Neutrogena Ultra Sheer Body Mist Sunscreen SPF 60	Johnson & Johnson	60	spray	avobenzone 3% oxybenzone 6%	homosalate 15% octisalate 5% octocrylene 10%
Neutrogena Ultra Sheer Dry-Touch SPF 55	Johnson & Johnson	55	lotion	avobenzone 3% oxybenzone 6%	homosalate 10% octisalate 5% octocrylene 2.8%
Neutrogena Ultra Sheer Dry-Touch SPF 70	Johnson & Johnson	70	lotion	avobenzone 3% oxybenzone 6%	homosalate 15% octisalate 5% octocrylene 2.8%
Neutrogena Ultra Sheer Dry-Touch SPF 85	Johnson & Johnson	85	lotion	avobenzone 3% oxybenzone 6%	homosalate 15% octisalate 5% octocrylene 4.5%
Neutrogena Ultra Sheer Face Sunscreen SPF 45	Johnson & Johnson	45	lotion	avobenzone 3% oxybenzone 6%	homosalate 10% octisalate 5% octocrylene 2.79%
Neutrogena Ultra Sheer Face Sunscreen SPF 60	Johnson & Johnson	60	lotion	avobenzone 3% oxybenzone 6%	homosalate 15% octisalate 5% octocrylene 2.79%
Neutrogena Waterguard Kids SPF 60	Johnson & Johnson	60	lotion	avobenzone 3% oxybenzone 5%	homosalate 15% octisalate 5% octocrylene 4%
Oil Free Lotion SPF 30	Prime Enterprises	30	lotion	oxybenzone 4%	homosalate 6% octinoxate 7.5% octisalate 5%
Ombrelle Clear Sport Gel SPF 30	Ombrelle	30	gel	avobenzone 3% oxybenzone 6%	octocrylene 10% octisalate 5%
Ombrelle Continuous Spray SPF 15	Ombrelle	15	spray	avobenzone 3%	octocrylene 10% octisalate 5%
Ombrelle Cream SPF 60	Ombrelle	60	cream	avobenzone 3.5% Mexoryl SX 3% Mexoryl XL 3% titanium dioxide 4.15%	octocrylene 10% Mexoryl XL 3% titanium dioxide 4.15%
Ombrelle Kids Lotion SPF 30	Ombrelle	30	lotion	avobenzone 3% Mexoryl SX 1% oxybenzone 5% titanium dioxide 3.3%	octocrylene 3.5% octisalate 5% titanium dioxide 3.3%
Ombrelle Kids SPF 30 Sensitive Skin	Ombrelle	30	lotion	Mexoryl SX 1% titanium dioxide 10.5%	titanium dioxide 10.5%
Ombrelle Kids SPF 45	Ombrelle	45	lotion	avobenzone 2% Mexoryl SX 3% oxybenzone 5% titanium dioxide 4.2%	octocrylene 3.5% octisalate 5% titanium dioxide 4.2%
Ombrelle Lip Balm SPF 30	Ombrelle	30	stick	avobenzone 3% Mexoryl SX 1% titanium dioxide 0.95%	octocrylene 10% titanium dioxide 0.95%
Ombrelle Lotion SPF 15	Ombrelle	15	lotion	avobenzone 2% Mexoryl SX 1%	octocrylene 10% enzacamene 3%

Product	Manufacturer	SPF Value	Dosage Form	UVA Absorber[a]	UVB Absorber[a]
Ombrelle Lotion SPF 30	Ombrelle	30	lotion	avobenzone 3% Mexoryl SX 1%	enzacamene 4% octocrylene 10% ensulizole 1.5%
Ombrelle Lotion SPF 45	Ombrelle	45	lotion	avobenzone 2% Mexoryl SX 3% titanium dioxide 3.6%	octocrylene 10% titanium dioxide 3.6%
Ombrelle Lotion Extreme	Ombrelle	30	lotion	avobenzone 3% Mexoryl SX 1% titanium dioxide 2.2%	octocrylene 10% titanium dioxide 2.2%
Ombrelle Sport Lotion SPF 30	Ombrelle	30	lotion	avobenzone 1.5% Mexoryl SX 0.5% titanium dioxide 2.5%	octocrylene 7% titanium dioxide 2.5%
Ombrelle Sport Lotion SPF 45	Ombrelle	45	lotion	avobenzone 1.5% Mexoryl SX 0.5% titanium dioxide 3.3%	octocrylene 7% titanium dioxide 3.3%
Ombrelle Stick SPF 60	Ombrelle	60	stick	avobenzone 3% Mexoryl XL 2% titanium dioxide 6.25%	octocrylene 10% Mexoryl XL 2% titanium dioxide 6.25%
Premium Sunscreen SPF 15	Norwood	15	lotion	avobenzone 3% oxybenzone 2%	ensulizole 2% octocrylene 10%
Shiseido Extra Smooth Cream SPF 38	Shiseido	38	cream	zinc oxide 9.3%	octinoxate 5.9% zinc oxide 9.3%
Shiseido Extra Smooth Lotion SPF 34	Shiseido	34	lotion	zinc oxide 9.3%	octinoxate 7.4% zinc oxide 9.3%
Shiseido Sun Protection Eye Cream SPF 32	Shiseido	32	cream	zinc oxide 9.3%	octinoxate 4.9% zinc oxide 9.3%
Shiseido Ultra Sun Protection Cream SPF 50	Shiseido	50	cream	zinc oxide 13.9%	octinoxate 7.4% zinc oxide 13.9%
Shiseido Ultra Sun Protection Lotion SPF 50	Shiseido	50	lotion	zinc oxide 13.9%	octinoxate 7.4% zinc oxide 13.9%
Solbar	Person & Covey	50	cream	oxybenzone 6%	octocrylene 10% octinoxate 7.5%
Sport Sunscreen Lotion SPF30	Fruit of the Earth	30	lotion	oxybenzone 5%	octinoxate 5% octisalate 3%
Spray Gel SPF 15	Prime Enterprises	15	gel	oxybenzone 2%	octinoxate 7.5% octisalate 5%
Sunscreen Continuous Spray SPF 15	Prime Enterprises	15	spray	avobenzone 2%	octisalate 5% octocrylene 2.5%
Sunscreen Continuous Spray for Kids SPF 30	Prime Enterprises	30	spray	oxybenzone 4%	homosalate 5% octinoxate 7.5% octisalate 5%
Sunscreen Lotion for Babies SPF 45	Fruit of the Earth	45	lotion	oxybenzone 6% titanium dioxide 1%	octinoxate 7.5% octisalate 5% octocrylene 9% titanium dioxide 1%
Sunscreen Lotion for Kids SPF 30	Fruit of the Earth	30	lotion	oxybenzone 5% titanium dioxide 1%	octinoxate 5% octisalate 5% octocrylene 4% titanium dioxide 1%
Sunscreen Lotion for Kids SPF 45	Prime Enterprises	45	lotion	oxybenzone 6%	octinoxate 7.5% octisalate 5% octocrylene 8%
Sunscreen Lotion SPF 4	Prime Enterprises	4	lotion		octinoxate 2%
Sunscreen Lotion SPF 8	Prime Enterprises	8	lotion	oxybenzone 2%	octinoxate 4%

Product	Manufacturer	SPF Value	Dosage Form	UVA Absorber[a]	UVB Absorber[a]
Sunscreen Lotion SPF 8	Fruit of the Earth	8	lotion	oxybenzone 1.5%	octinoxate 4.5%
Sunscreen Lotion SPF 15	Fruit of the Earth	15	lotion	oxybenzone 4%	octinoxate 7.5%
Sunscreen Lotion SPF 15	Prime Enterprises	15	lotion	oxybenzone 2%	octinoxate 5% octisalate 3%
Sunscreen Lotion SPF 30	Fruit of the Earth	30	lotion	oxybenzone 5% titanium dioxide 1%	octinoxate 7.5% octisalate 5% octocrylene 4% titanium dioxide 1%
Sunscreen Lotion SPF 30	Norwood	30	lotion	avobenzone 2% oxybenzone 2%	homosalate 10.5% octocrylene 2% octisalate 5%
Sunscreen Lotion SPF 30	Prime Enterprises	30	lotion	avobenzone 2% oxybenzone 2%	homosalate 7.5% octocrylene 2.5% octisalate 5%
Sunscreen Lotion SPF 45	Norwood	45	lotion	avobenzone 3% oxybenzone 6% titanium dioxide 4%	octocrylene 12% titanium dioxide 4%
Sunscreen Lotion SPF 50	Prime Enterprises	50	lotion	avobenzone 3% oxybenzone 4%	homosalate 10% octocrylene 2.5% octisalate 5%
Sunscreen Sport Gel SPF 30	Prime Enterprises	30	gel	oxybenzone 4%	octinoxate 7.5% octisalate 5%
Sunscreen Sport Spray SPF 30	Prime Enterprises	30	spray	oxybenzone 4%	homosalate 5% octinoxate 7.5% octisalate 5%
Sunscreen Spray for Kids SPF 45	Prime Enterprises	45	spray	oxybenzone 6%	octocrylene 8% octinoxate 7.5% octisalate 5%
Sunscreen Spray for Kids SPF 50	Prime Enterprises	50	spray	avobenzone 3% oxybenzone 4%	homosalate 10% ensulizole 1% octisalate 5% octocrylene 2.5%
Sunthera 3 Baby Lotion	Fruit of the Earth	60	lotion	avobenzone 5% oxybenzone 6% titanium dioxide 2.3%	homosalate 15% octisalate 6% titanium dioxide 2.3%
Sunthera 3 Continuous Spray SPF 60	Fruit of the Earth	60	lotion	avobenzone 5% oxybenzone 6%	homosalate 15% octisalate 6% octocrylene 4%
Sunthera 3 Kids Continuous Spray	Fruit of the Earth	50	spray	avobenzone 3% oxybenzone 6%	homosalate 15% octisalate 5%
Sunthera 3 Kids Lotion	Fruit of the Earth	60	lotion	avobenzone 5% oxybenzone 6% titanium dioxide 2.3%	homosalate 15% octisalate 6% titanium dioxide 2.3%
Sunthera 3 SPF 15 Lotion	Fruit of the Earth	15	lotion	avobenzone 2% titanium dioxide 0.66%	homosalate 3% octisalate 4% titanium dioxide 0.66%
Sunthera 3 SPF 30 Lotion	Fruit of the Earth	30	lotion	avobenzone 2% oxybenzone 4% titanium dioxide 2%	homosalate 4% octisalate 4% octocrylene 1.9% titanium dioxide 2%
Sunthera 3 SPF 60 Lotion	Fruit of the Earth	60	lotion	avobenzone 5% oxybenzone 6% titanium dioxide 2.3%	homosalate 15% octisalate 6% titanium dioxide 2.3%

Product	Manufacturer	SPF Value	Dosage Form	UVA Absorber[a]	UVB Absorber[a]
Vichy Broad Spectrum Lotion for Children SPF 35	Vichy	35	cream	avobenzone 2% Mexoryl SX 1.5% titanium dioxide 5%	octocrylene 10% titanium dioxide 5%
Vichy Lip Protection Stick	Vichy	15	stick	Mexoryl XL 0.5% titanium dioxide 4.6%	Mexoryl XL 0.5% octinoxate 7.5% titanium dioxide 4.6%
Vichy Protective Gel-Cream Body SPF 20	Vichy	20	cream		ensulizole 2% octocrylene 10%
Vichy Sun Protection Cream SPF 30	Vichy	30	cream	avobenzone 3% Mexoryl SX 1% Mexoryl XL 1.5% titanium dioxide 3.3%	octocrylene 10% Mexoryl XL 1.5% titanium dioxide 3.3%
Vichy Sun Protection Cream SPF 45	Vichy	45	cream	avobenzone 3% Mexoryl SX 1.5% Mexoryl XL 4% titanium dioxide 3.3%	octocrylene 5% Mexoryl XL 4% titanium dioxide 3.3%
Vichy Sun Protection Cream SPF 60	Vichy	60	cream	avobenzone 3% Mexoryl SX 2% Mexoryl XL 3% titanium dioxide 4.15%	octocrylene 10% Mexoryl XL 3% titanium dioxide 4.15%
Vichy Ultra-Fluid Protection SPF 20	Vichy	20	cream	avobenzone 3.5% Mexoryl SX 1% titanium dioxide 5%	octocrylene 10% titanium dioxide 5%
Vichy Ultra-Fluid Protection SPF 30	Vichy	30	cream	avobenzone 3% Mexoryl SX 1% Mexoryl XL 2% titanium dioxide 4%	octocrylene 8% Mexoryl XL 2% titanium dioxide 4%
Vichy Ultra Protection Stick SPF 60	Vichy	60	stick	avobenzone 3% Mexoryl XL 2% titanium dioxide 6.25%	oxtocrylene 10% titanium dioxide 6.25%
Weleda Children's Sunscreen	Weleda	18	cream	titanium dioxide 7.6% zinc oxide 0.4%	titanium dioxide 7.6% zinc oxide 0.4%

[a]**Ingredient Synonyms:**
avobenzone = butyl methoxydibenzoylmethane, Parsol 1789
ensulizole = enzulizole, phenylbenzimidazole-5-sulfonic acid
enzacamene = 4-methylbenzylidene camphor, Parsol 5000
meradimate = menthyl anthranilate
Mexoryl SX = terephthalyidene dicamphor sulfonic acid, ecamsule
Mexoryl XL = drometrizole trisiloxane, silatriazole
octinoxate = octylmethoxycinnamate, 2-ethylhexyl p-methoxycinnamate, Parsol MCX
octisalate = octyl salicylate, 2-ethylhexyl salicylate
oxybenzone = benzophenone-3

Product	Manufacturer	Active Ingredients
3M Avagard D Instant Hand Antiseptic	3M	ethyl alcohol 61%
Bactisan	Bentfield	ethyl alcohol 63%
DCT Hand Sanitizer	Diversified Chemical Technologies	ethyl alcohol 62%
Descoderm V	MedPro Defense	ethyl alcohol 80%
One Step Hand Sanitizer	Belvedere	ethyl alcohol 62%
Purell Advanced Sanitizer	Gojo	ethyl alcohol 70%
Purell Original	Gojo	ethyl alcohol 62%
Purell Sanitizing Wipes	Gojo	ethyl alcohol 62%
Purell with Aloe	Gojo	ethyl alcohol 62%

Product	Manufacturer	Dosage Form	Diphenhydramine Hydrochloride	Other Active Ingredients
Dormax	Nobel Pharm	capsule	50 mg	
Herbal Nerve	SunOpta	tablet		hops 50 mg skullcap 100 mg valerian 50 mg
Herbal Sleepwell	Swiss Herbal	tablet		hops 50 mg lemon balm 10 mg linden 10 mg passiflora incarnata 100 mg valerian 100 mg
Nytol Extra Strength Caplet	GlaxoSmithKline Consumer Healthcare	caplet	50 mg	
Nytol Extra Strength Tablets	GlaxoSmithKline Consumer Healthcare	tablet	50 mg	
Nytol Natural Source	GlaxoSmithKline Consumer Healthcare	tablet		valeriana officinalis (valerian root) 100 mg
Nytol Quick Gels	GlaxoSmithKline Consumer Healthcare	capsule	50 mg	
Nytol Tablets	GlaxoSmithKline Consumer Healthcare	tablet	25 mg	
Relax and Sleep Herbal Sedative Formula	Jamieson	capsule		catnip 100 mg hops 100 mg passiflora incarnata 100 mg valerian 200 mg
Simply Sleep	McNeil Consumer Healthcare	tablet	25 mg	
Sleep +	Genuine Health	capsule		L-5-hydroxytryptophan 100 mg hops 62.5 mg passiflora incarnata 125 mg lemon balm 50 mg skullcap 150 mg
Sleep Aid Extra Strength	Tanta	caplet	50 mg	
Sleep Aid Regular Strength	Tanta	caplet	25 mg	
Sleep-Eze	Medtech	caplet	25 mg	
Sleep-Eze D Extra Strength Caplets	Medtech	caplet	50 mg	
Sleep-Eze D Extra Strength Gelcaps	Medtech	capsule	50 mg	
Unisom Extra Strength	Paladin	tablet	50 mg	
Unisom Sleep Gels	Paladin	capsule	25 mg	
Unisom Sleep Gels Extra Strength	Paladin	capsule	50 mg	

Product	Manufacturer	Dosage Form	Active Ingredients
Butt It Out	Paradise Promotions	capsule	lobelia 130 mg
Habitrol 7 mg/day	Novartis Consumer Health	patch, extended release	nicotine 7 mg
Habitrol 14 mg/day	Novartis Consumer Health	patch, extended release	nicotine 14 mg
Habitrol 21 mg/day	Novartis Consumer Health	patch, extended release	nicotine 21 mg
Impulse Disposable Device	Jasper and Jasper	electronic cigarette	aroma glycerol water
Nicoderm Step 1/Clear	McNeil Consumer Healthcare	patch, extended release	nicotine 21 mg
Nicoderm Step 2/Clear	McNeil Consumer Healthcare	patch, extended release	nicotine 14 mg
Nicoderm Step 3/Clear	McNeil Consumer Healthcare	patch, extended release	nicotine 7 mg
Nicorette 2 mg	McNeil Consumer Healthcare	gum	nicotine polacrilex 2 mg
Nicorette 4 mg	McNeil Consumer Healthcare	gum	nicotine polacrilex 4 mg
Nicorette 5 mg Patch	McNeil Consumer Healthcare	patch, extended release	nicotine 5 mg
Nicorette 10 mg Patch	McNeil Consumer Healthcare	patch, extended release	nicotine 10 mg
Nicorette 15 mg Patch	McNeil Consumer Healthcare	patch, extended release	nicotine 15 mg
Nicorette Inhaler	McNeil Consumer Healthcare	inhaler with cartridges	nicotine 10 mg
Nicorette Lozenge	McNeil Consumer Healthcare	lozenge	nicotine polacrilex 2 mg
Nicorette Lozenge	McNeil Consumer Healthcare	lozenge	nicotine polacrilex 4 mg
Nicorette QuickMist	McNeil Consumer Healthcare	oral spray	nicotine 1 mg/spray
Revive Rechargeable Device	Jasper and Jasper	electronic cigarette	aroma glycerol water
Thrive Gum	Novartis Consumer Health	gum	nicotine polacrilex 2 mg
Thrive Gum	Novartis Consumer Health	gum	nicotine polacrilex 4 mg
Thrive Lozenge	Novartis Consumer Health	lozenge	nicotine bitartrate dihydrate 1 mg
Thrive Lozenge	Novartis Consumer Health	lozenge	nicotine bitartrate dihydrate 2 mg

Product	Manufacturer	Dosage Form	A (IU)	B$_1$ (mg)	B$_2$ (mg)	B$_3$ (mg)
Calcium Magnesium Drink	GFR Pharma	powder for solution				
Cod Liver Oil	Various Manufacturers	liquid	750 to 850			
Hemarexin (per 10 mL)	Sandoz	liquid		1	1	10
Hormodausse (per 10 mL)	Sandoz	liquid		2		7
Infantol Liquid (per 5 mL)	Church and Dwight	liquid	1600	1.25	2	10
Jamp Vitamin A, D And C Infant Drops	JAMP	liquid	1500			
Liquid Calcium-Magnesium and Vitamin D	Sisu	liquid				
Maltlevol-12 (per 45 mL)	Church and Dwight	liquid	6000	4.5	3	30
PediaVit	Euro-Pharm	liquid	1500			
PediaVit Minimum	Euro-Pharm	liquid	1500			
PediaVit Multi	Euro-Pharm	liquid	1500	0.5	0.6	4
PediaVit Plus	Euro-Pharm	liquid	1500			
Poly-Vi-Sol	Mead Johnson	liquid	1500	0.5	0.6	4
Polyvitamins Drops for Infants	Pharmetics	liquid	1500	0.5	0.6	4
Somarexin (per ampul)	Lab Lalco	liquid		4.5	2	40
Tri-Vi-Sol Drops	Mead Johnson	liquid	1500			
Trivitamins Drops for Infants	Pharmetics	liquid	1500			
Wampole Vitamin Syrup	JAMP	syrup		0.04	0.06	0.44

B₉ (mg)	B₁₂ (µg)	C (mg)	D (IU)	E (IU)	Elemental Calcium (mg)	Elemental Iron (mg)	Other Active Ingredients
			100		300		magnesium 150 mg
			75 to 85				
							sodium 3.65 mg
	2.3					5	
1.2		80	400				
		30	400				
			6.67		16		magnesium 12 mg
3	14		400	25		33.75	
		30	400				
		30	400				fluoride 0.25 mg
		30	400	5			
		30	400				fluoride 0.5 mg
		30	400				
		30	400				
3	10					16	
		30	400				
		30	400				
						0.33	

Product	Manufacturer	Dosage Form	A (IU)	B_1 (mg)	B_2 (mg)	B_3 (mg)
Alive Children's Multivitamin Gummy	Nature's Way	gummy	833	0.25	0.28	3.33
Alive Adult Multivitamin Gummy	Nature's Way	gummy	1667	0.25	0.28	3.33
B Complex	Jamieson	tablet		18	6	45
B Complex	Santé Naturelle	tablet		25	30	50
B Complex 100 Timed Release	Jamieson	tablet		100	100	100
B Complex 50	Jamieson	tablet		50	50	50
B Complex 75	Jamieson	tablet		75	75	75
B Complex plus C	Jamieson	tablet		5	5	50
B Compound 75	Swiss Herbal	tablet		75	75	75
B Compound with Vitamin C	Swiss Herbal	tablet		10	10	50
Balanced B	Adams Labs	tablet		50	50	50
Balanced B 100 Complex	Vitality	tablet		100	100	100
Balanced B 50 Complex	General Nutrition Canada	capsule		50	50	50
Balanced B 50 Complex, Timed Release	Vitality	tablet		50	50	50
Balanced B Complex	Adams Labs	capsule		25	25	25
Balanced Vitamin B Complex	General Nutrition Canada	tablet		50	50	50
Beta-carotene 25 000 IU with Vitamins C & E	Jamieson	tablet				
Beta-carotene with C, E & Selenium	Swiss Herbal	capsule				
Beta-carotene with Vitamin D	Swiss Herbal	capsule				
Bioplex	Santé Naturelle	tablet		50	50	50

Pantothenic Acid (mg)	B_6 (mg)	B_{12} (µg)	Folic Acid (mg)	C (mg)	D (IU)	E (IU)	Elemental Calcium (mg)	Elemental Iron (mg)	Other Active Ingredients
1.66	0.67	2	0.133	20	133	5			biotin 100 µg choline bitartrate 6.67 µg inositol 6.67 µg iodine 25 µg zinc 2.5 mg
3.33	1	4	0.133	25	5	7.5			biotin 100 µg choline bitartrate 20 µg inositol 13.33 µg iodine 0.05 mg zinc 2.5 mg
10.5	4.2	6	0.675						biotin 195 µg choline bitartrate 6 mg inositol 7 mg
60	35	25	1						biotin 60 µg choline bitartrate 50 mg inositol 50 mg
100	100	100	0.4						biotin 100 µg choline bitartrate 100 mg inositol 100 mg
50	50	50	0.4						biotin 50 µg choline bitartrate 50 mg inositol 50 mg
75	75	75	0.6						biotin 75 µg choline bitartrate 75 mg inositol 75 mg
25	5	10	0.05	250					biotin 10 µg choline bitartrate 50 mg inositol 50 mg p-aminobenzoic acid 15 mg
75	75	75	0.075						biotin 75 µg choline bitartrate 75 mg inositol 75 mg
25	10	10	1	500					biotin 10 µg choline bitartrate 50 mg inositol 50 mg
50	50	50	0.05						biotin 50 µg
100	100	100	0.4						
50	50	50	0.4						biotin 50 µg choline bitartrate 50 mg inositol 50 mg
50	50	50	0.4						biotin 50 µg
25	25	25	0.05						biotin 25 µg
50	50	50	0.4						biotin 50 µg choline bitartrate 50 mg inositol 50 mg
				250		100			ß-carotene 25 000 IU
				250		400			ß-carotene 10 000 IU selenium 25 µg
					1000				ß-carotene 25 000 IU
50	50	50	1						biotin 50 µg choline bitartrate 50 mg inositol 50 mg

Product	Manufacturer	Dosage Form	A (IU)	B₁ (mg)	B₂ (mg)	B₃ (mg)
Bugs Bunny and Friends Complete Multiple Vitamins	Bayer Consumer	tablet, chewable	1600	1.5	1.5	8
Cal 500 D	Europharm	tablet				
Cal Extra	Multi-Pro	tablet				
Cal Mag 2:1 with Vitamin D & Zinc	Swiss Herbal	tablet				
Cal Mag Citrate 300 with Vitamin D & Zinc	Swiss Herbal	tablet				
Cal Mag Citrate with Vitamin D & Zinc	Swiss Herbal	capsule				
Calcite D 500	Riva	tablet				
Calcium & Magnesium 2:1	Sisu	tablet				
Calcium & Magnesium Citrate with Vitamin D	Sisu	tablet				
Calcium & Magnesium Extra-Fort	Bio-Santé	tablet				
Calcium & Magnesium Supplement	Pharmetics	tablet				
Calcium & Magnesium with Vitamin D	Pharmetics	tablet				
Calcium & Magnesium with Vitamin D & Zinc	Pharmetics	tablet				
Calcium & Vitamin D	Various Manufacturers	tablet				
Calcium 600 & D	Riva	tablet				
Calcium 600 with Vitamin D	Pharmetics	tablet				
Calcium 650 with Vitamin D₃	Jamieson	caplet				
Calcium Citrate with Vitamin D	Pharmetics	tablet				
Calcium Citrate with Vitamin D	Jamieson	caplet				
Calcium Complete with Magnesium	General Nutrition Canada	capsule				
Calcium Complete with Magnesium & Vitamin C	General Nutrition Canada	caplet				
Calcium D-500	Trianon	tablet				
Calcium Magnesium	General Nutrition Canada	tablet				
Calcium Magnesium	Jamieson	caplet				
Calcium Magnesium & Vitamin D	Pharmetics	tablet				
Calcium Magnesium & Zinc with Copper	General Nutrition Canada	tablet				
Calcium Magnesium 1:1 with Vitamin D	Sisu	capsule				
Calcium Magnesium plus Vitamin D & Zinc	Santé Naturelle	tablet				
Calcium Magnesium with Vitamin D₃	Jamieson	caplet				
Calcium Magnesium with Zinc	Jamieson	caplet				
Calcium Plus	Pharmetics	tablet	1333			
Calcium plus Vitamin D	Lee-Adams	tablet				
Calcium with Magnesium & Vitamin D	General Nutrition Canada	tablet				
Calcium with Vitamin D	General Nutrition Canada	tablet				

Pantothenic Acid (mg)	B₆ (mg)	B₁₂ (µg)	Folic Acid (mg)	C (mg)	D (IU)	E (IU)	Elemental Calcium (mg)	Elemental Iron (mg)	Other Active Ingredients
10	1	3	0.1	50	400	10	160	4	biotin 30 µg copper 1 mg phosphorus 125 mg
					125		500		
					200		333	4	magnesium 167 mg zinc 10 mg
					200		300		magnesium citrate 150 mg zinc citrate 5 mg
					200		300		magnesium 300 mg zinc 10 mg
					100		150		magnesium oxide 150 mg zinc citrate 5 mg
					125		500		
							350		magnesium 175 mg
					100		275		magnesium 137.5 mg
							316		magnesium 160 mg
							140		magnesium 75 mg
					175		333		magnesium 166.5 mg
					175		333		magnesium 166.5 mg zinc 2.4 mg
					200		500		
					125		600		
					125		600		
					200		650		
					200		315		
					50		250		
							300		magnesium 150 mg
				100			400		magnesium 200 mg
					125		500		
							333		magnesium 167 mg
							333		magnesium 167 mg
							350		magnesium 175 mg
							333		copper 0.334 mg magnesium 133 mg zinc 5 mg
					100		100		magnesium 100 mg
					135		350		magnesium 175 mg zinc 10 mg
					133		333		magnesium 167 mg
							333		magnesium 167 mg zinc 20 mg
				33.3	133.3		333	3.3	magnesium 166.7 mg
					125		500		
					66.6		333.3		magnesium 166.6 mg
					200		650		

Product	Manufacturer	Dosage Form	A (IU)	B$_1$ (mg)	B$_2$ (mg)	B$_3$ (mg)
Calcium with Vitamin D	Pharmetics	tablet				
Calmag D	Gerbex	capsule				
Cal-Mag Vitamin C & Zinc	Swiss Herbal	tablet				
Caltrate with Vitamin D Soft Chews	Pfizer Consumer Healthcare	square chew				
Caltrate 600 with Vitamin D	Pfizer Consumer Healthcare	tablet				
Caltrate Plus Chewables	Pfizer Consumer Healthcare	tablet, chewable				
Caltrate Plus Tablets	Pfizer Consumer Healthcare	tablet				
Caltrate Select	Pfizer Consumer Healthcare	tablet				
Carbocal D 400	Euro-Pharm	tablet				
Carbocal D 1000	Euro-Pharm	tablet				
Carthamex	M. Vachon	capsule				
Centrum	Pfizer Consumer Healthcare	tablet	1000	2.25	3.2	15
Centrum Advantage	Pfizer Consumer Healthcare	tablet	500	1.25	2.5	7.5
Centrum Cardio	Pfizer Consumer Healthcare	tablet	1000	0.7	0.875	10

Pantothenic Acid (mg)	B₆ (mg)	B₁₂ (µg)	Folic Acid (mg)	C (mg)	D (IU)	E (IU)	Elemental Calcium (mg)	Elemental Iron (mg)	Other Active Ingredients
					125		250		
					133		333		magnesium 167 mg
				25			300		magnesium oxide 300 mg zinc gluconate 15 mg
					200		600		
					200		600		
					200		600		copper 1 mg magnesium 50 mg manganese 1.8 mg zinc 7.5 mg
					200		600		copper 1 mg magnesium 50 mg manganese 1.8 mg zinc 7.5 mg
					400		600		
					400		500		
					1000		500		
	0.5								safflower oil 912 mg
10	3	14	0.4	90	400	25	175	10	ß-carotene 3000 IU biotin 45 µg copper 2 mg iodine 150 µg magnesium 50 mg phosphorus 125 mg
5	2.5	50	0.3	125	400	100	200	2	ß-carotene 900 IU biotin 22.5 µg chromium 50 µg copper 0.5 mg iodine 75 µg magnesium 50 mg manganese 2.5 mg molybdenum 22.5 µg phosphorus 125 mg potassium 20 mg selenium 25 µg zinc 3.75 mg
3.75	2	1.5	0.2	60	100	11.75	14.25	2.5	ß-carotene 1000 IU biotin 31.25 µg chromium 20 µg copper 0.5 mg iodine 50 µg magnesium 50 mg manganese 1 mg selenium 15 µg vitamin K₁ 15 µg zinc 2.5 mg

Product	Manufacturer	Dosage Form	A (IU)	B_1 (mg)	B_2 (mg)	B_3 (mg)
Centrum for Men	Pfizer Consumer Healthcare	tablet	1000	4.2	4.6	16
Centrum for Women	Pfizer Consumer Healthcare	tablet	1000	3.85	3.85	14
Centrum Forte	Pfizer Consumer Healthcare	tablet	1000	2.25	3.2	15
Centrum Junior Complete	Pfizer Consumer Healthcare	tablet	1000	1	1	10
Centrum Materna	Pfizer Consumer Healthcare	tablet	1000	1.4	1.4	18

Pantothenic Acid (mg)	B₆ (mg)	B₁₂ (µg)	Folic Acid (mg)	C (mg)	D (IU)	E (IU)	Elemental Calcium (mg)	Elemental Iron (mg)	Other Active Ingredients
12.5	5.5	21.6	0.4	180	800	40	300	6	ß-carotene 1500 IU copper 0.9 mg chromium 35 µg iodine 150 µg lutein 1000 µg lycopene 600 µg magnesium 84 mg manganese 5.5 mg selenium 55 µg vitamin K, 25 µg zinc 11 mg
11	5	21.6	0.4	150	800	28	400	7.5	ß-carotene 1000 IU copper 0.9 mg chromium 25 µg iodine 150 µg lutein 1000 µg lycopene 600 µg magnesium 64 mg manganese 5 mg selenium 55 µg vitamin K, 20 µg zinc 8 mg
10	5	20	0.4	90	600	50	200	10	ß-carotene 3000 IU biotin 45 µg chromium 35 µg copper 1 mg iodine 150 µg lutein 500 µg magnesium 50 mg manganese 5 mg molybdenum 45 µg potassium 80 mg selenium 55 µg zinc 7.5 mg
5	1	2	0.1	75	400	10	250	5	biotin 30 µg copper 0.5 m iodine 150 µg magnesium 50 mg zinc 3 mg
6	1.9	2.6	1	85	400	30	250	27	ß-carotene 2500 IU biotin 30 µg calcium 250 mg chromium 30 µg copper 1 mg iodine 220 µg magnesium 50 mg manganese 2 mg molybdenum 50 µg selenium 30 µg zinc 7.5 mg

Product	Manufacturer	Dosage Form	A (IU)	B_1 (mg)	B_2 (mg)	B_3 (mg)
Centrum Performance	Pfizer Consumer Healthcare	tablet	1000	4.5	5.1	15
Centrum Select	Pfizer Consumer Healthcare	tablet	1000	2.25	3.2	15
Centrum Select Chewables	Pfizer Consumer Healthcare	tablet, chewable	1000	2.25	3.2	15
Chelated Cal-Mag with Vitamin C, D and Zinc	Swiss Herbal	tablet				
Children's Chewable Multivitamin	Vita Health	tablet	1395	1.5		8
Children's Chewable Multivitamin plus Iron	Vita Health	tablet	1395	1.5	1.5	8
Children's Chewable Multiple Vitamin & Minerals	SunOpta	tablet	2000	1	1.5	5
Children's Chewable Multivitamin	Jamieson	tablet	2000	1	1.5	5
Children's Chewable Vitamins	Pharmetics	tablet	1600	1.5	1.5	8
Children's Chewable Vitamins with Iron	Pharmetics	tablet	1600	1.5	1.5	8
Children's Choice Multivitamin	Swiss Herbal	tablet, chewable	5000	1.5	1.5	10

Pantothenic Acid (mg)	B$_6$ (mg)	B$_{12}$ (µg)	Folic Acid (mg)	C (mg)	D (IU)	E (IU)	Elemental Calcium (mg)	Elemental Iron (mg)	Other Active Ingredients
10	6	20	0.6	120	400	60	162	8	ß-carotene 2000 IU biotin 40 µg chromium 25 µg copper 1.4 mg iodine 150 µg magnesium 50 mg manganese 4 mg molybdenum 50 µg nickel 5 µg potassium 80 mg selenium 55 µg tin 10 µg vanadium 10 µg zinc 7.5 mg
10	8	25	0.6	90	400	75	200	4	ß-carotene 3000 IU biotin 45 µg chromium 100 µg copper 1 mg iodine 150 µg lutein 500 µg magnesium 50 mg manganese 5 mg molybdenum 45 µg potassium 80 mg selenium 55 µg zinc 7.5 mg
10	8	25	0.4	90	600	75	200	4	ß-carotene 3000 IU biotin 45 µg chromium 100 µg copper 1 mg iodine 150 µg lutein 500 µg magnesium 50 mg manganese 5 mg molybdenum 45 µg phosphorus 125 mg selenium 55 µg zinc 7.5 mg
				25	200		350		magnesium 175 mg zinc 10 mg
	1	3	0.1	50					
	1	3	0.1	50	400			4	
5	1	5	0.05	75	200	7.5	65	2	ß-carotene 500 IU copper 0.5 mg iodine 50 µg magnesium 32.5 mg zinc 1 mg
5	1	5	0.05	75	200	7.5	65	2	ß-carotene 300 IU biotin 5 µg copper 0.5 mg iodine 50 µg magnesium 32.5 mg zinc 1 mg
	1	3	0.1	50	400				
	1	3	0.1	50	400			4	
10	1	10		75	400	10			

Product	Manufacturer	Dosage Form	A (IU)	B_1 (mg)	B_2 (mg)	B_3 (mg)
Children's Choice Multivitamin with Iron	Swiss Herbal	tablet, chewable	5000	1.5	1.5	10
Children's Multiple Vitamins Plus Minerals	General Nutrition Canada	tablet	833.3	1.67	1.67	6.67
Choline	Swiss Herbal	tablet				
Citracal	Bayer Consumer	tablet				
Cod Liver Oil Capsule	Various Manufacturers	capsule	1250 to 2500			
Complexe B Compose 100	Bio-Santé	tablet		100	100	100
Complexe B Compose 50	Bio-Santé	tablet		50	50	50
Cool B	Sisu	capsule				500
Cool B50	Sisu	capsule		50	50	50
Diamine	Euro-Pharm	tablet		1.5	1.7	20
Dol Mite Powder (per 1.5 g)	Swiss Herbal	powder				
Dol Mite Tablet	Swiss Herbal	tablet				
Ester Aces	Sisu	capsule				
Ester C	Sisu	capsule	3333			
Euro-Cal D	Euro-Pharm	tablet				
Extra Once A Day	SunOpta	tablet	5000	25	25	25
Féminex 500	Santé Naturelle	tablet	1500			
Féminex Calcium 500	Santé Naturelle	tablet	1500			

Pantothenic Acid (mg)	B$_6$ (mg)	B$_{12}$ (µg)	Folic Acid (mg)	C (mg)	D (IU)	E (IU)	Elemental Calcium (mg)	Elemental Iron (mg)	Other Active Ingredients
10	1	10		75	400	10		4	
5	1.67	3.33	0.13	30	133.3	10		4	ß-carotene 833.3 IU biotin 33.3 µg choline 0.33 mg inositol 1.67 mg iodine 33 µg
									choline 500 mg
					200		315		
					100 to 270				
100	100	100	5						biotin 100 µg choline bitartrate 100 mg inositol 100 mg
50	50	50	5						biotin 50 µg choline bitartrate 50 mg inositol 50 mg
		300	0.3						
50	50	50	0.4						biotin 50 µg
10	10	6	1	100					biotin 300 µg
							270		magnesium 146 mg
							158		magnesium 80 mg
				250		200			ß-carotene 10 000 IU selenium 50 µg
	5			250					zinc 5 mg
					125		500		
25	25	25	0.8	150	400	50	130	15	ß-carotene 10 000 IU biotin 25 µg choline bitartrate 25 mg chromium 20 µg copper 1 mg dl-methionine 25 mg inositol 25 mg iodine 100 µg magnesium 65 mg manganese 2 mg molybdenum 20 µg potassium 15 mg selenium 20 µg vanadium 20 µg zinc 10 mg
	1	4.5	0.03	50	130	8	500	5	magnesium 25 mg
	1	4.5	0.3	50	130	8	500		magnesium 25 mg

Product	Manufacturer	Dosage Form	A (IU)	B$_1$ (mg)	B$_2$ (mg)	B$_3$ (mg)
Feminex Multi	Santé Naturelle	tablet	500	2.5	3	20
Flintstones Gummies	Bayer Consumer	gummy	1600			
Flintstones Multiple Vitamins	Bayer Consumer	tablet, chewable	1600	1.5	1.5	8
Flintstones Multiple Vitamins Complete	Bayer Consumer	tablet, chewable	1600	1.5	1.5	8
Flintstones Multiple Vitamins plus Iron	Bayer Consumer	tablet, chewable	1600	1.5	1.5	8
Flintstones Multiple Vitamins with Extra C	Bayer Consumer	tablet, chewable	1600	1.5	1.5	8
Flintstones Sour Gummies	Bayer Consumer	gummy	1600			
Folic Acid with Vitamin B$_{12}$	SunOpta	tablet				
Formula Forte Seniors	Pharmetics	tablet	3000	2.25	3.2	40
Formula HSN	General Nutrition Canada	tablet		2	2	2

Pantothenic Acid (mg)	B₆ (mg)	B₁₂ (µg)	Folic Acid (mg)	C (mg)	D (IU)	E (IU)	Elemental Calcium (mg)	Elemental Iron (mg)	Other Active Ingredients
5	5	12.5	0.3	75	200	50	100		ß-carotene 5000 IU biotin 25 µg chlorine 36 mg choline bitartrate 15 mg chromium 50 µg copper 1 mg dl-methionine 7.5 mg inositol 15 mg iodine 75 µg magnesium 50 mg manganese 2.5 mg molybdenum 12.5 µg nickel 2.5 µg phosphorus 62.5 mg potassium 40 mg selenium 12.5 µg silicon 5 µg tin 5 µg vanadium 5 µg zinc 7.5 mg
	2	6	0.1	20	200	10			
	1	3	0.1	50	400				
10	1	3	0.1	50	400	10	160	4	biotin 30 µg copper 1 mg (as cupric oxide) phosphorus 125 mg (as calcium phosphate dibasic)
	1	3	0.1	50	400			4	
	1	3	0.1	250	400				
	2	6	0.1	20	200	10			
		1000	1						
10	3	25	0.4	90	400	45	200	4	ß-carotene 3000 IU biotin 45 µg chlorine 72 mg chromium 100 µg copper 2 mg iodine 150 µg magnesium 100 mg manganese 5 mg molybdenum 25 µg nickel 5 µg phosphorus 125 mg potassium 80 mg selenium 25 µg silicon 10 µg tin 10 µg vanadium 10 µg zinc 15 mg
10	5	4	0.13	33.3	66.7	10	150	2	ß-carotene 1800 IU biotin 67 µg choline 25 mg dl-methionine 3.3 mg inositol 10 mg iodine 75 µg magnesium 30 mg manganese 3.3 mg phosphorus 115 mg selenium 8.3 µg silicon 2 mg zinc 5 mg

Product	Manufacturer	Dosage Form	A (IU)	B_1 (mg)	B_2 (mg)	B_3 (mg)
Forza 10	Euro-Pharm	tablet	4000	2	2	20
Halibut Liver Oil	Various Manufacturers	capsule	10 000			
Halibut Liver Oil	Various Manufacturers	capsule	5000			
Hi Potency B Compound	Swiss Herbal	tablet		50	50	50
Hi Potency Cod Liver Oil	Swiss Herbal	capsule	3000			
Hi Potency Stress B 60 with C	Lee-Adams	tablet		60	60	100
HVP Chelated Magnesium plus Vitamin D	Swiss Herbal	tablet				
HVP Chelated Selenium plus C & E	Swiss Herbal	tablet				
Hydroxy Cal with Boron	Sisu	capsule				
Inositol	General Nutrition Canada	tablet				186
Iron Copper B_{12}, C & Folic Acid	Swiss Herbal	tablet				
Lecithin Capsules	Adams Labs	capsule				
Liquid B Complex	General Nutrition Canada	capsule		50	50	50
Maximum Once A Day	SunOpta	tablet	5000	75	75	75
Mega B 100 Timed Release	SunOpta	tablet, sustained release		100	100	100
Mega B 50	SunOpta	capsule		50	50	50
Mega B 50 Vitamin B Complex	SunOpta	tablet		50	50	50

Pantothenic Acid (mg)	B$_6$ (mg)	B$_{12}$ (µg)	Folic Acid (mg)	C (mg)	D (IU)	E (IU)	Elemental Calcium (mg)	Elemental Iron (mg)	Other Active Ingredients
10	2	5	0.1	70	400	15			
					400				
					400				
50	50	50	1						biotin 50 µg choline bitartrate 50 mg inositol 50 mg
					300				
100	60	60	1	500					biotin 60 µg choline bitartrate 60 mg inositol 60 mg
					200				magnesium 150 mg
				100		50			selenium 200 µg
				50	100		125		boron 0.5 mg copper 0.5 mg magnesium 60 mg manganese 1 mg zinc 2.5 mg
									inositol 51 mg
		25	0.4	100				30	copper 2 mg
					150				lecithin 260 mg
50	50	50	0.4						biotin 50 µg choline bitartrate 50 mg inositol 50 µg
75	75	75	1	250	400	100	150	15	ß-carotene 10 000 IU biotin 75 µg choline bitartrate 75 mg chromium 50 µg copper 2 mg dl-methionine 50 mg inositol 75 mg iodine 100 µg magnesium 75 mg manganese 5 mg molybdenum 50 µg potassium 50 mg selenium 100 µg vanadium 50 µg zinc 20 mg
100	100	100	10						biotin 100 µg choline bitartrate 100 mg inositol 100 mg
50	50	50	0.4						biotin 50 µg choline bitartrate 50 mg inositol 50 mg
50	50	50	1						biotin 50 µg choline bitartrate 50 mg inositol 50 mg

Product	Manufacturer	Dosage Form	A (IU)	B_1 (mg)	B_2 (mg)	B_3 (mg)
Mega-Vim	Jamieson	tablet	5000	75	75	75
Megakids	General Nutrition Canada	tablet	5000	2.5	2	15
Multi Forte	Nutricorp	tablet	2000	2.25	3.2	40
Multi Mineral	Swiss Herbal	tablet				
Multi Mineral with Vitamin D	Adams Labs	tablet				
Multiple Vitamins	Adams Labs	tablet	5000	3	2.5	20
Multiple Vitamins	GFR Pharma	tablet	5000	1.5	2	20
Multiple Vitamins plus Iron	Pharmetics	tablet	10 000	2	2	20
Multiple Vitamins with Iron	Adams Labs	tablet	5000	3	2.5	20
Multiple Vitamins with Iron	GFR Pharma	tablet	5000	3	2.5	20
Multiple Vitamins with Minerals	Adams Labs	tablet	10 000	3	5	25

Pantothenic Acid (mg)	B₆ (mg)	B₁₂ (µg)	Folic Acid (mg)	C (mg)	D (IU)	E (IU)	Elemental Calcium (mg)	Elemental Iron (mg)	Other Active Ingredients
75	75	75	0.4	250	400	150	150	4	ß-carotene 1500 IU biotin 75 µg chromium 10 µg copper 1 mg iodine 100 µg lutein 300 µg magnesium 75 mg manganese 1 mg molybdenum 1 µg potassium 25 mg selenium 10 µg vanadium 1 µg zinc 10 mg
10	1	2	0.4	100	200	50	200	4	biotin 30 µg magnesium 10 mg
10	3	9	0.4	90	400	30	175	10	ß-carotene 3000 IU biotin 45 µg chlorine 36 mg chromium 25 µg copper 2 mg iodine 150 µg lutein 250 µg magnesium 100 mg manganese 5 mg molybdenum 25 µg potassium 40 mg selenium 25 µg silicon 10 µg tin 10 µg vanadium 10 µg zinc 15 mg
							250		chromium 50 µg copper 1 mg iodine 75 µg magnesium 195 mg manganese 1 mg zinc 7.5 mg
					400		150	5	copper 1 mg iodine 100 µg magnesium 60 mg manganese 1 mg phosphorus 70 mg potassium 50 mg zinc 0.1 mg
	1	3		40	400				
	2	6	0.1	60	400	10			
	2	6	0.4	100	400	15		4	
	1	3		40	400			4	
	1	3		50	400			4	
5	1	3		75	400		125	5	copper 1 mg iodine 150 µg

Product	Manufacturer	Dosage Form	A (IU)	B_1 (mg)	B_2 (mg)	B_3 (mg)
Multi-Vi-Min	Naka	capsule	4000	25	25	25
Multi-vitamins & Minerals	GFR Pharma	tablet	5000	2.25	2.6	20
Multivitamins & Minerals For Men	Pharmetics	tablet		2.25	2.25	20
Multivitamins & Minerals For Women	Pharmetics	tablet		1.5	1.7	14
Neo Cal D_3	Néolab	tablet				
Neo Cal-D-500	Néolab	tablet				
Neo-Tinic A	Néolab	tablet	2000	5	3	20
Nu-Cal D	Odan	tablet				
Nu-Cal D 200	Odan	tablet				
Nu-Cal D 400	Odan	tablet				
Nu-Cal D One a Day	Odan	tablet				
Nutrol A	M. Vachon	capsule	10000			
Nutrol C 500	M. Vachon	tablet				
Nutrol C 1000	M. Vachon	tablet				
Nutrol E 200	M. Vachon	capsule				
Occuvite Plus with Lutein	Bausch & Lomb	tablet				

Pantothenic Acid (mg)	B₆ (mg)	B₁₂ (µg)	Folic Acid (mg)	C (mg)	D (IU)	E (IU)	Elemental Calcium (mg)	Elemental Iron (mg)	Other Active Ingredients
25	25	25	0.5	75	200	25	62.5	5	biotin 25 µg choline 25 µg chromium 12.5 µg inositol 25 µg magnesium 50 mg manganese 500 µg molybdenum 12.5 µg potassium 5 mg selenium 12.5 µg zinc 5 mg
10	3	9	0.4	90	400	30	162	10	biotin 45 µg chlorine 27.2 mg chromium 25 µg copper 2 mg iodine 150 µg magnesium 100 mg manganese 5 mg molybdenum 25 µg phosphorus 125 mg potassium 30 mg selenium 25 µg zinc 15 mg
10	3	9	0.4	90	400	45			ß-carotene 10000 IU chromium 150 µg iodine 150 µg magnesium 100 mg manganese 3.3 mg molybdenum 41.7 µg potassium 37.5 mg selenium 87.5 µg zinc 15 mg
10	2	10	0.4	60	200	25	400	10	ß-carotene 1000 IU magnesium 50 mg
					100	250			
					125	500			
	3	5	1	100	400		160	60	ß-carotene 4000 IU
					125	500			
					200	500			
					400	500			
					800	500			
				500					
				1000					
						200			
				200		40			ß-carotene 500 IU lutein 2 mg selenium 55 µg zinc 40 mg

Product	Manufacturer	Dosage Form	A (IU)	B_1 (mg)	B_2 (mg)	B_3 (mg)
Once A Day	SunOpta	tablet	10 000	5	10	20
One A Day Advance Adult	Bayer Consumer	tablet	2500	1.5	1.7	20
One A Day Advance Adult 50 Plus	Bayer Consumer	tablet	3000	4.5	3.4	20
One A Day Men	Bayer Consumer	tablet	4000	2.25	2.55	20
One A Day Resolution	Bayer Consumer	tablet		1.9	2.1	25

Pantothenic Acid (mg)	B$_6$ (mg)	B$_{12}$ (µg)	Folic Acid (mg)	C (mg)	D (IU)	E (IU)	Elemental Calcium (mg)	Elemental Iron (mg)	Other Active Ingredients
15	5	15	0.1	150	400	15	125	15	biotin 10 µg choline bitartrate 20 mg chromium 10 µg copper 1 mg dl-methionine 20 mg inositol 20 mg iodine 100 µg magnesium 50 mg manganese 1 mg potassium 10 mg selenium 10 µg vanadium 10 µg zinc 2 mg
10	2	6	0.4	60	400	30	130	18	ß-carotene 2500 IU biotin 30 µg chlorine 34 mg chromium 10 µg copper 2 mg iodine 150 µg magnesium 100 mg manganese 2.5 mg molybdenum 10 µg potassium 37.5 mg selenium 10 µg zinc 15 mg
20	6	25	0.4	120	400	60	220		ß-carotene 3000 IU biotin 30 µg chlorine 34 mg chromium 10 µg copper 2 mg iodine 150 µg magnesium 100 mg manganese 2.5 mg molybdenum 10 µg potassium 37.5 mg selenium 10 µg zinc 15 mg
10	3	9	0.4	90	400	45			ß-carotene 1000 IU chlorine 34 mg chromium 150 µg copper 2 mg iodine 150 µg magnesium 100 mg manganese 3.3 mg molybdenum 42 µg potassium 37.5 mg selenium 87.5 µg zinc 15 mg
12.5	2.5	7.5	0.4	60	400	30	300	14	ß-carotene 1250 IU chromium 150 µg copper 2 mg magnesium 50 mg manganese 2 mg selenium 70 µg zinc 15 mg

Product	Manufacturer	Dosage Form	A (IU)	B_1 (mg)	B_2 (mg)	B_3 (mg)
One A Day Weightsmart	Bayer Consumer	tablet		1.9	2.1	25
One A Day Women	Bayer Consumer	tablet	2000	1.5	1.7	14
Only Minerals	Sisu	capsule				
Only One	Sisu	tablet	1500	30	30	50
Palafer CF	GlaxoSmithKline Consumer Healthcare	capsule				
Platinum Years	General Nutrition Canada	tablet	2500	17.5	17.5	17.5
Potassium plus Magnesium & B_6	Swiss Herbal	tablet				

Pantothenic Acid (mg)	B₆ (mg)	B₁₂ (µg)	Folic Acid (mg)	C (mg)	D (IU)	E (IU)	Elemental Calcium (mg)	Elemental Iron (mg)	Other Active Ingredients
12.5	2.5	7.5	0.4	60	200	20	300	14	ß-carotene 1250 IU chromium 150 µg copper 2 mg magnesium 50 mg manganese 2 mg selenium 70 µg zinc 15 mg
10	2	10	0.4	60	200	25	400	10	ß-carotene 500 IU magnesium 50 mg
							50		chromium 50 µg copper 0.5 mg iodine 100 µg magnesium 25 mg manganese 5 mg molybdenum 8 µg potassium 50 mg selenium 30 µg silicon 1 mg vanadium 12 µg zinc 2.5 mg
30	30	50	0.4	150	200	30	125	4	ß-carotene 10 000 IU biotin 25 µg choline bitartrate 50 mg chromium 100 µg copper 1 mg dl-methionine 50 mg inositol 50 mg iodine 100 µg magnesium 50 mg manganese 3 mg molybdenum 10 µg potassium 10 mg selenium 50 µg vanadium 10 µg zinc 5 mg
			0.5	200				100	
10	17.5	15	0.2	100	200	50	100	5	ß-carotene 5000 IU biotin 15 µg chlorine 36 mg choline 25 µg chromium 50 µg copper 1 mg inositol 25 µg iodine 25 µg magnesium 50 mg manganese 1.5 mg molybdenum 12.5 µg nickel 2.5 µg potassium 40 mg selenium 12.5 µg silicon dioxide 1000 µg zinc 7.5 mg
	25								magnesium oxide 50 mg potassium gluconate 167 mg

Product	Manufacturer	Dosage Form	A (IU)	B$_1$ (mg)	B$_2$ (mg)	B$_3$ (mg)
Premium Multi-Cap with the Right C	SunOpta	capsule		25	25	25
Premium Multi-Cap with the Right C Iron Free	SunOpta	capsule		25	25	25
Premium Multi-One with Niacinamide	SunOpta	tablet	7500	50	50	50
Prenatal Supplement	General Nutrition Canada	caplet	1000	5	5	8.5
Prenatal	Jamieson	caplet	1000	3	3.75	22
Prenatal/Postpartum Vitamins & Minerals	Pharmetics	tablet	1500	3	3.4	20

Pantothenic Acid (mg)	B₆ (mg)	B₁₂ (µg)	Folic Acid (mg)	C (mg)	D (IU)	E (IU)	Elemental Calcium (mg)	Elemental Iron (mg)	Other Active Ingredients
	25	25	0.5	75	200	50	125	10	ß-carotene 5000 IU chromium 50 µg iodine 50 µg magnesium 50 mg manganese 1.5 mg molybdenum 25 µg potassium 25 mg selenium 50 µg vanadium 25 µg zinc 5 mg
25	25	25	0.5	75	200	50	125		ß-carotene 5000 IU chromium 50 µg iodine 50 µg magnesium 50 mg manganese 1.5 mg molybdenum 25 µg potassium 25 mg selenium 50 µg vanadium 25 µg zinc 5 mg
50	50	50	0.5	150	400	50	125	15	ß-carotene 2500 IU biotin 50 µg choline 50 mg chromium 25 µg copper 1 mg inositol 50 mg iodine 100 µg magnesium 60 mg manganese 2 mg molybdenum 25 µg potassium 10 mg selenium 50 µg vanadium 25 µg zinc 10 mg
7.5	5	5	0.5	30	100	12.5	250	9	ß-carotene 5000 IU copper 0.5 mg iodine 93 µg magnesium 50 mg phosphorus 193.75 mg zinc 7.5 mg
10	10	10	1	150	200	30	200	30	ß-carotene 1800 IU biotin 30 µg chromium 25 µg copper 1 mg iodine 150 µg magnesium 100 mg manganese 5 mg zinc 20 mg
10	10	12	1	100	250	30	250	60	ß-carotene 1500 IU biotin 30 µg chromium 25 µg copper 2 mg iodine 150 µg magnesium 50 mg manganese 5 mg molybdenum 25 µg selenium 25 µg zinc 25 mg

Product	Manufacturer	Dosage Form	A (IU)	B_1 (mg)	B_2 (mg)	B_3 (mg)
Pretal	Jaapharm	tablet	1500	3	3.4	20
Redoxon-B	Bayer Consumer	tablet, effervescent		15	15	50
Redoxon Lemon/Orange	Bayer Consumer	tablet, effervescent				
Replavite	WN Pharmaceuticals	tablet		1.5	1.7	20
Selenium Plus	Sisu	capsule				
Selenium plus Beta-Carotene & Vitamins C & E	Jamieson	tablet				
Senior Multi-One Formula	Swiss Herbal	capsule		25	25	25
Solotron	General Nutrition Canada	tablet	9000	30	30	30
Stress B Complex with Vitamins C & E & Iron	Pharmetics	tablet		10	10	100
Stress B Complex with Vitamins C & E, Zinc & Copper	Pharmetics	tablet		10	10	100
Stress Formula	JAMP	capsule		35	15	50
Stress Formula with Iron	JAMP	capsule		35	15	50
Stress Formula with Zinc	JAMP	capsule		35	15	50

Pantothenic Acid (mg)	B$_6$ (mg)	B$_{12}$ (µg)	Folic Acid (mg)	C (mg)	D (IU)	E (IU)	Elemental Calcium (mg)	Elemental Iron (mg)	Other Active Ingredients
10	10	12	1	100	250	30	250	20	ß-carotene 1500 IU biotin 30 µg chromium 25 µg copper sulfate 2 mg iodine 150 µg magnesium oxide 50 mg manganese sulfate 5 mg molybdenum 25 µg zinc oxide 25 mg
23	10	10		1000					biotin 150 µg magnesium 100 mg
				1000	300				
10	10	6	1	100					biotin 300 µg
									l-methionine 1.4 mg selenium 200 µg
				60		10			ß-carotene 5000 IU selenium 50 µg
25	25	25	0.5	75	200	50	125		ß-carotene 5000 IU biotin 10 µg chromium 50 µg copper gluconate 1 mg iodine 50 µg magnesium 50 mg manganese gluconate 1.5 mg molybdenum citrate 25 µg potassium citrate 25 mg selenium 50 µg vanadium 25 µg zinc 5 mg
30	30	30	0.4	200	400	30		18	ß-carotene 1000 IU biotin 30 µg choline bitartrate 30 mg chromium 25 µg copper gluconate 2 mg inositol 30 µg iodine 150 µg magnesium oxide 50 mg manganese gluconate 5 mg molybdenum 25 µg nickel sulfate 5 µg potassium citrate 10 mg selenium 25 µg silicon dioxide 10 µg tin 10 µg vanadium 10 µg zinc 30 mg
20	5	12	0.4	500		30		18	biotin 45 µg
20	5	12	0.4	500		30			biotin 45 µg copper sulfate 3 mg zinc sulfate 23.9 mg
20	5	10		500					
20	5	10		500				10	
20	5	10		500					zinc sulfate 24 mg

Product	Manufacturer	Dosage Form	A (IU)	B$_1$ (mg)	B$_2$ (mg)	B$_3$ (mg)
Stress Plex	Jamieson	tablet		3	2.5	12
Stressease	Jamieson	caplet		35	35	50
Stresstabs for Men	Pfizer Consumer Healthcare	tablet		15	15	20
Stresstabs for Women	Pfizer Consumer Healthcare	tablet		15	15	20
Stresstabs Plus	Pfizer Consumer Healthcare	tablet			15	
Stresstabs Z-Bec	Pfizer Consumer Healthcare	tablet		30	10	20
Super B Complex	Sisu	capsule		25	25	75
Super Daily	Lee-Adams	tablet	8000	10	10	100
Super Once A Day Timed Release	SunOpta	tablet, sustained release	10 000	50	50	50
Super Stress Mega B plus Vitamin C	SunOpta	tablet		50	50	50
Super Vita Vim	Jamieson	tablet	5000	30	30	50
Synergistic Selenium plus Vitamin C & E	SunOpta	caplet				

Pantothenic Acid (mg)	B$_6$ (mg)	B$_{12}$ (µg)	Folic Acid (mg)	C (mg)	D (IU)	E (IU)	Elemental Calcium (mg)	Elemental Iron (mg)	Other Active Ingredients
5	3	10	0.05	250					biotin 10 µg choline bitartrate 5 mg inositol 5 mg zinc gluconate 5 mg
20	15	30	1	500		30	150		biotin 15 µg magnesium oxide 75 mg zinc gluconate 5 mg
20	10	25	0.4	500		30			biotin 30 µg copper 1 mg lycopene 1 mg selenium 70 µg zinc oxide 7.5 mg
20	10	25	0.4	500		30		18	biotin 30 µg
	25	50	0.8	500		200			lycopene 2mg selenium 70 µg
25	10	25	0.5	600		45			copper 3 mg zinc sulfate 23.9 mg
125	51.5	100	0.2						biotin 100 µg choline 125 mg inositol 50 mg
50	10	15	0.75	250	400		125	10	biotin 10 µg choline bitartrate 50 mg copper 1 mg inositol 50 mg iodine 150 µg magnesium 50 mg manganese 1 mg potassium 15 mg zinc 1.5 mg
50	50	50	0.2	150	400	50	125	15	biotin 50 µg choline bitartrate 50 mg chromium 25 µg copper 1 mg inositol 50 mg iodine 100 µg magnesium gluconate 100 mg manganese 1 mg phosphorus 50 mg potassium gluconate 50 mg selenium 25 µg zinc 10 mg
50	50	50	1	1000					biotin 50 µg choline bitartrate 50 mg inositol 50 mg
50	50	50	0.4	200	400	60	150	4	ß-carotene 1500 IU biotin 30 µg chromium 10 µg copper 1 mg iodine 100 µg magnesium 75 mg manganese 1 mg molybdenum 1 µg potassium 25 mg selenium 10 µg vanadium 1 µg zinc 10 mg
				100		25			selenium 200 µg

Product	Manufacturer	Dosage Form	A (IU)	B_1 (mg)	B_2 (mg)	B_3 (mg)
Synergistic Zinc & Copper plus Beta-Carotene	SunOpta	caplet				
Time Released Balanced B	Lee-Adams	tablet, sustained release		50	50	50
Time Released Women's Ultra Mega	General Nutrition Canada	caplet	4300	40	40	40
Timed Release Mega Men	General Nutrition Canada	tablet, sustained release	2500	15	15	15
Timed Release Stress B with C	General Nutrition Canada	caplet		100	100	100
Timed Release Swiss One 50 with B Vitamins	Swiss Herbal	caplet		50	50	50
Timed Release Ultra Mega	General Nutrition Canada	tablet, delayed action	9750	75	75	75

Pantothenic Acid (mg)	B$_6$ (mg)	B$_{12}$ (µg)	Folic Acid (mg)	C (mg)	D (IU)	E (IU)	Elemental Calcium (mg)	Elemental Iron (mg)	Other Active Ingredients
									ß-carotene 5000 IU copper 1 mg zinc 20 mg
50	50	50	0.4						biotin 50 µg
40	40	40	0.2	100	200	50	250	13.5	ß-carotene 700 IU biotin 40 µg choline bitartrate 5 mg chromium 50 µg copper 1 mg inositol 5 µg iodine 75 µg magnesium 100 mg manganese 2.5 mg potassium 5 mg selenium 50 µg silicon dioxide 1 mg zinc 7.5 mg
15	15	15	0.2	150	100	50	137.5		ß-carotene 2500 IU biotin 125 µg choline bitartrate 5 mg copper 1 mg inositol 5 mg iodine 75 µg magnesium 50 mg manganese 2.5 mg phosphorus 105 mg potassium 15 mg selenium 12.5 µg silicon 5 µg zinc 25 mg
100	100	500	0.4	500					biotin 50 µg choline bitartrate 50 mg inositol 50 mg
50	50		0.4	100	400	75	125	18	ß-carotene 10 000 IU biotin 50 µg choline 50 mg chromium 25 µg copper 2 mg dl-methionine 50 mg inositol 50 mg iodine 225 µg magnesium 100 mg manganese 5 mg potassium 25 mg selenium 25 µg zinc 10 mg
75	75	75	0.4	200	400	100	125	18	ß-carotene 250 IU biotin 75 µg choline bitartrate 75 mg chromium 10 µg copper 1 mg inositol 75 µg iodine 150 µg manganese 6.1 mg molybdenum 10 µg potassium 10 mg selenium 10 µg zinc 15 mg

Product	Manufacturer	Dosage Form	A (IU)	B$_1$ (mg)	B$_2$ (mg)	B$_3$ (mg)
Timed Release Ultra Mega Gold	General Nutrition Canada	tablet, slow release	5000	50	50	50
Timed Release Ultra Mega Gold without Iron	General Nutrition Canada	tablet, slow release	5000	50	50	50
Total One Maternity Multivitamin with Minerals	Swiss Herbal	caplet		25	25	50
Ultra Mega Softgels	General Nutrition Canada	capsule	2500	25	25	25

Pantothenic Acid (mg)	B_6 (mg)	B_12 (μg)	Folic Acid (mg)	C (mg)	D (IU)	E (IU)	Elemental Calcium (mg)	Elemental Iron (mg)	Other Active Ingredients
50	50	50	0.2	250	200	150	125	7	biotin 50 μg choline 25 mg chromium 50 μg copper 1 mg inositol 25 mg iodine 50 μg magnesium 25 mg manganese 5 mg potassium 10 mg selenium 25 μg zinc 7.5 mg
50	50		0.2	250	200	150	125		biotin 50 μg choline 25 mg chromium 50 μg copper 1 mg inositol 25 mg iodine 50 μg magnesium 25 mg manganese 5 mg potassium 5 mg selenium 25 μg zinc 7.5 mg
30	50	50	1		400	50	200	60	ß-carotene 10 000 IU biotin 100 μg calcium ascorbate 100 mg choline bitartrate 25 mg chromium 25 μg copper 2 mg dl-methionine 22 mg inositol 25 mg iodine 50 μg magnesium 100 mg manganese 5 mg molybdenum 25 μg potassium 50 mg selenium 25 μg
25	25	25	0.2	150	200	150	100		ß-carotene 2500 IU biotin 25 μg choline 25 mg copper 1 mg inositol 25 μg iodine 75 μg magnesium 25 mg manganese 5 mg potassium 15 mg selenium 25 μg zinc 7.5 mg

Product	Manufacturer	Dosage Form	A (IU)	B$_1$ (mg)	B$_2$ (mg)	B$_3$ (mg)
Ultravite Forte 25	Nutravite	tablet	2000	2.25	3.2	40
Vitalux Healthy Eyes	Novartis Pharmaceuticals	tablet	1500	1.13	1.6	17.5
Vitalux Plus Omega-3	Novartis Pharmaceuticals	capsule				
Vitalux-S	Novartis Pharmaceuticals	tablet				
Vitalux-S Plus Omega-3	Novartis Pharmaceuticals	tablet				
Vitalux Time Release	Novartis Pharmaceuticals	tablet			20	
Vitalux AREDS	Novartis Pharmaceuticals	tablet				
Vitamin A & D	Various Manufacturers	capsule	10 000			

Pantothenic Acid (mg)	B$_6$ (mg)	B$_{12}$ (µg)	Folic Acid (mg)	C (mg)	D (IU)	E (IU)	Elemental Calcium (mg)	Elemental Iron (mg)	Other Active Ingredients
10	3	9	0.4	90	400	30	175	10	ß-carotene 3000 IU biotin 45 µg chlorine 36 mg chromium 25 µg copper 2 mg iodine 150 µg magnesium oxide 100 mg manganese 5 mg molybdenum 25 µg nickel sulfate 5 µg phosphorus 125 mg potassium 40 mg selenium 25 µg silicon 10 µg tin 10 µg vanadium 10 µg zinc oxide 15 mg
5	4	12.5	0.25	150	200	50	81		ß-carotene 5000 IU biotin 22.5 µg chlorine 36 mg chromium 50 µg copper 1 mg iodine 75 µg lutein 10 mg magnesium oxide 25 mg manganese 2.5 mg molybdenum 12.5 µg phosphorus 62.5 mg potassium 40 mg selenium 12.5 µg silicon 5 µg tin 5 µg zeaxanthin 1 mg zinc oxide 20 mg
				125		100			ß-carotene 2387 IU copper 0.25 mg fish oil 263 mg lutein 10 mg zeaxanthin 0.5 mg zinc 6.25 mg
				250		200			copper 1 mg lutein 5 mg zinc 40 mg
				125		100			copper 0.25 mg fish oil 263 mg lutein 2.5 mg zeaxanthin 0.5 mg zinc 6.25 mg
				300		100			ß-carotene 5000 IU copper 2 mg lutein 4 mg selenium 50 µg zeaxanthin 0.2 mg zinc gluconate 40 mg
				250		200			ß-carotene 12 500 IU copper 1 mg lutein 5 mg zinc 40 mg
					400				

Product	Manufacturer	Dosage Form	A (IU)	B_1 (mg)	B_2 (mg)	B_3 (mg)
Vitamin B Complex plus Vitamin C 300 mg	GFR Pharma	tablet		35	15	50
Vitamin B Complex plus Vitamin C 550 mg	GFR Pharma	capsule		15	10	50
Vitamin B Complex with Vitamin C 300	Pharmetics	tablet		35	15	50
Vitamin C Powder with Calcium, Magnesium & Potassium	Sisu	powder				
Vitamin E 400 with Selenium	General Nutrition Canada	capsule				
Vitamin E with Selenium	Jamieson	caplet				
Vitamins B, E & C with Zinc	Lee-Adams	tablet		15	10.2	100
Wampole Complete Multi Pre- and Post-Natal	JAMP	tablet	1500	3	3.4	20
Wampole Complete Multi-Adult	JAMP	tablet	4000	2.25	2.6	20
Wampole Complete Multi-Adult 50+	JAMP	tablet	4000	1.5	1.7	20

Pantothenic Acid (mg)	B$_6$ (mg)	B$_{12}$ (µg)	Folic Acid (mg)	C (mg)	D (IU)	E (IU)	Elemental Calcium (mg)	Elemental Iron (mg)	Other Active Ingredients
20	5	10		300					
10	5	10		550					
20	5	10		300					
				1262			240		magnesium 153 mg potassium 53 mg
						400			selenium 100 µg
						200			selenium 25 µg
33	11	6		600		45			zinc sulfate 22.5 mg
10	10	12	1	100	250	30	250	60	ß-carotene 1500 IU biotin 30 µg chromium 25 µg copper 2 mg iodine 150 µg magnesium 50 mg manganese 5 mg molybdenum 25 µg zinc 25 mg
10	3	9	0.4	90	400	30	162	10	ß-carotene 1000 IU biotin 45 µg chlorine 27.2 mg chromium 25 µg copper 2 mg iodine 150 µg magnesium 100 mg manganese 5 mg molybdenum 25 µg nickel 5 µg phosphorus 125 mg potassium 30 mg selenium 25 µg silicon 10 µg tin 10 µg vanadium 10 µg zinc 15 mg
10	3	14	0.2	90	400	25	200	9	ß-carotene 2000 IU biotin 30 µg chlorine 72 mg chromium 100 µg copper 2 mg iodine 15 µg magnesium 100 mg manganese 2.5 mg molybdenum 25 µg nickel 5 µg phosphorus 150 mg potassium 80 mg selenium 25 µg silicon 10 µg tin 10 µg vanadium 10 µg zinc 15 mg

Product	Manufacturer	Dosage Form	A (IU)	B_1 (mg)	B_2 (mg)	B_3 (mg)
Women's Timed Release Ultra Mega without Iron	General Nutrition Canada	tablet, sustained release	4300	40	40	40

Pantothenic Acid (mg)	B₆ (mg)	B₁₂ (µg)	Folic Acid (mg)	C (mg)	D (IU)	E (IU)	Elemental Calcium (mg)	Elemental Iron (mg)	Other Active Ingredients
40	40	40	0.2	100	200	50	250		ß-carotene 700 IU biotin 40 µg choline 5 mg chromium 50 µg copper 1 mg inositol 5 µg iodine 75 µg magnesium 100 mg manganese 2.5 mg potassium 5 mg selenium 50 µg silicon dioxide 1 mg zinc 7.5 mg

Product	Manufacturer	Dosage Form	Active Ingredients
Acti-B$_{12}$	Sandoz	liquid	hydroxocobalamin 50 µg/mL
Apo-Cal 250	Apotex	tablet	calcium carbonate 625 mg
Apo-Cal 500	Apotex	tablet	calcium carbonate 1250 mg
Apo-Ferrous Gluconate	Apotex	tablet	ferrous gluconate 300 mg
Apo-Ferrous Sulfate	Apotex	tablet	ferrous sulfate 300 mg
Apo-K	Apotex	tablet	potassium chloride 600 mg
Aquasol E Drops	Columbia	drops	vitamin E 50 IU/mL
Arovit A Capsules	Bio-Santé	capsule	vitamin A 10 000 IU
Baby D Drops	Ddrops Company	liquid	vitamin D$_3$ 400 IU/drop
Beta Carotene 10 000 IU	Various Manufacturers	tablet	ß-carotene 10 000 IU
Beta Carotene 10 000 IU	Various Manufacturers	capsule	ß-carotene 10 000 IU
Beta Carotene 25 000 IU	Various Manufacturers	tablet	ß-carotene 25 000 IU
Beta Carotene 25 000 IU	Various Manufacturers	capsule	ß-carotene 25 000 IU
Beta Carotene Pro Vitamin A 10 000 IU	Jamieson	tablet	ß-carotene 10 000 IU
Biotin 50 µg	Swiss Herbal	tablet	biotin 50 µg
Biotin 250 µg	Jamieson	tablet	biotin 250 µg
Biotin 300 µg	General Nutrition Canada	tablet	biotin 300 µg
Biotin 300 µg	Swiss Herbal	tablet	biotin 300 µg
Biotin 500 µg	General Nutrition Canada	tablet	biotin 500 µg
Buffered Vitamin C 500 mg	Swiss Herbal	tablet	ascorbic acid 500 mg
Buffered Vitamin C 1000 mg	General Nutrition Canada	caplet	ascorbic acid 1000 mg
Calcium	Various Manufacturers	tablet	calcium lactate 650 mg
Calcium 350 mg	General Nutrition Canada	tablet	calcium carbonate 875 mg
Calcium 350 mg	Swiss Herbal	tablet	calcium citrate 350 mg
Calcium 350 mg	Jamieson	tablet, chewable	calcium 350 mg (as carbonate, citrate, fumarate, glutarate, malate and succinate)
Calcium 650 mg	Jamieson	tablet, chewable	calcium 650 mg (as carbonate, citrate, fumarate, glutarate, malate and succinate)
Calcium Carbonate 1250 mg	Various Manufacturers	tablet	calcium carbonate 1250 mg
Calcium Carbonate 1500 mg	Various Manufacturers	tablet	calcium carbonate 1500 mg
Calcium Citrate 250 mg	General Nutrition Canada	tablet	calcium citrate 250 mg
Calcium D Pantothenate 100 mg	Swiss Herbal	tablet	calcium d-pantothenate 100 mg
Calcium Liquid	Pharmetics	liquid	calcium 20 mg/mL
Calcium Oyster Shell 500 mg	Novopharm	tablet	calcium carbonate 1250 mg
Calcium-Sandoz Forte 500 mg	Novartis Consumer Health	tablet, effervescent	calcium 500 mg (as carbonate and gluconolactate)
Caltrate 600	Wyeth Consumer Healthcare	tablet	calcium carbonate 1500 mg
Chelated Chromium 200 µg	General Nutrition Canada	tablet	chromium 200 µg
Chelated Chromium 200 µg	Jamieson	tablet	chromium 200 µg
Chelated Zinc 10 mg	Jamieson	tablet	zinc gluconate 10 mg
Chelated Zinc 50 mg	Swiss Herbal	tablet	zinc gluconate 50 mg
Chromium 200 µg	General Nutrition Canada	tablet	chromium 200 µg
Chromium 400 µg	General Nutrition Canada	tablet	chromium 400 µg
Chromium 500 µg	Swiss Herbal	tablet	chromium 260 µg
Chromium GTF 200 µg	Jamieson	tablet	chromium 200 µg

Product	Manufacturer	Dosage Form	Active Ingredients
Chromium GTF 200 µg	Quest	tablet	chromium 200 µg
Ci-Cal	Euro-Pharm	tablet	calcium citrate 250 mg
Ddrops	Ddrops Company	liquid	vitamin D_3 1000 IU/drop
Ddrops Booster	Ddrops Company	liquid	vitamin D_3 600 IU/drop
D Vi Sol Solution	Mead Johnson	drops	vitamin D_3 400 IU/mL
D-Pantothenic Acid 100 mg	Swiss Herbal	tablet	pantothenic acid 100 mg
D-Pantothenic Acid 250 mg	Swiss Herbal	tablet	pantothenic acid 250 mg
D-Pantothenic Acid 500 mg	Swiss Herbal	tablet	pantothenic acid 500 mg
Erdol	Odan	drops	vitamin D_2 207 IU/drop
Ester C 500	WN Pharmaceuticals	tablet	ascorbic acid 500 mg
Ester C 600	WN Pharmaceuticals	tablet	ascorbic acid 600 mg
Ester C 1000	WN Pharmaceuticals	tablet	ascorbic acid 1000 mg
Ester C Chewables	WN Pharmaceuticals	tablet	ascorbic acid 250 mg
Euro-B_1	Euro-Pharm	tablet	vitamin B_1 50 mg
Euro-D 400	Euro-Pharm	capsule	vitamin D_3 400 IU
Euro-D 800	Euro-Pharm	capsule	vitamin D_3 800 IU
Euro-D 1000	Euro-Pharm	capsule	vitamin D_3 1000 IU
Euro-Cal	Euro-Pharm	tablet	calcium carbonate 500 mg
Euro-Fer Capsules	Euro-Pharm	capsule	ferrous fumarate 300 mg
Euro-Fer Suspension	Euro-Pharm	liquid	ferrous fumarate 60 mg/mL
Euro-Ferrous Sulfate	Euro-Pharm	tablet	ferrous sulfate 300 mg
Euro-K 600	Euro-Pharm	tablet	potassium chloride 600 mg
Fer-in-Sol	Mead Johnson	liquid	ferrous sulfate 30 mg/mL
Ferodan Infant Drops	Odan	liquid	ferrous sulfate 75 mg/mL
Ferodan Syrup	Odan	syrup	ferrous sulfate 30 mg/mL
Ferodan Tablets	Odan	tablet	ferrous sulfate 300 mg
Ferrous Gluconate 300 mg	Various Manufacturers	tablet	ferrous gluconate 300 mg
Ferrous Sulfate 300 mg	Various Manufacturers	tablet	ferrous sulfate 300 mg
Folic Acid 0.4 mg	Various Manufacturers	tablet	folic acid 0.4 mg
Folic Acid 1 mg	Sisu	capsule	folic acid 1 mg
Folic Acid 1 mg	Various Manufacturers	tablet	folic acid 1 mg
GNC C-Complex Formula 500 mg	General Nutrition Canada	capsule	ascorbic acid 500 mg
GNC Chewable Citrus Free Vitamin C	General Nutrition Canada	tablet	ascorbic acid 500 mg
GNC Chewable Vitamin C 100 mg	General Nutrition Canada	tablet, chewable	ascorbic acid 100 mg
GNC Chewable Vitamin C 500 mg	General Nutrition Canada	tablet, chewable	ascorbic acid 500 mg
GNC Natural Source Beta-Carotene	General Nutrition Canada	capsule	ß-carotene 6 mg
GNC Natural Source Ultra E 1000	General Nutrition Canada	capsule	vitamin E 1000 IU
GNC Natural Source Ultra E 400	General Nutrition Canada	capsule	vitamin E 400 IU
GNC Natural Source Vitamin E 100 IU	General Nutrition Canada	capsule	vitamin E 100 IU
GNC Natural Source Vitamin E 400 IU	General Nutrition Canada	capsule	vitamin E 400 IU
GNC Natural Source Vitamin E 600 IU	General Nutrition Canada	capsule	vitamin E 600 IU
GNC Natural Source Vitamin E 1000 IU	General Nutrition Canada	capsule	vitamin E 1000 IU
GNC One Gram Vitamin C 1000 mg	General Nutrition Canada	tablet/capsule	ascorbic acid 1000 mg

Product	Manufacturer	Dosage Form	Active Ingredients
GNC One Half Gram Vitamin C	General Nutrition Canada	tablet	ascorbic acid 500 mg
GNC Selenium 50 µg	General Nutrition Canada	tablet	selenium 50 µg
GNC Selenium 100 µg	General Nutrition Canada	tablet	selenium 100 µg
GNC Timed Release Iron	General Nutrition Canada	tablet, sustained release	ferrous fumarate 18 mg
GNC Timed Release Vitamin C 500 mg	General Nutrition Canada	capsule	ascorbic acid 500 mg
GNC Timed Release Vitamin C 500 mg	General Nutrition Canada	tablet, sustained release	ascorbic acid 500 mg
GNC Timed Release Vitamin C 1500 mg	General Nutrition Canada	tablet, sustained release	ascorbic acid 1500 mg
GNC Vitamin C 500 mg	General Nutrition Canada	tablet	ascorbic acid 500 mg
Gramcal	Novartis Consumer Health	tablet, effervescent	calcium 1000 mg
Hi Potency Cal 650 mg	Swiss Herbal	tablet	calcium carbonate 1625 mg
Hi Potency KIB$_6$ 17 mg	Swiss Herbal	tablet	pyridoxine hydrochloride 17 mg
Hi Potency Magnesium Oxide 835 mg	Swiss Herbal	tablet	magnesium oxide 835 mg
Hi Potency KIB$_6$ 500 µg	Swiss Herbal	tablet	cyanocobalamin 500 µg
Iron 50 mg Timed Disintegrating	Jamieson	tablet, sustained release	ferrous gluconate 430 mg
Kamu Vitamin C 500 mg	Jamieson	tablet	ascorbic acid 500 mg
Kids D drops	Ddrops Company	liquid	vitamin D$_3$ 400 IU/drop
K-Lyte	WellSpring	tablet, effervescent	potassium citrate 2500 mg
Maglucate Tablets	Pharmascience	tablet	magnesium gluconate 500 mg
Magnesium 50 mg	Jamieson	tablet	magnesium 50 mg (as citrate, fumarate, glutamate, malate, oxide and succinate)
Magnesium 100 mg	Jamieson	tablet	magnesium 100 mg (as citrate, fumarate, glutamate, malate, oxide and succinate)
Magnesium 100 mg	Various Manufacturers	capsule	magnesium citrate 150 mg
Magnesium 250 mg	General Nutrition Canada	tablet	magnesium 250 mg (as glycerophosphate, malate and oxide)
Magnolex Capsules	Santé Naturelle	capsule	magnesium glucoheptonate 15 mg
Magnolex Liquid	Santé Naturelle	liquid	magnesium chloride 2.37 mg/mL
Magnorol Capsules	M. Vachon	capsule	magnesium glucoheptonate 20 mg
Magnorol Sirop	M. Vachon	syrup	magnesium glucoheptonate 4.5 mg/mL
Manganese 25 mg	Natural Factors	tablet	manganese 25 mg
Manganese Amino Acid Chelate 15 mg	Swiss Herbal	tablet	manganese 15 mg
Mixed E Tocopherol	Sisu	capsule	vitamin E 400 IU
Neo Cal 500	Néolab	tablet	calcium carbonate 1250 mg
Neo Fer 300 mg	Néolab	capsule	ferrous fumarate 300 mg
Niacin 50 mg	Adams	tablet	niacin 50 mg
Niacin 50 mg	Valeant	tablet	niacin 50 mg
Niacin 100 mg	Various Manufacturers	tablet	niacin 100 mg
Niacin 500 mg	Various Manufacturers	tablet	niacin 500 mg
Niacinamide 100 mg	Various Manufacturers	tablet	niacinamide 100 mg
Niacinamide 500 mg	Various Manufacturers	tablet	niacinamide 500 mg
Novo-Ferrous Gluconate	Novopharm	tablet	ferrous gluconate 300 mg

Product	Manufacturer	Dosage Form	Active Ingredients
Nutrol A	M. Vachon	capsule	vitamin A 10 000 IU
Nutrol C 500 mg	M. Vachon	tablet, chewable	ascorbic acid 500 mg
Nutrol C 1000 mg	M. Vachon	tablet, sustained release	ascorbic acid 1000 mg
Nutrol E 200	M. Vachon	capsule	vitamin E 200 IU
Organex E 200	Santé Naturelle	capsule	vitamin E 200 IU
Organex E 800	Santé Naturelle	capsule	vitamin E 800 IU
Oystershell Calcium 250 mg	General Nutrition Canada	tablet	calcium carbonate 625 mg
Palafer Capsules	GlaxoSmithKline Consumer Health	capsule	ferrous fumarate 300 mg
Palafer Suspension	GlaxoSmithKline Consumer Health	suspension	ferrous fumarate 60 mg/mL
Pantothenic Acid 100 mg	Swiss Herbal	tablet	d-pantothenic acid 100 mg
Pantothenic Acid 100 mg	General Nutrition Canada	tablet	d-pantothenic acid 100 mg
Pantothenic Acid 250 mg	Swiss Herbal	tablet	d-pantothenic acid 250 mg
Pantothenic Acid 250 mg	General Nutrition Canada	tablet	d-pantothenic acid 250 mg
Pantothenic Acid 500 mg	Swiss Herbal	capsule	d-pantothenic acid 500 mg
Pantothenic Acid 500 mg	General Nutrition Canada	capsule	d-pantothenic acid 500 mg
PediaFer	Euro-Pharm	liquid	ferrous sulfate 75 mg/mL
PediaFer Solution	Euro-Pharm	liquid	ferrous sulfate 30 mg/mL
PMS Ferrous Sulfate Drops	Pharmascience	drops	ferrous sulfate 75 mg/mL
PMS Ferrous Sulfate Solution	Pharmascience	liquid	ferrous sulfate 30 mg/mL
PMS Ferrous Sulfate Tablets	Pharmascience	tablet	ferrous sulfate 300 mg
Potassium 50 mg	Jamieson	tablet	potassium gluconate 50 mg
Potassium 50 mg	Santé Naturelle	tablet	potassium gluconate 50 mg
Potassium Chelated	Swiss Herbal	tablet	potassium 50 mg
Pyridoxine Hydrochloride 25 mg	Swiss Herbal	tablet	pyridoxine hydrochloride 25 mg
Pyridoxine Hydrochloride 100 mg	Adams	tablet	pyridoxine hydrochloride 100 mg
Pyridoxine Hydrochloride 100 mg	Swiss Herbal	tablet	pyridoxine hydrochloride 100 mg
Pyridoxine Hydrochloride 250 mg	Adams	tablet	pyridoxine hydrochloride 250 mg
Pyridoxine Hydrochloride 250 mg	Swiss Herbal	tablet	pyridoxine hydrochloride 250 mg
Redoxon Lemon/Orange	Bayer Consumer	tablet, effervescent	ascorbic acid 1000 mg
Riboflavin 100 mg	Swiss Herbal	tablet	riboflavin 100 mg
Riva D	Riva	capsule	vitamin D_3 400 IU
Selenium 50 µg	Various Manufacturers	tablet	selenium 50 µg
Selenium 100 µg	Various Manufacturers	tablet	selenium 100 µg
Selenium 200 µg	Various Manufacturers	tablet	selenium 200 µg
Slow-Fe	Novartis Consumer Health	tablet, sustained release	ferrous sulfate 160 mg
Slow-K	Novartis	tablet	potassium chloride 600 mg
Super C 500 mg	Natural Factors	tablet	ascorbic acid 500 mg
Thiamine Hydrochloride 50 mg	Various Manufacturers	tablet	thiamine hydrochloride 50 mg
Timed Release C 1000 mg	Jamieson	tablet, sustained release	ascorbic acid 1000 mg
Timed Release D-Pantothenic Acid 1000 mg	Swiss Herbal	tablet, sustained release	d-pantothenic acid 1000 mg

Product	Manufacturer	Dosage Form	Active Ingredients
Timed Release Ester C	General Nutrition Canada	tablet, sustained release	ascorbic acid 1000 mg
Timed Release Potassium	General Nutrition Canada	tablet, sustained release	potassium gluconate 100 mg
Timed Release Vitamin C	General Nutrition Canada	tablet, sustained release	ascorbic acid 1000 mg
Vicks Vitamin C Drops	Procter & Gamble	lozenge	ascorbic acid 25 mg
Vitamin A 10 000 IU	Various Manufacturers	capsule	vitamin A 10 000 IU
Vitamin A 10 000 IU	Jamieson	capsule	vitamin A 10 000 IU
Vitamin A 10 000 IU	SunOpta	capsule	vitamin A 10 000 IU
Vitamin A 10 000 IU	Swiss Herbal	capsule	vitamin A 10 000 IU
Vitamin A 10 000 IU	Various Manufacturers	tablet	vitamin A 10 000 IU
Vitamin B_1 50 mg	Various Manufacturers	tablet	thiamine hydrochloride 50 mg
Vitamin B_1 100 mg	Various Manufacturers	tablet	thiamine hydrochloride 100 mg
Vitamin B_2 100 mg	Various Manufacturers	tablet	riboflavin 100 mg
Vitamin B_6 25 mg	Various Manufacturers	tablet	pyridoxine hydrochloride 25 mg
Vitamin B_6 50 mg	Various Manufacturers	tablet	pyridoxine hydrochloride 50 mg
Vitamin B_6 100 mg	Sisu	capsule	pyridoxine hydrochloride 100 mg
Vitamin B_6 100 mg	Various Manufacturers	tablet	pyridoxine hydrochloride 100 mg
Vitamin B_6 250 mg	SunOpta	capsule	pyridoxine hydrochloride 250 mg
Vitamin B_6 250 mg	Various Manufacturers	tablet	pyridoxine hydrochloride 250 mg
Vitamin B_{12} 25 µg	Various Manufacturers	tablet	cyanocobalamin 25 µg
Vitamin B_{12} 50 µg	Jamieson	tablet	cyanocobalamin 50 µg
Vitamin B_{12} 100 µg	Jamieson	tablet	cyanocobalamin 100 µg
Vitamin B_{12} 250 µg	Various Manufacturers	tablet	cyanocobalamin 250 µg
Vitamin B_{12} 500 µg	General Nutrition Canada	tablet	cyanocobalamin 500 µg
Vitamin B_{12} 500 µg	Swiss Herbal	tablet	cyanocobalamin 500 µg
Vitamin B_{12} 1000 µg	General Nutrition Canada	tablet	cyanocobalamin 1000 µg
Vitamin B_{12} 1000 µg	Swiss Herbal	tablet	cyanocobalamin 1000 µg
Vitamin B_{12} 1000 µg	Sisu	capsule	cyanocobalamin 1000 µg
Vitamin B_{12} 1000 µg	SunOpta	strip	cyanocobalamin 1000 µg
Vitamin B_{12} 1200 µg	Jamieson	tablet, sustained release	cyanocobalamin 1200 µg
Vitamin C 100 mg	Various Manufacturers	tablet	ascorbic acid 100 mg
Vitamin C 100 mg Orange	Various Manufacturers	tablet	ascorbic acid 100 mg
Vitamin C 250 mg	Various Manufacturers	tablet	ascorbic acid 250 mg
Vitamin C 250 mg	Various Manufacturers	tablet, chewable	ascorbic acid 250 mg
Vitamin C 250 mg Orange	Various Manufacturers	tablet, chewable	ascorbic acid 250 mg
Vitamin C 250 mg with Non-medicinal Echinacea & Lemon Bioflavonoids	General Nutrition Canada	capsule	ascorbic acid 250 mg
Vitamin C 500 mg	Various Manufacturers	tablet	ascorbic acid 500 mg
Vitamin C 500 mg	Various Manufacturers	tablet, chewable	ascorbic acid 500 mg
Vitamin C 500 mg	Various Manufacturers	tablet, chewable	ascorbic acid 500 mg
Vitamin C 500 mg Timed Release	Various Manufacturers	capsule, sustained release	ascorbic acid 500 mg

Product	Manufacturer	Dosage Form	Active Ingredients
Vitamin C 500 mg Timed Release	Various Manufacturers	tablet, sustained release	ascorbic acid 500 mg
Vitamin C 500 mg Tropical Fruit	Jamieson	tablet, chewable	ascorbic acid 500 mg
Vitamin C 600 mg	General Nutrition Canada	tablet	ascorbic acid 600 mg
Vitamin C 600 mg	Sisu	capsule	ascorbic acid 600 mg
Vitamin C 1000 mg	Various Manufacturers	tablet	ascorbic acid 1000 mg
Vitamin C 1000 mg	Swiss Herbal	tablet	ascorbic acid 1000 mg
Vitamin C 1000 mg Timed Release	Various Manufacturers	tablet, sustained release	ascorbic acid 1000 mg
Vitamin C 1500 mg	Jamieson	tablet, sustained release	ascorbic acid 1500 mg
Vitamin C 1500 mg Timed Release	Swiss Herbal	tablet, sustained release	ascorbic acid 1500 mg
Vitamin C Crystals 1000 mg	Swiss Herbal	powder	ascorbic acid 1000 mg/g
Vitamin D 400 IU	Various Manufacturers	tablet	vitamin D_3 400 IU
Vitamin D 1000 IU	Jamieson	tablet	vitamin D_3 1000 IU
Vitamin D 1000 IU	Various Manufacturers	tablet	vitamin D_3 1000 IU
Vitamin E 100 IU	Various Manufacturers	capsule	vitamin E 100 IU
Vitamin E 100 IU Natural	Adams	capsule	vitamin E 100 IU
Vitamin E 200 IU	Various Manufacturers	capsule	vitamin E 200 IU
Vitamin E 200 IU Natural Source	Various Manufacturers	capsule	vitamin E 200 IU
Vitamin E 400 IU	General Nutrition Canada	tablet, chewable	vitamin E 400 IU
Vitamin E 400 IU	Various Manufacturers	capsule	vitamin E 400 IU
Vitamin E 400 IU	Jamieson	caplet	vitamin E 400 IU
Vitamin E 400 IU Natural Source	Various Manufacturers	capsule	vitamin E 400 IU
Vitamin E 400 IU Synthetic	Adams	capsule	vitamin E 400 IU
Vitamin E 800 IU	Various Manufacturers	capsule	vitamin E 800 IU
Vitamin E 1000 IU	Various Manufacturers	capsule	vitamin E 1000 IU
Zinc 10 mg	Various Manufacturers	tablet	zinc gluconate 10 mg
Zinc 25 mg	Jamieson	tablet	zinc gluconate 25 mg
Zinc 30 mg	General Nutrition Canada	tablet	zinc gluconate 30 mg
Zinc 30 mg	Sisu	capsule	zinc citrate 30 mg
Zinc 50 mg	Various Manufacturers	tablet	zinc gluconate 50 mg
Zinc 50 mg	Jamieson	tablet, sustained release	zinc gluconate 50 mg
Zinc 50 mg	Swiss Herbal	capsule	zinc citrate 50 mg
Zinc 100 mg	General Nutrition Canada	tablet	zinc gluconate 100 mg

Poison Control Centres

Alberta
Poison and Drug Information Service
Foothills Hospital
1403–29th St NW
Calgary AB T2N 2T9
Tel: 1-800-332-1414
Tel: 403-944-1414
Fax: 403-944-1472

British Columbia
B.C. Drug and Poison Information Centre
1081 Burrard St
Vancouver BC V6Z 1Y6
Tel: 1-800-567-8911 (remainder of Province)
Tel: 604-682-5050 (Lower Mainland)
Fax: 604-806-8262

Manitoba
Manitoba Poison Control Centre
Children's Hospital
840 Sherbrook St
Winnipeg MB R3A 1S1
Tel: 204-787-2591
Fax: 204-787-5008

New Brunswick
Clinidata division of Sykes Assistance Services Corporation
Poison Information Centre
774 Main St 6th floor
Moncton NB E1C 9Y3
Tel: 911 (within New Brunswick)
Fax: 506-867-3259

Newfoundland
Poison Information Centre
The Janeway Child Health Centre
300 Prince Philip Dr
St. John's NL A1B 3V6
Tel: 709-722-1110
Fax: 709-726-0830

Northwest Territories
Telecare Health Line
Tel: 1-888-255-1010

Nova Scotia
Poison Information Centre
The IWK Health Centre
PO Box 3070
Halifax NS B3J 3G9
Tel: 1-800-565-8161 (Nova Scotia and Prince Edward Island)
Tel: 902-470-8161 (remainder of Provinces)
Fax: 902-470-7213

Nunavut
Baffin (Qikiqtani) Regional Hospital
Box 1000
Iqaluit NU X0A 0H0
Tel: 867-975-8600
Fax: 867-975-8634

Cambridge Bay (Ikaluktutiak) Health Centre
Box 53
Cambridge Bay NU X0B 0C0
Tel: 867-983-4500
Fax: 867-983-4509
Rankin Inlet (Kangiqliniq) Health Centre
Bag 008
Rankin Inlet NU X0C 0G0
Tel: 867-645-8300
Fax: 867-645-8389

Ontario
Ontario Poison Centre
The Hospital for Sick Children
555 University Ave
Toronto ON M5G 1X8
Tel: 1-800-268-9017
Tel: 416-813-5900
Fax: 416-813-7489

Prince Edward Island
Poison Information Centre
The IWK Health Centre
PO Box 3070
Halifax NS B3J 3G9
Tel: 1-800-565-8161

Quebec
Centre antipoison du Québec
Pavillon Jeffery Hale
1270, chemin Sainte-Foy, 4e étage
Quebec QC G1S 2M4
Tel: 1-800-463-5060
Fax: 418-654-2747

Saskatchewan
Poison and Drug Information Service
Foothills Hospital
1403–29th St NW
Calgary AB T2N 2T9
Tel: 1-866-454-1212

Yukon Territory
Emergency Department
Whitehorse General Hospital
5 Hospital Rd
Whitehorse YT Y1A 3H7
Tel: 867-393-8700
Fax: 867-393-8762

Pharmaceutical Manufacturers

2G Pharma Inc.
6-2400 Dundas St. West, Suite #724
Mississauga, ON   L5K 2K8
Tel: 905-271-2122
Email: info@2gpharma.com

3M Canada Inc.
Administrative Office
300 Tartan Drive
London, ON   N5V 4M9
Tel: 1-888-364-3577
 Fax: 1-800-479-4453

Abbott Diabetes Care
7115 Millcreek Drive
Mississauga, ON   L5N 3R3
Tel: 1-888-519-6890
Fax: 1-800-760-6691
Website: www.abbottdiabetescare.ca

Abbott Nutrition
8401 Trans-Canada Highway
Saint-Laurent, QC   H4S 1Z1
Tel: 514-832-7000
1-800-361-7852
Fax: 514-832-7800
Abbott Nutrition Information for Health Care Professionals
Tel: 1-866-767-7411, ext 1
Fax: 514-832-7871

Abundance Naturally
4090 Ridgeway Driveway, Unit #5
Mississauga, ON   L5L 5X5
Tel: 905-412-3055
1-888-481-8446
Fax: 905-412-3060
Website: www.abundancenaturally.com

Adams Labs Ltd.
Suite 100- 6111 Royalmount Ave
Montréal, QC   H4P 2T4

Adrien Gagnon (AG) Natural Health Ltd
369 Charles-Peguy East
La Prairie, QC   J5R 3E8
Tel: 450-659-7723
1-888-686-8888
Fax: 450-659-4119
Website: www.agnaturalhealth.ca

Advantage CKN (Distributor)
151 Esna Park Drive, Unit 4
Markham, ON   L3R 3B1
Tel: 905-475-9623
Fax: 905-475-5439
Website: www.ckn-inc.com

Advanced Vision Research Inc.
660 Main Street
Woburn, MA 01801 USA
Tel: 781-932-8327
1-800-579-8327
Fax: 781-935-5075

Afexa Life Sciences
9604 20th Avenue
Edmonton, AB   T6N 1G1
Tel: 780-432-0022
1-888-280-0022
Fax: 780-432-7772

Airplus Footcare
an Implus Footcare, LLC brand
2001 T.W. Alexander Drive
Durham, NC 27709-3925 USA
Phone: 1-800-446-7587

ANI Biotech Oy
Tiilitie 3
FI-01720 VANTAA
Finland
Tel: +358 (0)20 155 7510
Fax: +358 (0)20 155 7517
Email: info@anibiotech.f

Atlas (Laboratoires Atlas)
9600 Boul. Des Sciences
Montréal, QC   H1J 3B6
Tel: 514-254-7188
Fax: 514-254-3006

Alba Botanica
see Purity Life Health Products, Ltd.,
see Pure Source,Inc.,
see Tallgrass Distribution

Akorn Pharmaceuticals
1430 Birchmount Rd.
Toronto, ON   M1P 2E8
Tel: 416-615-0185
1-800-461-1200
Fax: 416-631-8272
1-800-313-8696

Alberto-Culver Canada
506 Kipling Ave
Etobicoke, ON   M8Z 5E2
Tel: 416-251-3741
1-888-252-3786
Fax: 416-251-3062

Alcon Canada Inc.
2665 Meadowpine Boulevard
Mississauga, ON   L5N 8C7
Tel: 905-826-6700
1-800-268-4574
Fax: 905-826-1448
Website: www.alcon.ca

Allergan Canada Inc.
85 Enterprise Blvd. Suite 500
Markham ,ON   L6G 0B5
Tel: 1-800-668-6424
Fax: 905-940-1902
Website: www.allergan.ca

Alva-Amco Pharmacal Inc.
7711 Merrimac Avenue
Niles, Illinois 60714-3423 USA
1-847-663-0700

AMD-Ritmed Inc.
1200, 55th Ave,
Lachine, QC   H8T 3J8
Tel: 514-633-1111
Fax: 514-633-1186
1-888-441-2120
1-888-434-4988 (Fax:)
Website: www.amdritmed.com

AMG Medical Inc.
8505 Dalton
Montréal, QC   H4T 1V5
Tel: 1 800 361 2210
Fax: 1 800 295 6572
Website: www.amgmedical.com
Website: www.amgphysiologic.com

ANB Canada (Associated National Brokerage) (Distributor)
199 Matthew Boyd Cres.
Newmarket, ON   L3X 3C7
Tel: 905-953-9777
1-800-953-2140
Fax: 905-953-8124
Website: www.anbcanada.com

Ansell Canada Inc.
105 Lauder St.
Cowansville, QC   J2K 2K8
Tel: 450-266-1850
Fax: 450-266-6150
1-888-267-3555
Website: www.ansell.com

Anurex
8740 S.W. 21st Street
Ft. Lauderdale, FL 33324 USA
MALITEK INTERNATIONAL Inc. (Distributor)
Tel: 905-841-3731
Fax: 905-841-8821

Apotex Inc.
150 Signet Dr.
Weston, ON   M9L 1T9
Tel: 416-749-9300
Fax: 416-401-3849
1-800-268-4623

Apothecary Products, Inc.
11750 12th Ave South
Burnsville, MN 55337-1295 USA
Tel: 1-800-328-2742
Fax: 1-800-328-1584

Apothecus Inc.
220 Townsend Square
Oyster Bay, NY 11771-1532   USA
Tel: 516-624-8200
Fax: 516-624-8201
1-800-227-2393

Aptalis Pharma
597 Laurier Blvd.
Mont-Saint-Hilaire, QC   J3H 6C4
Tel: 450-467-5138
Fax: 450-464-9979
1-800-565-3255
Website: www.aptalispharma.com

AstraZeneca Canada Inc.
1004 Middlegate Rd.
Mississauga, ON   L4Y 1M4
Tel: 905-277-7111
Fax: 905-270-3248
1-800-668-6000

Aton Pharma Inc.
see Valeo Pharma Inc.

Attends Healthcare Products
P.O. Box 192
Richmond Hill, ON   L4B 4R7
Tel: 252-752-1100
1-800-428-8363
Fax: 1-800-933-8433
Email: info@attends.com

Aurium Pharma Inc.
7577 Keele Street, Suite 102
Concord, ON   L4K 4X3
Tel: 905-669-9057
1-877-728-7486
Fax: 905-669-0781

Auto Control Medical Inc.
Millcreek Drive, Unit 5
Mississauga, ON L5N 5R8
Tel: 905-814-6350
Fax: 905-814-6355
1-800-461-0991
Website: www.autocontrol.com

Avon Canada Inc.
5500 Trans-Canada Hwy.
Pointe-Claire, QC H9R 1B6
Tel: 514-695-3371

Axia Canada
Natrica USA
149 South Barrington Ave
Lon Angeles, Califormia
90049, USA
Tel: 310-430-4488
Fax: 410-440-3822
Website: www.axia3.ca

Axxess Pharma Inc.
20 Valleywood Dr., Unit 105
Markham, ON L3R 6G1
Tel: 905-513-0000
1-888-654-0004
Fax: 905-513-1040

Banana Boat Company, The
6363 Northam Dr.
Mississauga, ON L4V 1N5
Tel: 905-677-6211
Fax: 905-677-7965
1-888-786-8477

Barrett Health Inc.
38 Scott Road
Chelsea, QC J9B 1R5
Tel: 1-877-427-1924
Fax: 819-827-8120

Bausch & Lomb Canada Inc.
520 Applewood Crescent
Vaughan, ON L4K 4B4
Tel: 905-695-7700
1-888-459-5000
Fax: 905-695-7656
Website: www.bausch.ca

Bayer Inc.
(Consumer Care Division and Diabetes Healthcare Division)
77 Belfield Rd.
Toronto, ON M9W 1G6
Tel: 416-248-0771
Fax: 1-800-567-1710
1-800-622-2937

Becton Dickinson Canada Inc.
2100 Derry Road West Suite 100
Mississauga, ON L5N 0B3
Tel: 905-288-6000
1-866-979-9408
Fax:1- 800-565-0897
Website: www.bd.com/ca

Beiersdorf Canada Inc.
4727 Levy Street
St. Laurent, QC H4R 2P9
Tel: 514-956-4330
Fax: 514-956-4346
Website: www.beiersdorf.ca

Belvedere International Inc.
5675 Keaton Crescent
Mississauga, ON L5R 3G3
Tel: 905-568-0700
Fax: 905-568-0711

Bill Beauty & Health Products Ltd.
20 Melford Drive, Unit 1-4
Scarborough, ON M1B 2X6
Tel: 416-298-1228
1-866-857-1228
Fax: 416-298-2208
Website: www.billbeauty.com

Bioelectronics Inc.
4539 Metropolitan Ct.
Frederick, MD 21704   USA
Tel: 301-874-4890
1-866-757-2284
Fax: 301- 874-6935

Bio Film Inc.
3225 Executive Ridge
Vista, CA 92081 USA
Tel: 760-727-9030
Fax: 760-727-8080

Biomation (Distributor)
335 Perth St.
P.O. Box 156
Almonte, ON K0A 1A0
Tel: 613-256-2821
1-888-667-2324
Fax: 613-256-5872

Bionime Canada Corp
10865 Rancho Bernardo Road
Suite #100
San Diego, California
92127 USA
Tel: 858-481-8485
Fax: 858-481-8472
1-888-481-8485
Website: www.bionimecanada.com

Bio-Santé (Laboratoires Bio-Santé Inc.)
2675 Boulevard Ford
Chateauguay, QC J6J 4Z2
Tel: 450-698-3581
Fax: 450-698-0609

Biotherm Canada
2115 Crescent St.
Montréal, QC H3G 2C1
Tel: 514-335-8000
Fax: 514-287-9393
Website: www.biotherm.ca

Blairex Laboratoires Inc.
1600 Brian Drive P.O. Box 2127
Columbus, IN 47202-2127
Tel: 812-378-1864
1-800-252-4739

Blistex Ltd.
5915 Airport Rd.
Suite 908
Mississauga, ON L4V 1T1
Tel: 905-678-2521
Fax: 905-678-2099

Body Shop Canada Ltd., The
510- 1 Yorkdale Road
Toronto, ON M6A 3A1
Tel: 1-800-387-4592

Boehringer Ingelheim Canada Ltd.
(Consumer Health Care)
5180 South Service Rd.
Burlington, ON L7L 5H4
Tel: 905-639-6000
Fax: 905-639-5293
1-800-263-9107

Boiron Canada Inc.
1300 René-Descartes
Saint-Bruno-de-Montarville, QC
J3V 0B7
Tel: 450-723-2066
1-800-461-2066
Website: www.boiron.ca

Braintree Laboratories Inc.
60 Columbian Street
Braintree, Massachusetts
02185-0929 USA
Tel: 781-843-2202
1-800-874-6756
Fax: 781-843-7932

Braun
see Procter & Gamble Inc.

Burt's Bees Canada Inc.
146 Regis Cres S.
Toronto, ON M3J 1Y8
Tel: 416-630-3295

Canderm Pharma Inc.
5353 Thimens Blvd.
St-Laurent, QC H4R 2H4
Tel: 514-334-3835
Fax: 514-334-7078
Website: www.canderm.com

Carestream Medical Ltd.
Units 14/15 – 211 Schoolhouse St.
Coquitlam, BC V3K 4X9
Tel: 1-888-310-2186
Fax: 1-888-310-2187
Website: www.carestream.com

Carter-Horner Inc.
see Church & Dwight Ltd.

CB Fleet
Fleet Laboratories
4615 Murray Place
Lynchburg, Virginia
USA 24502
Tel: 434-528-4000

Century Pharmaceuticals Inc.
10377 Hague Road
Indianapolis, Indiana
USA 46256

Chattem (Canada) Inc.
2220 Argentia Rd.
Mississauga, ON L5N 2K7
Tel: 905-821-4975
Fax: 905-821-0544

Church & Dwight Ltd.
6600 Kitimat Rd.
Mississauga, ON L5N 1L9
Tel: 905-826-6200
Fax: 905-826-0389
1-800-387-2130

CIBA Vision Canada
2150 Torquay Mews
Mississauga, ON L5N 2M6
Tel: 905-821-4774
Fax: 905-821-8106
Website: www.cibavision.ca

Clarins Canada Inc.
815 Desserte Est, Autoroute 13
Laval, QC H7W 5N4
Tel: 450-688-0144

Clement-Clarke International Ltd.
Edinburgh Way
Harlow, Essex
CM20 2TT   UK
Tel: +44 (0) 1279 414 969
Fax: +44 (0) 1279 456 304

Clif Bar & Company
1610 5th Street
Berkeley, CA 94710-1715   USA
1-800-254-3227

Clinical Products, LLC
2200 Westport Plaza Dr., Suite 316,
St. Louis ,MO 63146 USA
1-800-887-2919

Clinique Laboratories, Dist.
161 Commander Blvd.
Agincourt, ON   M1S 3K9

Colgate Oral Pharmaceuticals Inc.
see Colgate-Palmolive Canada Inc.

Colgate-Palmolive Canada Inc.
Two Morneau Sobeco Centre, 6th Floor
895 Don Mills Road
Toronto, ON   M3C 1W3
Tel: 416-421-6000
 1-800-268-6757

Coloplast Canada
3300 Ridgeway Drive, Unit 12
Mississauga, ON   L5L 5Z9
Tel: 1-877-820-7008

Columbia Laboratories Canada Inc.
33-2000 Thurston Drive
Ottawa, ON   K1G 4K7
Tel: 613-247-7000
 1-888-266-6682
Fax: 613-260-9000

Combe Inc.
1101 Westchester Ave.
White Plains, NY 10604-3597 USA
1-800-873-7400

ConvaTec Canada
Customer Relations Centre
1425 Trans-Canada Highway, Suite 250
 Dorval, QC   H9P 2V3
Tel: 1-800-465-6302
Fax: 1-800-437-1777
Website: www.convatec.com

Coopersurgical Inc.
95 Corporate Drive
Trumbull, CT 06611 USA
Tel: 1-800-243-2974

Coopercare Division
Monarch McLaren
329 Deerhide Crescent
Toronto, ON   M9M 2Z2
Tel: 416-741-9675
Fax: 416-741-2873

Cormair Canada
A Division of L'Oreal Canada Inc
1500 University Street
Suite 600
Montréal, QC   H3A 3S7
Tel: 1-800-363-3834

Coty Canada Inc.
1255 Trans Canada Hwy., Ste. 200
Dorval, QC   H9P 2V4
Tel: 514-421-5050
Fax: 514-421-9848

CV Technologies
see Afexa Life Sciences

D-Drops Company
501 Rowntree Dairy Road, Unit 3,
Woodbridge, ON   L4L 8H1
Tel: 905-851-8898

Dermal Therapy Research Inc. DTR
3 Sprucedale Court
London, ON   N5X 2N9
Tel: 519-439-6633
1-800-668-8000
Fax: 226-663-6180
Website: www.dermaltherapy.com/canada

Dermtek Pharmaceuticals Ltd.
1600 Trans Canada Hwy., Ste. 200
Dorval, QC   H9P 1H7
Tel: 514-685-3333
1-800-465-8383
Fax: 514-685-8828
Website: www.dermtek.com

The Dial Corporation
3515 Quilter Court
Burlington, ON   L7M 3C3
Tel: 905-319-9249
Fax: 905-319-9266

Dioptic Laboratories
Division of Akorn Pharmaceuticals
1405 Denison St.
Markham, ON   L3R 5V2
Tel: 905-513-6393
Fax: 905-415-1440
1-800-465-3845
Website: www.dioptic.com

Diversified Chemical Technologies Inc.
15477 Woodrow Wilson
Detroit, Michigan
48238 USA
Tel: 313-867-5444
Fax: 313-867-3831

Dominion Pharmacal
see Pharmascience Inc.

Dormer Laboratories Inc.
91 Kelfield St., Unit 5
Rexdale, ON   M9W 5A3
Tel: 416-242-6167
Fax: 416-242-9487
1-877-436-7637
1-800-363-5040
Website: www.dormer.com

Douglas Laboratories
552 Newbold Street
London, ON   N6E 2S5
Tel: 519-439-84241-
1-866-856-9954
Fax: 519-432-0071
1-888-220-9441

Dr. Harold Katz LLC
750 N. Highland Ave.
Los Angeles, CA 90038 USA
Tel: 323-993-8320
1-800-973-737)
Fax: 323-993-8327
Website: www.therabreath.com

Dreambrands Inc.
11645 North Cave Creek Road
Phoenix, Arizona
85020 USA
Tel: 602-354-7640
Website: www.dreambrands.net

Duchesnay Inc.
950, Boulevard Michele-Bohec
Blainville, QC   J7C 5E2
Tel: 450-433-7734
Fax: 450-433-2211
1-888-588-8508

Duramed Pharmaceuticals Inc.
A Subsidary of Barr Pharmaceuticals, Inc.
223 Quaker Road
Pomona, NY
10970 USA
Medical info: 1-888-550-6060

Durex Canada
Division SSL Canada Inc.
100 Courtland Ave.
Concord, ON   L4K 3T6
Tel: 905-669-6877
Fax: 905-669-9662
1-800-267-8700
Website: www.durex.com

EastMed Inc.
1721 Lower Water St.
Halifax, NS   B3J 1S5
1-800-560-5690
Website: www.eastmed.ca

Efamol Ltd.
see Flora Manufacturing & Distribution Ltd

Eli Lilly
see Lilly

Empi
Division of DJO Canada Inc.
6485 Kennedy Rd
Mississauga, ON   L5T 2W4
Tel: 1-866-866-5031
Fax: 1-866-866-5032

Encore Medical Products
2300 Plantside Drive
Louisville, KY 40299   USA
1-800-221-6603

Epien Medical Inc.
4225 White Bear Parkway, Suite 600
St. Paul, Minnesota
55110 USA
Tel: 651-653-3380
1-888-884-4675
Fax: 651-653-8569

Erfa Canada Inc.
8250 Décarie - suite 110
Montréal, QC   H4P 2P5
Tel: 514-931-3133
Fax: 514-931 7330

Estee Lauder Cosmetics Ltd.
161 Commander Blvd.
Agincourt, ON   M1S 3K9
Tel: 416 292-1111

Ethix Medical Inc.
1460 Dr. Penfield, Suite 1104
Montréal, QC H3G 1B8
Tel: 514-935-5593
1-888-88-Ethix (38449)
Fax: 514-221-2142

Euro-Pharm Canada Inc.
9400, boul. Langelier
Montréal, QC H1P 3H8
Tel: 514-323-8757
Toll free: 1-888-929-0835
Fax: 514-323-6325

Farleyco Marketing Inc (Distributor)
30 East Wilmot Street,
Richmond Hill, ON L4B 1A4
Tel: 905-709-2650
Fax: 905-709-8731

FemCap Inc.
14058 Mira Montana Drive
Del Mar, CA
USA 92014
Tel: 858-481-8837
Fax: 858-792-2624

Ferring Inc.
200 Yorkland Boulevard, Suite 800
North York, ON M2J 5C1
Tel: 416-490-0121
Fax: 416-493-1692

Flora Manufacturing & Distribution Ltd
7400 Fraser Park Drive
Burnaby, BC V5J 5BG
Tel: 902-678-2727
1-888--436-6697
Website: www.florahealth.com

Forest Laboratories UK Ltd.
Riverbridge House, Anchor Boulevard
Crossways Business Park
Dartford, Kent
DA2 6SL, UK
Tel: +44(0) 1322-421800
Website: www.forest-labs.co.uk

Formedica Inc.
7109, Trans-Canada
Montréal, QC H4T 1A2
Tel: 514-336-4821
Fax: 514-336-2418

Fruit of the Earth
6090 White Hart Lane
Mississauga, ON L5R 3Y4
Tel: 905-568-2511

Galderma Canada Inc.
105 Commerce Valley Drive West,
Suite 300
Thornhill, ON L3T 7W3
Tel: 905-762-2500
Fax: 905-762-2505
1-800-467-2081

General Nutrition Canada
6299 Airport Rd, Ste. 201
Mississauga, ON L4V 1N3

Generex Pharmaceuticals
Generex Biotechnology Corporation
33 Harbour Square, Suite 202
Toronto, ON M5J 2G2
1-800-391-6755

Genuine Health
317 Adelaide St. W.
Suite #501
Toronto, ON M5V 1P9
Tel: 416-977-8765
1-877-500-7888
Fax: 1-877-500-7999

Gerber Products Inc.
Contact: NUK USA
2 University Plaza Suite 500
Hackensack, NJ
07601 USA
Phone: 1-888-685-1238

Gerbex Inc. (Les Produits Gerbex)
7345, Boulevard LaFramboise
Saint-Hyacinthe, QC J2R 1E3
Tél: 450-796-5868
Fax: 450-796-1705

Germiphene Corporation Inc.
1379 Colborne Street East
Brantford, ON N3T 5M1
Tel: 519-759-7100
1-800-265-9931
Fax: 519-759-1625
Website: www.germiphene.com

GFR Pharma
11450-201A Street
Maple Ridge, BC V2X 0Y4
Tel: 604-460-8440
1-877-560-8440
Fax: 604-648-8221
Website: www.gfrpharma.com

Gillette Canada Inc.
see Procter and Gamble Inc.

GlaxoSmithKline Consumer Healthcare
2030 Bristol Circle
Oakville, ON L6H 5V2
Tel: 905-829-2030
Fax: 905-829-6064
1-800-268-4600

Gojo Corporate Headquarters
1 Gojo Plaza, Suite 500
P.O. Box 991
Akron, Ohio 44309-0991 USA
Tel: 330-255-60001
1- 800-321-9647
Fax: 330-255-6119

Graceway Pharmaceuticals
252 Pall Mall Street, Suite 302
London, ON N6A 5P6
Tel: 1-866-272-1661
Fax: 519-432-8097

GT Urological LLC.
1313 - 5th Street S.E., Suite 221
Minneapolis, MN
55414 USA
Tel: 612-379-3578
Fax: 612-379-3579

H. J Sutton Industries
8701 Jane St. Unit C
Concord, ON L4K 2M6
Tel: 905-660-4311

Haw Par Corporation Ltd.
Cdn. Dist.: Le Kiu Importing Co. Ltd.
P.O. Box 4129
Vancouver, BC V6B 3Z6
Tel: 604-681-6111

Heiko
See VitalScience Corp.
93 Woodstream Blvd. Unit 93
Woodbridge, ON L4L 7Y7
Tel: 905-264-9697
1-800-231-4751
Fax: 905-264-7393
Website: www.VitalScienceCorp.com

Helix Biopharma Inc.
305 Industrial Parkway South, Unit 3
Aurora, ON L4G 6X7
Tel: 905-841-2300 ext. 286
Fax: 905-841-2244
Website: www.helixbiopharma.com

Herbes Universelles
7, 70e Av. O.
Blainville, QC J7C 1R7
Tel: 514-435-7514

Heritage Brands
Cdn. Dist.: Associated National Brokerage Inc.
120 Harry Walker Parkway N.
Newmarket, ON L3Y 7B2

Hilary's Salesmaster Distribution Ltd.
145 Idema Rd.
Markham, ON L3R 1A9
Tel: 905-475-5446
Fax: 905-475-0377

Holista Health Canada Inc.
2000 Brigantine Drive
Coquitlam, BC V3K 7B5
Tel: 1-800-204-4372
Fax: 1-888-668-4252
Website: www.holista.ca

Hollister Ltd.
95 Mary St.
Aurora, ON L4G 1G3
Tel: 905-727-4344
1-800-263-7400
Fax: 905-727-1614

Home Diagnostics Inc.
see Nipro Diagnostics Inc

Homeocan
3025, boul. de l'Assomption
Montréal, QC H1N 2H2
Tel: 514-256-6303
Fax: 514-256-9256
1-800-556-0824
Website: www.homeocan.ca

HRA Pharma
see: Bayer Inc
Toronto Office
77 Belfield Road
Toronto, ON M9W 1G6
Tel: 416-248-0771
1-800-622-2937

Hyde
see Mentholatum Company of Canada Ltd.

Hydralyte Canada
2400 Canoe Avenue
Coquitlam, BC V3K 8C2
Tel: 604-552-3610
Fax: 604-552-3036
Website: www.hydralytecanada.com

Hylands Homeopathic Canada
381-A, route 139
Sutton, QC   J0E 2K0
Tel: 450-538-6636
Fax: 450-538-6638
1-800-363-8933

Idelle Labs, Ltd.
83 Wooster Heights Road
Danbury, Connecticut
06810 USA
Tel: 203-797-9350

I-Med Pharma Inc. (Distributor)
1601 St Regis Blvd
Dollard-Des-Ormeaux, QC   H9B 3H7
Tel: 514-685-8118
1-800-461-1008
Fax: 514- 685-8998
Website: www.imedpharma.com

Insight Pharmaceuticals Inc.
150 - 1170 Wheeler Way
Langhorne, Pennsylvania
USA 19047
Tel: 800-344-7239

Institut Rosell Inc.
8480 Boul Saint-Laurent
Montréal, QC   H2P 2M6
Tel: 514-381-5631
1-800-452-4364
Fax: 514-383-4493

International Dermatologicals Inc.
1940 Lonsdale Ave., Ste. 217A
Vancouver, BC   V7M 2K2
Tel: 604-980-2511
Fax: 604-985-2336

i-Test
see Wholesale Medical Network Inc. (Distributor)

Jaapharm Canada Inc.
200 Trowers Rd., Unit 1
Woodbridge, ON   L4L 5Z7
Tel: 905-851-7885
1-800-465-9587
Fax: 905-856-5838

Jamieson Laboratories Ltd.
4025 Rhodes Dr.
Windsor, ON   N8W 5B5
Tel: 519-974-8482
Fax: 519-974-4742
1-800-265-5088
Website: www.jamiesonvitamins.com

Johnson & Johnson Inc.
88 Mcnabb Street
Markham, ON   L3R 5L2
Tel: 905-968-2000
1-800-387-6577
Fax: 905-968-2400

Johnson & Johnson - Merck Consumer Pharmaceuticals of
Canada
88 Mcnabb Street
Markham, ON   L3R 5L2
Tel: 905-968-2000
1-800-387-6577
Fax: 905-968-2400

KAO Brands Company
2535 Spring Grove Ave
Cincinnati, OH 45214 USA
Tel: 1-800-572-2391

Kimberly Clark Inc.
50 Burnhamthorpe W.
Mississauga, ON   L5B 3C2
Tel: 905-277-6500

KineSys Pharmaceutical Inc.
415- 3771 Jacombs Road
Richmond, BC   V6V 2L9
Tel: 1-888- 546-3797
Website: www.kinesys.com

King Pharmaceuticals Canada, Inc.
2915 Argentia Road, Suite 7
Mississauga, ON   L5N 8G6
Tel: 905-812-9911
1-877-374-7361

La Roche-Posay Canada (Laboratoires)
4895 Hickmore
Montréal, QC   H4T 1K5
Tel: 514-342-0880
Website: www.laroche-posay.ca

Laboratoires Druide Inc.
154 Oneida Drive,
Pointe-Claire, QC   H9R 1A8
Tel: 514-426-7227
Fax: 514-426 7233
Website: www.druide.ca

Laboratoire Lalco Inc.
1540 Nationale Street
Lachenaie, QC J6W 6M1
Tel: 514-522-3187
1-800 361-810
Fax: 450-492-1096
Website: www.lalco.ca

Laderma Inc.
see Farleyco Marketing (distributor)

LaCorium Health
6111 Broken Sound Parkway, NW
Suite #365
Boca Raton, Florida
33487, USA
Tel: 561-241-5415
Website: www.lacorium

Lansinoh Laboratories, Inc.
333 North FairFax: Street, Suite 400
Alexandria, VA 22314 USA
Tel: 1-800-292-4794

Lee-Adams Laboratories
see Adams Labs Ltd.

Les Produits Gerbex Inc.
see Gerbex

Lifescan Canada
4170 Still Creek Dr., Ste. 300
Burnaby, BC V5C 6C6
Tel: 604-293-2266
Fax: 604-293-1619
1-800-663-5521
Website: www.lifescan.com
Website: www.onetouch.ca

Lifesource
see Auto Control Medical Inc.

Lilly Canada Inc.
3650 Danforth Ave.
Toronto, ON M1N 2E8
1-800-268-4446
Fax: 416-699-7352

Little Remedies
see Prestige Brands Inc.

LivCorp Inc
3310 South service Road
Suite #202
Burlington, ON L7N 3M6
Tel: 905-639-7878
Fax: 905-639-7864
Website: livrelief.com

Lofthouse of Fleetwood
see TFB & Associates Limited

L'Oreal Canada
2115, rue Crescent

Montréal, QC H3G 2C1
Tel: 514-287-4800

Luna Fertility Indicator Inc.
PO Box 18028
Vancouver, BC V6M 4L3
Tel: 604-244-0056
1-888-818-5862
Fax: 604-270-7795
Website: www.lunafertility.com

M. Vachon
Le Groupe M. Vachon Inc.
8700 boul. de la Rive-Sud C.P. 100
Lévis, QC G6V 6N6
Tel: 418-837-2426
1-800-463-4319
Fax: 418-835-6043

Mansfield Medical Inc.
5775 Andover
Montréal, QC H4T 1H6\
Tel: 514-739-3633
1-800-361-6240
Fax: 514-342-1632
Website: www.mansfieldmedical.com

Mary Kay Cosmetics Ltd.
2020 Meadowvale Blvd.
Mississauga, ON L5N 6Y2
Tel: 905-858-0020
Fax: 905-858-8407

Mayer Laboratories Inc.
1950 Addison Street, Suite #101
Berkeley, California
94704, USA
Tel: 1-800-426-6366
Website: www.mayerlabs.com

McNeil Consumer Healthcare
890 Woodlawn Rd. W.
Guelph, ON N1K 1A5
Tel: 519-836-6500
Fax: 519-826-6200
1-800-265-7323

Mead Johnson Nutritionals
333 Preston St., Ste. 700
Ottawa, ON K1S 5N4
Tel: 613-567-3536
Fax: 613-239-3996
1-800-263-7464
Website: www.meadjohnson.ca

Medel
see Wholesale Medical Network Inc. (Distributor)

Medela Canada Inc.
4090B Sladeview Cres. Unit #2
Mississauga, ON L5L 5Y5
Tel: 1-800-435-8316
Fax: 1-800-995-7867
Website: www.medela.com

MediBrands Inc.
see ANB Canada (Distributor)

Medical Developments International Inc.
see Carestream Medical Ltd.

Medical Futures Inc.
29 16 Sims Crescent
Richmond Hill, ON L4B 2P1
Tel: 1-866-789-2090
Fax: 1-877 731-2873
Website: www.medfutures.com

Medican Pharma Inc.
1120 Victoria N.
Kitchener, ON N2B 3T2
Tel: 519-741-2199
Fax: 519-741-0499
1-800-727-2076

Medicis Canada Ltd.
226 543 Richmond Street West
Toronto, ON M5V 1Y6
Tel: 1-800-661-3376

Medisense Canada Inc.
see Abbott Diabetes Care

Medline Industries, Inc.
One Medline Place
Mundelein, Illinois 60060 USA
Tel: 905-465-8800
1-800-396-6996
Fax: 905-465-9241

MedPro Defense Inc.
see AMG Medical

Medtech Labs Inc.
see Prestige Brands Inc.

Mega Electronics Inc.
see Biomation

Mentholatum Co. of Canada Ltd.
20 Lewis St.
Fort Erie, ON L2A 5M6

Tel: 905-871-1665
Fax: 905-871-2535
1-800-663-7246

Merck Frosst Canada Ltd.
16711 Trans-Canada Hwy
Kirkland, QC H9H 3L1
Tel: 514-428-8600
1-800-567-259
Website: www.merckfrosst.ca

Microlife Inc.
424 Skinner Blvd., Suite B
Dunedin, Florida
34698 USA
Tel: 727-738-8846
Fax: 727-738-0878
Website: www.microlife.com

Milex
see CooperSurgical Inc.

Molnlycke Healthcare
2010 Winston Park Dr., Ste. 100
Oakville, ON L6H 5R7
Tel: 905-829-1502
Fax: 905-829-8858
1-800-494-5134
Website: www.molnlycke.com

Multi-Pro Distributions Inc.
8480 Champ d'eau
St-Leonard, QC H1P 1Y3
Tel: 514-955-1128

Naka Herbs & Vitamins Ltd.
53 Queen's Plate Dr., Unit #3
Etobicoke, ON M9W 6P1
Tel: 416-741-6969
Website: www.nakaherbs.com

Nasmark Inc.
5650 Tomken Rd., Unit 12
Mississauga, ON L4W 4P1
Tel: 905-602-0867
Fax: 905-602-0868
1-800-268-5040

Natural Factors Nutritional Products Ltd.
1550 United Boulevard
Coquitlam, BC V3K 6Y2
Tel: 604-777-1757
1-800-663-8900
Fax: 604-777-4777
Website: www.naturalfactors.com

Nature Made
see Pharmavite Corporation

Nature's Sunshine Canada Ltd.
90 Walker Dr., Unit 1
Brampton, ON   L6T 4H6
Tel: 905-458-6100
 Website: www.naturessunshine.ca

Nature's Way Products Inc.
1375 N. Mountain Springs Parkway
Springville, Utah
84663 USA
Tel: 801-489-1500
1-800-962-8873
Fax: 801-489-1700
Website: www.naturesway.com

Neolab
5476 Upper Lachine Rd.
Montréal, QC H4A 2A4
Tel: 514-481-0226

Nestlé Canada Inc.
25 Sheppard Ave. W.
North York, ON   M2N 6S8
Tel: 416-512-9000
Fax: 416-218-2654

Nicar Inc, (Laboratoires)
10 Gaston Dumoulin, Suite 500
Blainville, QC   J7C 0A3
Tel: 450-979-4000
1-888-567-9683
Fax: 450-433-0387
1-866-933-0387
Website: www.nicar.ca

Nipro Diagnostics Inc
2400 NW 55th. Court
Fort Lauderdale, FL
33309, USA
Tel: 954-677-9201
1-800-342-7226
Website: www.niprodiagnostics.com

Norwood Packaging Ltd.
8519-132nd St., R.R. 4
Surrey, BC V3W 4N8
Tel: 604-599-0370

Nova Biomedical Canada, Ltd.
17-2900 Argentia Road
Mississauga, ON L5N 7X9
Tel: 905-567-7700
Fax: 905-567-5496
1-800-263-5999
Website: www.novabiomedical.com

Novartis Consumer Health Canada Inc.
2233 Argentia Rd., Ste. 205
Mississauga, ON   L5N 2X7
Tel: 905-812-4100
Fax: 905-821-4936

Novartis Ophthalmic
Novartis Pharmaceuticals Canada Inc.
385 Bouchard Blvd.
Dorval, QC   H9S 1A9
1-866- 393-6337

Novo Nordisk Canada Inc.
300-2680 Skymark Avenue,
Mississauga, ON L4W 5L6
Tel: 905-629-4222
1-800-465-4334
Fax: 905-629-8662
Website: www.novonordisk.ca

Novopharm Ltd.
see Teva Canada

Nspire Health Inc.
1830 Lefthand Circle
Longmont, CO
80501USA
Tel: 303-666-5555
 1-800-574-7374
Fax: 303-666-5588

Numark Labs Inc.
164 Northfield Ave.
Edison, NJ 08837 USA
Tel: 1-800-338-8079

Nutravite
157A Rutland Rd. South
Kelowna, BC   VIX 2Z3
Tel: 1-800-416-4474
Fax: 1-800-805-6581
Website: www.nutravite.com

Nutricorp International
4025 Rhodes Drive
Windsor, ON N8W 5B5

Nutrimmune Technologies
20 Kingland Cres
North York, ON   M2J 2B7
Tel: 416-847-0027

Nutripur Inc.
86 des Entreprises, suite 101
Boisbriand, QC J7G 2T3
Tel: 450-435-2040
Fax: 450-435-5659
Website: www.nutripur.com

Nycomed Canada Inc.
435 North Service Rd. West
1st Floor
Oakville, ON L6M 4X8
Tel: 905-469-9333
1-800-367-3331
Fax: 905-469-4883
Website: www.nycomed.ca

Odan Laboratories Ltd.
325 Stillview Ave
Pointe-Claire, QC H9R 2Y6
Tel: 514-428-1628
Fax: 514-428-9783
1-800-387-9342
Website: www.odanlab.com

Ombrelle Canada
4895 Hickmore
Montréal, QC H4T 1K5
Tel: 514-342-0880
1-888-966-2735
Website: www.ombrelle.ca

Omega Laboratories Ltd
11177 Hamon Street
Montréa,l QC H3M 3E4
Tel: 514-335-0310
1-800-363-0584
Fax:514- 339-1407

Omron Canada Inc.
885 Milner Avenue
Toronto, ON M1B-5V8
Tel: 416-286-6465
Fax: 416-286-6159
Website: www.omron.ca

O'My Products Inc.
188 Pemberton Ave
North Vancouve,r BC V7P 2R5
Tel: 604-990-9700
Fax: 604-990-8286
Website: www.omyinternational.com

Oral-B Laboratories Inc,
A Division of Procter & Gamble Inc.
4711 Yonge Street 12th Floor
Toronto, ON M2N 6K8
Tel: 1-800-566-7252

Origin BioMed Inc.
5162 Duke St., Suite 300
Halifax, NS B3J 1N7
Tel: 902-423-5745
1-800-234-7256
Fax:902-492-0013
Website: www.originbiomed.com

OvumOptics Inc.
123 Wildflower Lane
P.O. Box 2050
Hanna, Alberta T0J 1P0
Tel: 403-578-3055
1-888-632-9378

Owen Mumford Inc.
1755 West Oak Commons Court
Marietta, Georgia
30062 USA
Tel: 1-800-421-6936
Fax: 770-977-2866

Paladin Labs Inc.
6111 Royalmount Ave., Ste. 102
Montréal, QC H4P 2T4
Tel: 514-340-1112
Fax: 514-344-4675
1-800-376-7830
Website: www.paladin-labs.com

Paradise Promotions Ltd.
P.O. Box 394,
Novar, ON P0A 1R0
1-800-332-9964

Pari Respiratory Equipment Inc.
2943 Oak Lake Blvd.
Midothian, Virginia
23112 USA
Tel: 804-253-7274
Fax: 804-253-0260
Website: www.pari.com

PendoPharm
A Division of Pharmascience Inc.
5950 chemin de la Côte-de-Liesse
Montréal, QC H4T 1E2
Tel: 514-340-1114
1-866-926-7653
Fax: 514-733-9684
1-866-926-7654
Website: www.pendopharm.com

Person & Covey Inc.
616 Allen Ave
Glendale, CA
91201USA
Tel: 1-800-423-2341

Pfizer Consumer Healthcare Inc.
5975 Whittle Rd.
Mississauga, ON L4Z 3M6
Tel: 905-507-7000
1-800-387-8647
Website: www.pfizer.ca

Pharmascience Inc.
6111 Royalmount Ave., Ste. 100
Montréal, QC H4P 2T4
Tel: 514-340-1114
1-800-363-8805
Fax: 514-342-7764
Website: www.pharmascience.com

Pharmasystems Inc.
361 Steelcare Rd. West, Unit 10
Markham, ON   L3R 3V8
Tel: 905-475-2500
1-888-475-2500
Fax: 905-475-7155
1-888-475-7155
Website: www.pharmasystems.com

Pharmavite Corporation
8510 Balboa Blvd.
Northridge, California
USA 91325
Tel: 818-221-6200
Fax: 818-221-6611
Website: www.naturemade.com

Pharmetics Inc.
3695 Autoroute Des Laurentides
Laval, QC   H7L 3H7
Tel: 450-682-5672

Philips Avent Inc.
see Philips Electronics Ltd

Philips Electronics Ltd
281 Hillmount Road
Markham, Ontario L6C 2S3
Main Telephone: 905-201-4100
Tel: 1-800-542-8368
Main Fax: 905-887-4241

Philips Respironics Inc.
see Auto Control Medical (Distributor)

Physiologic
see AMG Medical Inc.
Website: www.amgphysiologic.com

Pierre Fabre Canada Inc.
1400 Marie-Victorin, Suite 207
St-Bruno-de-Montarville QC   J3V 6B9

Polymer Technology Systems Inc.
7736 Zionsville Rd
Indianapolis, Indiana
46268 USA
Tel: 317-870-5610
Fax: 317-870-5608
Website: www.cardiochek.com

Pos-T-Vac, Inc.
1701 N 14th P.O. Box 1436
Dodge City KS
67801 USA
Tel: 1-866-523-7328
Fax: 620-227-8474
Website: www.postvac.com

PowerBar Foods Inc.
2150 Shattuck Ave.
Berkeley, California
94704 USA
Tel: 510-843-1330
Website: www.powerbar.com

President's Choice
22 St-Clair Ave., E. 8th Floor
Toronto, ON   M4T 2S8
Tel: 416-967-2501
1-888-495-5111

Prestige Brands Inc.
90 N Broadway
Irvington, NY 10533   USA
1-800-754-2253
1-800-754-8853

Prime Enterprises Inc.
16363 Nw 49th Ave.
Miami Lakes Florida
33014-6316   USA
Tel: 305-625-4929

Procter & Gamble Inc.
P.O. Box 355 Stn A
Toronto, ON   M5W 1C5
Tel: 416-730-4711
1-800-983-4237
Fax: 416-730-4415
Website: www.pg.com

Prodemdis Enr.
4355 Sir Wilfrid Laurier Blvd.
St-Hubert, QC   J3Y 3X3
Tel: 450-443-6666
1-888-826-6322
Fax: 450-443-4466
Website: www.confab.ca

Profoot Inc.
74 20th St Fl 2
Brooklyn, NY
11232-1101 USA
Tel: 718-965-8600
Fax: 718-965-9729
Website: www.profootcare.com

Purdue Pharma
575 Granite Court
Pickering, ON L1W 3W8
Tel: 905-420-6400
1-800-387-5349
Fax:905-420-2503
Website: www.purdue.ca

Pure Source, Inc. (Distributor)
7018 HWY 24 South - RR # 7
Guelph, ON   N1H 6J4
Tel:1- 800-265-7245

Purity Life Health Products (Distributor)
6 Commerce Cres.
Acton, ON L7J 2X3
Tel: 519-853-3511
Fax: 519-853-0917
1-800-265-2615
Website: www.puritylife.com

Quantum Health Inc
see Purity Life Health Products (Distributor)
Website: www.quantumhealth.com

Quest Vitamins
see Purity Life Health Products (Distributor)
Website: www.questvitamins.com

ratiopharm Inc.
6755 Mississauga Rd
4th Floor
Mississauga,ON   L5N 7Y2
Tel: 905 858-9612
 1-800-266-2584
Fax: 905- 858-9610
1-800-881-5175
Website: www.ratiopharm.ca

Reckitt Benckiser (Canada) Inc.
Unit #2 1680 Tech Avenue
Mississauga, ON L4W 5S9
Tel: 905-283-7000
Fax: 905- 283-7001

Rennich Industries Ltd.
23 Scandia Point N.W
Calgary, AB   T3L 1T6
Tel: 403-241-2548
1-866-748-2548

Revlon Canada Inc.
1590 South Gateway Rd
Mississauga, ON L4W 0A8
Tel:905-276-4500

RGR Pharma Ltd.
103 Crystal Harbour Dr.
LaSalle, ON   N9J 3R6
Tel: 519-734-6600

Ricola
Lindt & Sprüngli (Canada) Inc.
181 University Avenue, Suite 900
Toronto, ON   M5H 3M7
Tel: 416-351-8566 ext. 284
Fax: 416-351-8507

Riemann & Co. A/S
Dk-3400 Hilleroed
Denmark
Fax: +45 47 18 20 01
Website: www.riemann.com

Riva Laboratories Inc.
660 Industriel Blvd.
Blainville, QC   J7C 3V4
Tel: 450-434-7482
 1-800-363-7988
Fax: 450-434-2500
Website: www.labriva.com

Robert et Fils Inc.
1212 Louvain Ouest
Montréal, QC   H4N 1G5
Tel: 514-274-2568
1-800-361-0324
Fax: 514-274-7894
1-800-488-7894
Website: www.robertetfils.com

Roche Diagnostics
201 Armand-Frappier Blvd.
Laval, QC   H7V 4A2
Tel: 450-686-7050
Fax: 450-686-7009
1-800-361-2070
Website: www.rochediagnostics.ca

Rochester Medical Inc.
One Rochester Medical Dr
Stewartville, MN
USA   55976-1647
Tel: 507-533-9309
Fax: 507-533-4232

Rolmex International Inc.
1351 Rue Gay-Lussac
Boucherville QC J4B 7K1
Tel: 450-655-5239

Rougier Pharma
A Division of ratiopharm Inc.
17 800 Lapointe St.
Mirabel, QC J7J 1P3
Tel: 1-866-207-0161
Fax: 450-433-0991
Website: www.rougier.com

S.C. Johnson Canada
1 Webster Street
Brantford, ON N3T 5R1
1-877-506-7352

Sandoz Canada Inc.
145 Jules-Leger St.
Boucherville, QC J4B 7K8
Tel: 450-641-4903
Fax: 514-596-1460
1-800-361-3062

sanofi-aventis
2150 St. Elzear Blvd. West
Laval, QC H7L 4A8
Tel: 514-331-9220
1-800-363-6364
Website: www.sanofi-aventis.ca

Santé Naturelle
see Adrien Gagnon (AG) Natural Health Ltd.

Sato Pharma Canada
Unit 190 - 3751 Shell Road
Richmond, BC V6X 2W2
Tel: 604-207.9185
Website: www.satocanada.com

SCA Personal Hygiene Products
1275 North Service Rd West, ste 612
Oakville, ON L6M 3G4
Tel: 1-800-510-8023
Consumer Information:
Tel: 1-800-360-8362
Website: www.tena.ca

Schering-Plough Canada Inc.
16750, route Transcanadienne
Kirkland, QC H9H 4M7
Tel: 514-426-7300
Toll free:1-800-361-2353
Website: www.schering-plough.ca

Scott Chemical Canada
275 Finchdene Square
Scarborough ON M1X 1C7

Shiseido America Inc.
900 Third Avenue
New York NY
USA 10022

Sisu Inc.
102-7635 North Fraser Way
Burnaby, BC V5J 0B8
Tel: 604-420-6610
1-800-663-4163
Fax: 604-420-6640
1-888-420-6640
Website: www.sisu.com

Smith & Nephew Inc.
2250 Alfred Nobel Blvd., Suite 300
St. Laurent, QC H4S 2C9
Tel: 514-956-1010
1-800-636-0772
Fax: 514-956-1414
1-800-671-9140
Website: www.wound.smith-nephew.com

Source Medical Inc.
1000 Tesma Way
Vaughan, ON L4K 5R8
Tel: 905-417-2900
Website: www.sourcemedical.com

SRS Medical Inc.
8672 154th Ave. NE, Bldg. P
Redmond, WA 98052, USA
Tel: 800-345-5642
Fax: 800-886-2774
Website: www.srsmedical.com

Stella Pharmaceutical Canada Inc.
407-220 Duncan Mill Rd.
Don Mills, ON M3B 3J5
Tel: 416-443-0636
1-800-263-7546
Fax: 416-443-8504
Website: www.stellapharmaceutical.com

SteriMax Inc.
2735 Matheson Boulevard East, Suite 1
Mississauga, ON L4W 4M8
Tel: 905-890-0661
1-800-881-3550
Fax: 905-890-0508
1-877-546-7667

Stiefel Canada Inc.
6635 Henri-Bourassa Blvd. W.
Montréal, QC H4R 1E1
Tel: 514-332-3800
1-800-363-2862
Fax: 514-332-1961
1-800-561-1898

SunOpta Inc.
see also Purity Life Health Products
2838 Bovaird Dr. West
Brampton, ON L7A OH2
Tel: 905-455-2528
Website: www.sunopta.com

Superior Medical Inc.
520 Champagne Dr
Toronto, ON M3J 2T9
Tel: 416-635-9797
1-800-268-7944
Fax: 416-635-8931
Website: www.superiormedical.com

Swiss Herbal Remedies Ltd.
35 Fulton Way
Richmond Hill, ON L4B 2N4
Tel: (905) 886-9500
1-800-268-9879
Fax: 905-886-5434
Website: www.swissherbal.ca

Taiga BioActives Inc.
6-2616 16th Street NE
Calgary, AB T2E 7J8
Tel: 403-717-0776
Website: www.taigabioactives.com

Tallgrass Distribution
40 E. 5th Avenue
Vancouver, BC V5T 1G8
Tel: 604-709-0101
Toll Free: 1-800-616-5900

Tanning Research Labs
108 Newbold Court
London, ON N6E 1Z7
Tel: 519-649-4942

Tanta Pharmaceuticals Inc.
1009 Burns St. E.
Whitby, ON L1N 6A6
Tel: 905-430-8440
1-800-668-2682
Fax: 905-430-8449
Website: www.tanta.ca

Taro Pharmaceuticals Inc.
130 East Dr.
Bramalea ON L6T 1C3
Tel: 905-791-8276
1-800-268-1975
Fax: 905-791-5008
Website: www.taro.ca

TCD (Trans CanaDerm)
see Stiefel Canada Inc.

TENDER CANADA INC.
19 Alliance Blvd., Unit 10
Barrie ON L4M 5B5
Tel: 705-722-3400
Fax: 705-722-5795
Website: www.tendercorp.com

Teva Canada Ltd.
30 Novopharm Court
Toronto ON M1B 2K9
Tel: 416-291-8876
1-800-268-4127
Fax: 416-291-1874
Website: www.tevacanada.com

TFB & Associates Limited
600 Alden Rd., Ste. 102
Markham ON L3R 0E7
Tel: 905-940-0889
Fax: 905-940-0913

Thea (Spectrum-Thea Pharmaceutical Ltd.)
see I-Med Pharma Inc. (Distributor)

ThermoFlash USA
Tel: +1 305 702 6440
Fax: +1 305 945 9446

Tom's of Maine
302 Lafayette Dr.
Kennebunk, Maine
USA 04043
Tel: 1-800-367-8667
Fax: 207-985-2196

Trans Research Labs Inc.
78 Kinkora Drive
Winnipeg, MB R3R 2L6
Tel: 1-866-335-3596
Website: www.transresearchlabs.com

Tremblay Harrison Inc
Wholesale Medical Network
9 Hearthstone Cres.
North York ON M2R 1G2
Tel: 1-866-829-7926
Fax: 416-654-7014
Website: www.tremblayharrison.com

Trianon Laboratories Inc.
660 Industriel Blvd.
Blainville QC J7C 3V4
Tel: 450-434-7482
Fax: 450-434-2500
1-800-363-7988
Website: www.labriva.com

Trillium Health Care Products Inc.
2337 Parkdale Ave.
Brockville, ON   K6V 5W5
Tel: 613-342-4436

Trophic Canada Ltd.
260 Okanagan Avenue East
Penticton, BC   V2A 3J7
Tel: 1-800-663-4136
Fax: 250-492-5066
Website: www.trophic.net

Trudell Medical International
725 Third St.
London, ON   N5V 5G4
Tel: 519-455-7060
Fax: 519-455-6239
1-800-465-3296
Website: www.trudellmed.com

Ultimark Products LLC.
307 E. Church Road
King of Prussia, PA
USA 19406
Tel: 610-592-0041
Fax: 610-592-0049

Unico Holdings Inc.
2201 Fourth Avenue North
Lake Worth, Florida
USA 33461
Tel: 561-582-3030

Unilever Canada
PO Box 38
Saint John, NB   E2L 3X1
Tel: 1-800-565-7273
Fax: 506-631-6424

University Medical Products
88 Maxwell
Irvine, CA
USA 92618-4641
Tel: 949-851-5353
1-800-535-0000

Valeant Canada Ltd.
4787 Rue Lévy
Montréal, QC H4R 2P9
Tel: 514-744-6792
1-800-361-4261
Fax: 514-744-1842
1-800-361-4266

Valeo Pharma Inc.
16,667 Hymus Blvd
Kirkland, QC H9H 4R9
Tel: 514-694-0150
1-866-694-0150
Fax: 514-694-0865
1- 888-694-0865

Vichy Canada
4895 Hickmore
Montréal, QC H4T 1K5
Tel: 514-342-0880
Website: www.vichy.ca

Vicks Canada
see Procter & Gamble Inc.

Vita Health Products Inc.
150 Beghin Ave.
Winnipeg, MB R2J 3W2
Tel: 204-661-8386
1-800-361-9975
Fax: 204-663-8386
Website: www.vitahealth.ca

Vitality Products Inc.
#304 - 837 West Hastings Street
Vancouver, BC   V6C 3N6
Tel: 604-683-6611
Fax: 604-662-8524
Website: www.vitality.ca

W.F. Young, Inc.
302 Benton Drive
East Longmeadow, Massachusetts
USA 01028
Tel: 413-526-9999
Fax: 413-526-8990
Website: www.wfyoung.com

W.K. Buckley
The Buckley's Company
205-2233 Argentia Road
Mississauga, ON L5N 2X7
Tel: 1-800-434-1034
Fax: 1-800-434-1035
Website: www.buckleys.com

Wakunaga of America Co., Ltd.
23501 Madero
Mission Viejo, CA
USA 92691
Tel: 949-855-2776
Website: www.kyolic.com

Watkins Inc.
150 Liberty Street
PO Box 5570
Winona, MN 55987-0570
USA
Tel: 507-457-3300
Fax: 507-452-6723

Waymar Pharmaceuticals Inc.
330 Marwood Dr., Unit 4
Oshawa, ON   L1H 8B4
Tel: 905-434-1814
Fax: 905-434-1816
1-800-810-8065

Weleda North America
1 Closter Rd PO Box 675
Palisades, NY
USA   10964
Tel: 1-800-241-1030
Fax: 1-800-280-4899
Website: www.weleda.ca

WellSpring Pharmaceutical Canada
400 Iroquois Shore Rd.
Oakville, ON   L6H 1M5
Tel: 905-337-4500
Fax: 905-337-7752
Website: www.wellspringpharm.com

Wholesale Medical Network Inc.
9 Hearthstone Crescent
Toronto, ON   M2R 1G2
Tel: 416-913-0042
1-866-759-9664

WN Pharmaceuticals Ltd.
2000 Brigantine Dr
Coquitlam, BC V3K 7B5
Tel: 778-284-7400
1-800-430-7898
Fax: 778-284-7401
1-888-597-2885
Website: www.wnpharmaceuticals.com

Wockhardt UK Ltd.
Ash Road North
Wrexham Industrial Estate
Wrexham
LL 13 9UF   UK
Tel: 01978 661261
Fax: 01978 660130
Website: www.wockhardt.co.uk

Xenex Laboratories Inc.
2402 Canoe Ave.
Coquitlam, BC   V3K 6C2

Tel: 1-800-663-1002
Fax: 1-888-552-4993
Website: www.xenexlabs.com

YouMedical
Van Breestraat 107bg
1071 ZJ Amsterdam
The Netherlands
T +31 20 679 8529
F +31 20 524 8759
Website: www.hemoclin.com

Youngflex Manufacturing Inc.
151 Nashdene Rd. Unit 7
Toronto, ON   M1V 4B9
Tel: 416-335-3039

ZEE Medical Canada Inc.
4170 Sladeview Cres., Unit 2
Mississauga, ON   L5L 0A1
Tel: 1-800-661-1491
Fax: 1-888-253-9944
Website: www.zeemedical.com

Index

F

G

H

l-arginine
  Herbal and Natural Health Products: Combination Products   101
Lassar's Paste   192, 200
Laxaco Herbal Laxative   97
Lax A Day   97
Laxative   97
Laxatives *see* **Gastrointestinal Products: Laxatives**
Laxcodyl   97
Lean+   159
lecithin
  Herbal and Natural Health Products: Combination Products   101
  Skin Care Products: Dermatitis and Dry Skin   191
  Vitamin and Mineral Products: Combinations, Solid   238
Lecithin Capsules   238
Leg Lastrap Brace   144
lemon balm
  Herbal and Natural Health Products: Combination Products   101
lemongrass oil
  Insect Repellents   134
Lenoltec No 1   7
leptandra
  Gastrointestinal Products: Laxatives   97
  Herbal and Natural Health Products: Combination Products   101
Levemir   73, 74
levonorgestrel
  Contraceptive Products: Emergency Contraceptives   29
licorice
  Cough, Cold and Allergy Products   48
  Gastrointestinal Products: Laxatives   95–96, 99
  Herbal and Natural Health Products: Combination Products   101
Lid-Care Towelettes   164
lidocaine
  Analgesic Products: External Analgesics   3
  Male Sexual Health Products: Premature Ejaculation   135
  Skin Care Products: Anesthetics   188
  Skin Care Products: First Aid   198–201
lidocaine hydrochloride
  Otic Products   180
  Skin Care Products: Anesthetics   188
Lidodan
  Ointment   188
  Viscous   188
Lidomyxin   180
Lifesource Digital Thermometer   118
LifeStyles   30
  4Play   30

Endurance (climax control lubricant)   30
Excite Combo   30
Her Passion (lubricated)   30
Large (lubricated)   30
Lubricated   30
Luscious Flavours (lubricated)   30
Mr. Big (lubricated)   30
Natural Feeling (lubricated)   30
Skin (lubricated)   30
Spermicidally Lubricated   30
Studded (lubricated)   30
Trio (lubricated)   30
True-Fit (lubricated)   30
Ultra Sensitive (lubricated)   30
Ultra Sensitive with Warming Lubricant   30
Ultrathin Large (lubricated)   30
Ultrathin (lubricated)   30
Xtra Pleasure (lubricated)   30
Xtra Pleasure with Ribs (lubricated)   30
Light Flow Nursing Pads   20
ligustilide
  Herbal and Natural Health Products: Combination Products   101
Li'l Goat's Milk Zinc Oxide Ointment   17
lindane
  Skin Care Products: Scabicides   206
linden flower
  Herbal and Natural Health Products: Combination Products   101
linoleic acid
  Herbal and Natural Health Products: Combination Products   100, 102
  Herbal and Natural Health Products: Single Entity Products   105
Lipactin   138
Lipclear Lysine Plus Ointment   138
Lipsorex   138
Liquid B Complex   238
Liquid Calcium-Magnesium and Vitamin D   222
Liquifilm Forte   163
lispro
  Diabetes Products: Insulin   73
Listerine
  Advanced Plus   140
  Antiseptic Original/Cool Mint/Fresh Burst   140
  Fluoride / Listerine Platinum   140
  Smart Rinse for Kids   140
  Tartar Control   140
  Total Care   140
  Total Care for Sensitive Teeth   140
  Ultraclean Anti-Cavity   140

S